W0050529

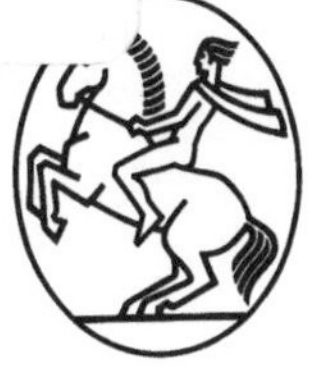

ACTA NEUROCHIRURGICA
SUPPLEMENTUM 33

Advances in Stereotactic and Functional Neurosurgery 6

Proceedings of the 6th Meeting of the European Society for Stereotactic and Functional Neurosurgery, Rome 1983

Edited by
J. Gybels, E. R. Hitchcock, Ch. Ostertag, G. F. Rossi, J. Siegfried, G. Szikla

SPRINGER-VERLAG
WIEN NEW YORK

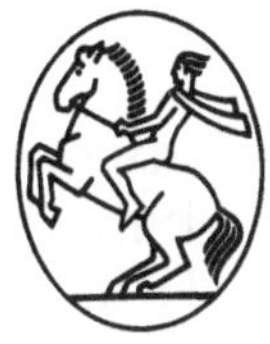

Professor JAN GYBELS

Department of Neurosurgery, Academisch Ziekenhuis, Leuven

Professor EDWARD R. HITCHCOCK

Midland Centre for Neurosurgery and Neurology and Queen Elizabeth Hospital, Birmingham

Priv.-Doz. CHRISTOPH OSTERTAG

Abteilung für Stereotaxie, Neurochirurgische Universitätsklinik, Freiburg i. Br.

Professor GIAN FRANCO ROSSI

Istituto di Neurochirurgia, Università Cattolica del Sacro Cuore, Rome

Professor JEAN SIEGFRIED

Neurochirurgische Klinik, Universitätsspital, Zürich

Professor GABOR SZIKLA

With 165 Figures

Library of Congress Cataloging in Publication Data. European Society for Stereotactic and Functional Neurosurgery. Meeting (6th: 1983: Rome, Italy) Advances in stereotactic and functional neurosurgery 6. (Acta neurochirurgica. Supplementum; 33) 1. Stereoencephalotomy—Congresses. 2. Epilepsy—Surgery—Congresses. 3. Brain—Tumors—Surgery—Congresses. 4. Pain—Surgery—Congresses. I. Gybels, J. (Jan) II. Title. III. Series. [DNLM: 1. Brain neoplasms—Surgery—Congresses. 2. Epilepsy—Surgery—Congresses. 3. Neurosurgery—Congresses. 4. Pain—Surgery—Congresses. 5. Stereotaxic technics—Congresses. W1 AC8661 no. 33/WL 368 E89 1983 a.] RD 594.E85. 1983. 617'.481. 83-26766

ISSN 0065-1419 (Acta Neurochirurgica/Suppl.)
ISSN 0720-7972 (Advances in Stereotactic and Functional Neurosurgery)
ISBN-13:978-3-211-81773-5 e-ISBN-13:978-3-7091-8726-5
DOI: 10.1007/978-3-7091-8726-5

It was while this Supplementum was in press, that the tragic news of Dr. Gabor Szikla's death reached us.

Not only was he President of the European Society for Stereotactic and Functional Neurosurgery and one of the most qualified representatives of this branch of neurosurgery, but was also mainly responsible for the editing of this Supplementum.

The coeditors dedicate this volume to his memory.

Contents

Section I. Epilepsy

Editors:
E. R. Hitchcock and G. F. Rossi

1. Diagnosis

A. Introduction

B. Reports

C. Communications

2. Surgical Treatment

A. Introduction

B. Communications

Section II. Cerebral Tumours

Editors:
CH. OSTERTAG and G. SZIKLA

Introductory Lecture

1. Stereotactic Biopsy

2. Stereotactic Focal Irradiation

I. Effects on Tumour and Brain

II. Clinical Results

III. Technical Aspects

Concluding Remarks of the Moderator

Section III. Pain

Editors:
J. Gybels and J. Siegfried

Introductory Lecture

I. Pelvic Cancer Pain (Somatogenic Pain)

II. Plexus Avulsion Pain (Neurogenic Pain)

III. Other Topics on Pain

Section IV. Miscellaneous

Editors:
G. F. Rossi and E. R. Hitchcock

Section IV: Miscellaneous

[illegible]

Section I

Epilepsy

1. Diagnosis

Acta Neurochirurgica, Suppl. 33, 3—5 (1984)

A. Introduction

Progress in Diagnosis in View of Surgical Treatment of the Epileptic Patient

G. F. Rossi[1]

The diagnostic informations which are necessary to the neurosurgeon facing the problem of treating the epileptic patient are many. First of all those necessary to decide whether surgery is indicated or not. Second, there are the diagnostic findings which help in the selection of the best type of treatment; indeed, as we shall see during the second part of the day, there are several different surgical modalities to treat epilepsy, each one based on different rationales or principles. Third, there are the findings used to plan the details of the selected surgical approach.

Some of the diagnostic informations are related to the etiology of the epilepsy; more precisely, to the nature of the disease primarily responsible for it. Others give us a picture of the severity of the epileptic syndrome. Others are related to the spatial organization of the epileptic process within the cerebrum; and so on.

Consequently, the means available to provide all the necessary diagnostic informations are many and of different nature. Some of them are well established procedures; others have been developed in recent times; others have been proposed quite recently and are regarded as still in development.

The main purpose of the first part of our session on epilepsy is to point out the most recent advances of some of these diagnostic procedures.

1. First of all, we shall take into consideration the clinical

[1] Istituto di Neurochirurgica, Università Cattolica del Sacro Cuore, Largo A. Gemelli, 8, I-00168 Roma, Italy.

manifestations of the seizure. It is the oldest of the diagnostic aids. An accurate analysis of all the motor, sensory, visceral and psychic components of the seizure, obviously coupled with a good knowledge of cerebral functional organization, is important to disclose which are the epileptic cerebral structures.

A relevant progress in this direction was made possible by combining analysis of the clinical seizure patterns with that of the simultaneously recorded electrocerebral activity, and particularly of the electrical activity directly recorded from the brain through stereotactically implanted electrodes. This integrated electro-clinical approach greatly increased the possibility of reliably inferring from the seizure pattern the cerebral site of origin and the main pathways of propagation of the ictal discharge. Actually, in certain cases, it changed our previous views, which were based exclusively on the analysis of the clinical manifestations of the epileptic attack.

2. The study of electro-cerebral activity certainly is the most widely used means to study epilepsy, both in the clinical environment and in the experimental laboratory. Direct recording from selected cortical and subcortical brain sites through stereotactically implanted electrodes—or stereo-EEG—greatly enhances the number and the reliability of the diagnostic informations. However, when looking at a record of the electrical activity from the brain of a patient suffering from a severe epileptic syndrome, one might be discouraged. This is particularly true when examining the interictal epileptic activity; the number of abnormal potentials, their morphological appearance, their spatial distribution and their temporal relations seem very complex. One needs to find a means of analyzing this seemingly multifarious material in such a way as to extract from it the informations which it contains.

Attempts to overcome this difficulty and to improve our knowledge of the physio-pathological meaning of the recorded electrocerebral events were made by using automatic analysis. The progress so far achieved in this field is remarkable. The use of this analysis of the epileptic potentials in consideration of surgical treatment will be the second subject discussed this morning.

3. Finally, we come to the third diagnostic approach, the one aiming at getting an insight into the organization of the epileptic process through the study of the brain metabolism. It can be regarded as the last born of the diagnostic approaches; actually, it is perhaps safer to regard it as a diagnostic approach still in gestation.

When closing the discussion on surgery of epilepsy at the last meeting of our Society, four years ago, I stressed that the ideal way to treat epilepsy should not be surgical, but the correction of the functional abnormality of the epileptic cerebral neurones without surgical brain manipulation. The achievement of this goal seems to a great extent dependent on knowledge of the metabolic disorders affecting the epileptized neurones. Therefore, the application of studies of cerebral metabolism to the epileptic brain, even if in their first stages of application, should be regarded as very promising. In any way, they are very stimulating and certainly worth consideration in a meeting like ours.

Acta Neurochirurgica, Suppl. 33, 7—15 (1984)

B. Reports

Localizing Value of the Clinical Manifestations of the Partial Seizures

J. Bancaud[1,2], **A. Bonis**[1,2], **C. Munari**[1,2], **G. Szikla**[1,2], **J. P. Chodkiewicz**[2], and **J. Talairach**[2]

Summary

This study of partial seizures recorded during stereo-EEG explorations in patients with severe drug resistant partial epilepsies intends to evaluate the localizing value of some clinical signs.

The term of "automatisms" includes many different symptoms: authors show that an oro-alimentary motor activity does not have the same significance than a restlessness. Actually, a mastication or chewing activity seems to be linked to an ictal involement of the amygdaloid nucleus. On the contrary, gestural activity, mainly complex, is related to the ictal dysfunctioning of the anterior part of the cingulate gyrus. Moreover, the occurrence of an automatic activity is not necessarily linked to an impairment of consciousness. The usefulness of a classification of partial seizures without a localizing value is discussed.

Keywords: Stereo-EEG; complex partial seizures; epilepsy; surgery of epilepsy; automatisms.

Introduction

Success or failure of neurosurgical interventions in partial epilepsies is strictly linked to the topographic definition of the so-called "epileptogenic" zone. Many criteria were used to define as precisely as possible this "epileptogenic" zone.

---

[1] Unité 97 de recherches sur l'épilepsie, INSERM, 2ter rue d'Alésia, F-75014 Paris, France.

[2] Service de Neurochirurgie B, Hôpital Sainte Anne, 1 rue Cabanis, F-75014 Paris, France.

Actually, the occurrence of the different ictal symptoms corresponds to the involvement by the ictal discharge of different cortical structures. Thus, on the basis of a careful analysis of the clinical signs, we may "visualise" the intracerebral trajectory of the electrical discharges.

The theoretical basis of this methodological approach has been recently described (Bancaud 1980)[3]. The aim of this paper is to show what may be the localizing value of some ictal clinical signs studied during stereo-EEG explorations. We deliberately choose two symptoms generally considered as characterizing the so-called "complex" partial seizures[8,11]: "automatic activities" and "impairment" of consciousness.

Patients and Methods

At our department, more than 800 patients underwent to a stereo-EEG exploration in view of a surgical treatment for severe, drug resistant partial epilepsies, since 1959.

The methodology of these investigations has been described in detail in several previous papers[5–7,26,28].

We will just mention that the stereo-EEG investigations are performed on the basis of previously collected data:

clinical (history of the patient, clinical evolution of the seizures, neurological examination)

electrical (mainly EEG recording of spontaneous seizures) and

anatomical (stereotactic neuroradiological investigations).

Thus the choice of the cortical structures to be explored by intracerebral depth-electrodes is defined on the basis of apparently consistent hypothesis on the localization of the "epileptogenic" area.

When the stereo-EEG data confirm the existence of an unique, relatively localized, epileptogenic zone, and if the surgical removal of this cerebral area may be realized without severe neurological impairment, the patients are submitted to a surgical intervention.

It is evident that the critical evaluation of the surgical results (Bonis 1979)[9] allows us to progressively improve this methodology.

We briefly expose some data concerning two groups of 120 patients presenting:

a) an ictal automatic activity;

b) an impairment of consciousness.

All data were collected during "acute" stereo-EEG explorations performed with 7 to 12 intracerebral multilead electrodes, on awake cooperative patients. During these investigations, patients were directly observed by two neurologists: their remarks were recorded on a tape recorder and transcribed on the stereo-EEG record. The patients were simultaneously filmed by two telecameras and recorded on videotape.

Results

I. Automatic Activities

A. Oro-alimentary Automatic Activities

1. Temporal Lobe Seizures

These "automatisms" occur in more than 80% of temporal lobe seizures. They are almost always of the motor type, as a chewing.

Oro-alimentary activities like chewing occur during the first 10 seconds in more than 35% of the seizures.

Ictal discharges affecting only the deep anterior temporal structures (amygdaloid nucleus, temporal pole, anterior part of Ammon's horn) may be associated only with an oro-alimentary automatic activity like chewing, without any loss of consciousness.

The electrical stimulation of the amygdaloid nucleus provokes this type of oro-alimentary automatic activities only in those patients presenting this manifestations during spontaneous seizures. In the same patients the electrical stimulation of Ammon's horn can provoke this activity only when the after-discharge involves the amygdaloid nucleus.

2. Frontal Lobe Seizures

During frontal lobe seizures without temporal lobe involvement, we never observed an early oro-alimentary automatic activity.

This activity may sometimes occur in the course, or rather at the end, of the seizures when the ictal discharge affects the temporal lobe and/or when it spread in both hemispheres.

B. Gestural Automatic Activities

1. Temporal Lobe Seizures

— Gestural automatic activities are observed in more than 60% of temporal lobe seizures.

— These activities are generally simple and they occur during the first 10 seconds of the seizures in less than 20% of temporal lobe seizures.

— These early gestural automatic activities are never linked to an ictal discharge affecting exclusively a single temporal lobe: they are related to the rapid ictal involvement of the homolateral frontal lobe, of the controlateral temporal lobe or of both.

— The temporal lobe seizures with gestural automatic activities are characterized by a clinical symptomatology more complex than temporal lobe seizures without gestural automatic activities.

2. Frontal Lobe Seizures

— Gestural automatic activities characterize more than 75% of frontal lobe seizures. They occur in more than 2/3 of patients presenting frontal lobe seizures.

When these activities appear early, in the first 10 seconds (20% of the seizures), the patients, presenting a global behavioral modification, are often restless.

— The ictal discharge mostly affects the medial frontal cortex, mainly the anterior part of the cingulate gyrus (area 24).

— In 60% of the frontal lobe seizures, the gestural automatic activities occur later than the firts 10 seconds and, in 25% of the seizures, this activity occurs in the post-ictal period.

II. Impairment of Consciousness

1. Temporal Lobe Seizures

Among 100 patients presenting temporal lobe seizures, 21 had only seizures without impairment of consciousness, 43 had only seizures with impairment of consciousness and 36 had both types of seizures.

In 60% of temporal lobe seizures, we do not observe any impairment of consciousness.

The lenght of the seizures with impairment of consciousness is double (> 90″) of those without impairment of consciousness (47″).

The seizures without impairment of consciousness have a relatively simple clinical semiology: predominantly oro-alimentary automatic activities as chewing, and subjective, mainly epigastric, early manifestations. We never observed any secondary generalization.

The clinical semiology of the seizures with impairment of consciousness is more complex; thymic and/or affective manifestations occur in more than 50% of them, associated with oro-alimentary automatic activities and, above all, gestural automatic activities. Moreover, these seizures are also characterized by lateralized somatomotor manifestations, followed in 20% by a secondary generalization.

During the seizures with impairment of consciousness the ictal discharge always affects extratemporal structures and particularly the homolateral frontal lobe and/or the controlateral temporal lobe. There is a direct chronological relationship between the involvement of these structures and the occurrence of the impairment of consciousness.

2. Frontal Lobe Seizures

— The impairment of consciousness characterizes 3/4 of the frontal lobe seizures in 75% of the patients presenting these seizures.

— Whatever is the origin of the seizures (in the frontal lobe, with impairment of consciousness) the ictal discharge always affects the anterior part of the cingulate gyrus.

— Among the clinical signs associated with the impairment of consciousness it is necessary to point out gestural automatic activities (early in 20%, late in 60% and post-ictal in 25% of the seizures).

Discussion

The first remark concerns our methodological approach: it is evident that we can not explore all cortical regions in our patients. Thus one may conceive that the ictal discharges sometimes can arise in other, not explored, cortical areas: in this occurrence the anatomo-electro-clinical correlations we study could be wrong. In this paper, we only take into account the data concerning the origin and the propagation of the ictal discharges in those patients in whom the operative results confirmed the localization of the epileptogenic area. These results can not be discussed in details: it should be mentioned however that in the last group of patients operated on for a temporal lobe epilepsy, the success rate was more than 90% (Bonis 1979)[9].

Since Jackson introduced the term of "automatism"[14], this expression is more and more widely used. In 1937, Gibbs *et al.*[13] introduced the term "psychomoter seizures" to encompass the psychic and motor manifestations. This increasingly popular term rapidly became synonymous with automatisms to describe a specific manifestation of an attack (Penry 1975)[23].

Shortly after, began the era of temporal lobectomies in the treatment of epilepsy[21]: because of the large number of "psychomotor seizures" described in patients with temporal lesions and because of the fact that stimulation of the temporal lobe may produce such symptoms, the anatomical definition "temporal lobe epilepsy" was preferred (Penfield and Erikson 1941)[21].

In 1970, Gastaut[11] proposed the term of "partial seizures with complex symptomatology", including in this definition the previously so called psychomotor and/or temporal lobe seizures. These partial seizures with complex symptomatology are mainly characterized by an impairment of consciousness and by automatisms (or psychomotor symptomatology).

Considering this association, it might seem appear established that an automatic activity could exist only when the conciousness is impaired. Thus, for Daly[10] "an automatism consists of a transient confusional state in which responsiveness is impaired or lost and for which the patient is amnesic".

Our methodological approach to a possible surgical therapy in epileptic patients, needs to establish precise correlations between the ictal clinical symptomatology and the intracerebral trajectory of the ictal discharge. In this perspective we use a "logical model" of interpretation of clinical signs characterizing a partial seizure: the seizure is considered as a sequence of different words (clinical symptoms) constituting a phrase (the seizure) (Bancaud 1980)[3]. The validity and the limits of such a model, which has been used for many years, have been recently discussed.

— It is well known in the literature that automatic behaviour, although a frequent symptom of temporal lobe epilepsy, can be linked with seizures arising from a variety of locations: frontal convexity (Penfield and Jasper 1954)[22], supplementary motor and parieto-occipital regions (Ajmone-Marsan and Ralston 1957)[2], cingulate gyrus (Talairach *et al.* 1973)[27], Stoffels *et al.* (1981)[25] etc. Moreover, automatisms may occur during "Petit Mal" absences (Penry and Dreifuss 1969)[24]. On the other hand, because of the complexity of automatisms, no universal agreement exists on their classification (Ajmone-Marsan and Ralston 1957[2], Penry and Dreifuss 1969[24], Gastaut and Broughton 1972[12]). Moreover, differents authors consider that in patients developing automatisms, the ictal discharge invariabily spreads to both temporal lobes, or to the temporo-parietal cortex, or, often, to the frontal cortex (Jasper 1964)[15] and can not be focal in the usual sense of unilateral or localized (Aird 1977)[1].

Our data seem show that all the automatic activities do not have the same localizing value: an oro-alimentary motor activity as chewing appears to be strictly linked with the ictal involvement of the amygdaloid nucleus, while a simple gestural activity is not related to a discharge only affecting the anterior deep temporal structures. Thus, a seizure only characterized at the onset by automatic chewing activity does not admit the same origin as a seizure starting with a complex behavioral restlessness[16]: both these manifestations are nevertheless considered as "automatic"[19].

Moreover we observed different seizures with an automatic chewing activity without any impairment of consciousness: during these seizures (related to a discharge localized in the anterior part of only one temporal lobe) the patient may answer questions and can describe later what happened. Therefore, an impairment of consciousness is not a necessary condition permitting the occurrence of some automatisms[17].

Some clinical signs, like motor activities, auditory hallucinations, visual manifestations etc.... have a generally admitted localizing value.

The automatisms are considered as characterizing the complex partial seizures: their anatomical substrate is considered to be the temporal or fronto-temporal regions[8]. A careful analysis of anatomo-electro-clinical correlations may permit to attribute a localizing value to some of these activities, instead of considering them as a homogeneous group of equivalent signs which they are actually not[18].

The variety of clinical signs characterizing temporal lobe seizures (Bancaud 1981)[4] does not allow to "automatically" attribute to the dysfunctioning of only this lobe different clinical symptoms as a gestural complex activity or an early impairment of consciousness[20].

Finally it is difficult to understand the usefulness of a classification of partial seizures based on the occurrence of a sign as impairment of consciousness. Its interpretation is very difficult since it seems to be related rather to the duration and to the extent of the discharge than to a particular localization of the seizures[17].

References

1. Aird, R. B., Some observations of clinical interest on the pathophysiology of epilepsy. In: Physiological aspects of clinical neurology (Rose, F. C., ed.), pp. 305—313. Oxford: Blackwell Scientific. 1977.
2. Ajmone-Marsan, C., Ralston, B., The epileptic seizures. Its functional morphology and diagnostic significance, 251 pp. Springfield, Illinois: Ch. C Thomas. 1957.

3. Bancaud, J., Introduction à l'étude des crises épileptiques partielles complexes chez l'homme. In: Progressi in Epilettologia (Canger, R., Avanzini, G., Tassinari, C. A., eds.), pp. 73—88. Lega Italiana contro l'epilessia, 29-30, 1980.
4. Bancaud, J., Epileptic attacks of temporal origin in man. Jap. J. EEG EMG, suppl. Sept. 1981, pp. 61—71.
5. Bancaud, J., Talairach, J., Macro-stéréo-électroencephalography in epilepsy. In: Handbook of EEG and Clinical Neurophysiology, vol. 10 (Bancaud, J., ed.), 10 B-3. Amsterdam: Elsevier Publ. 1975.
6. Bancaud, J., Talairach, J., Bonis, A., Schaub, C., Szikla, G., Morel, P., Bordas-Ferrer, M., La stéréo-électro-encéphalographie dans l'épilepsie, 351 pp. Paris: Masson et Cie. 1965.
7. Bancaud, J., Talairach, J., Geier, S., Scarabin, J. M., EEG et SEEG dans les tumeurs cérébrales et l'épilepsie, 351 pp. Paris: Edifor. !973.
8. Bancaud, J., Henriksen, O., Rubio-Donnadieu, F., Seino, M., Dreifuss, F. E., Penry, J. K., Purposal for revised clinical and electroencephalographic classification of epileptic seizures. Epilepsia *22* (1981), 490—501.
9. Bonis, A., Long term results of cortical excision based on stereotactic investigations in severe drug resistant epilepsies. In: Advances in Stereotactic and Functional Neurosurgery 4 (Gillingham, F. J., Gybels, J., Hitchcock, E. R., Rossi, G. F., Szikla, G., eds.), pp. 55—56. Acta Neurochir. Suppl. *30*. Wien-New York: Springer. 1979.
10. Daly, D. D., Ictal clinical manifestations of complex partial seizures. In: Advances in Neurology, vol. 11 (Penry, J. K., Daly, D. D., eds.), pp. 57—82. New York: Raven Press. 1975.
11. Gastaut, H., Clinical and electroencephalographical classification of epileptic seizures. Epilepsia *11* (1970), 101—113.
12. Gastaut, H., Broughton, R., Epileptic seizures. Springfield, Illinois: Ch. C Thomas. 1982.
13. Gibbs, F. A., Gibbs, E. L., Lennox, W. G., Epilepsy: a paroxysmal cerebral dysrythmic. Brain *60* (1937), 377—388.
14. Jackson, J. H., On temporal mental disorders after epileptic paroxysms. In: Selected Writings of John Hughlings Jackson, vol. 1 (Taylor, Y., ed.), pp. 119—134. London: Hodder and Stoughton. 1931.
15. Jasper, H. H., Some physiological mechanisms involved in epileptic automatisms. Epilepsia *5* (1964), 1—20.
16. Munari, C., Bancaud, J., Bonis, A., Buser, P., Talairach, J., Szikla, G., Philippe, A., Rôle du noyau amygdalien dans la survenue de manifestations oro-alimentaires au cours des crises épileptiques chez l'homme. Rev. EEG Neurophysiol. *3* (1979), 236—240.
17. Munari, C., Bancaud, J., Bonis, A., Stoffels, C., Szikla, G., Talairach, J., Impairment of consciousness in temporal lobe seizures: a stereoelectro-encephalographic study. In: Advances in Epileptology, XIth Epilepsy International Symposium (Canger, R., Angeleri, F., Penry, J. K., eds.), pp. 111—114. New York: Raven Press. 1980.

18. Munari, C., Bancaud, J., Stoffels, C., Talairach, J., Bonis, A., Manifestations automatiques dans les crises épileptiques partielles complexes d'origine temporale. Progressi in Epilettologia, Canger, R., Avanzini, G., Tassinari, C. A., eds., 1980, 115—117.
19. Munari, C., Bonis, A., Stoffels, C., Bossi, L., Talairach, J., Bancaud, J., Automatic activities during frontal and temporal lobe seizures: are they the same? Acta Neurol. Scand., suppl. 7, *62* (1980), 40—41.
20. Munari, C., Stoffels, C., Bossi, L., Brunet, P., Bonis, A., Bancaud, J., Talairach, J., Partial seizures with elementary or complex symptomatology: a valid classification for temporal lobe seizures? In: Advances in Epileptology: XIIIth Epilepsy Intern. Symposium (Akimoto, H., Kazamatzuri, A., Seino, M., Ward, A., eds.), pp. 25—27. New York: Raven Press. 1982.
21. Penfield, W., Erickson, T. C., Epilepsy and cerebral localization: a study of the mechanisms, treatment and prevention of epileptic seizures. Springfield, Illinois: Ch. C Thomas. 1941.
22. Penfield, W., Jasper, H., Epilepsy and the functional anatomy of the human brain, 896 pp. Boston: Little, Brown. 1954.
23. Penry, J. K., Perspectives in complex partial seizures. In: Advances in Neurology, vol. 11 (Penry, J. K., Daly, D. D., eds.), pp. 1—11. New York: Raven Press. 1975.
24. Penry, J. K., Dreifuss, F. E., Automatisms associated with the absence of petit mal epilepsy. Arch. Neurol. *21* (1969), 142—149.
25. Stoffels, C., Munari, C., Bonis, A., Bancaud, J., Talairach, J., Manifestations génitales et "sexuelles" lors des crises épileptiques partielles chez l'homme. Rev. EEG Neurophysiol. *10*, 4 (1981), 386—392.
26. Szikla, G., Bouvier, G., Hori, T., Petrov, V., Angiography of the human brain cortex. Atlas of vascular patterns and stereotactic cortical localization, 273 pp. Berlin-Heidelberg-New York: Springer. 1977.
27. Talairach, J., Bancaud, J., Geier, S., Bordas-Ferrer, M., Bonis, A., Szikla, G., Rusu, M., The cingulate gyrus and human behaviour. Electroenceph. clin. Neurophysiol. *34* (1973), 45—52.
28. Talairach, J., Bancaud, J., Szikla, G., Bonis, A., Geier, S., Vedrenne, C., Approche nouvelle de la neurochirurgie de l'épilepsie. Méthodologie stéréotaxique et résultats thérapeutiques. Neurochirurgie, suppl. 20, 240 pp. Paris: Masson et Cie. 1974.

Acta Neurochirurgica, Suppl. 33, 17—33 (1984)

Automatic Analysis of Electrocerebral Activity

H. G. Wieser[1]

With 10 Figures

Summary

An overview of different methods of automatic EEG analysis is presented from the clinical point of view. Correlation analysis and coherence functions have somewhat limited value because they assume "normality" or Gaussian distribution of the signals under consideration. Since the curves are more complex the "Average Amount of Mutual Information" (AAMI) technique may become more important in future investigations. Automatic EEG analysis lends itself well to the study of epileptic phenomena especially in terms of seizure origin and subsequent spread of discharges.

Keywords: Automatic EEG analysis.

With respect to the use of computers for EEG analysis Rémond and Storm van Leeuwen[17] have remarked that

"Machines can do nothing that humans aren't already doing or capable of doing if they set their minds to it and take enough time".

This statement is obviously false in its generality—as everyone, who has tried to fly to Rome without the use of a machine, will admit. But even in the restricted field of computerized EEG analysis we feel that this statement is not true.

The use of computers in EEG analysis aims at the following main goals:

[1] Department of Neurology/SEEG, University Hospital, CH-8091 Zürich, Switzerland.

Firstly, it should relieve the human EEG-er in his time-consuming and tiring work.

Secondly, and more importantly, it should discover things not visible to the naked eye.

Thirdly, a computer program is a complete description of how the results are arrived at. Therefore complete replication of evaluation techniques, and comparison of results between centers is possible. Moreover, based on the quantification processes, exact numerical descriptions of the EEG characteristics are available.

Furthermore, tasks can be carried out, which are virtually impossible without computers. The detailed analysis of interrelations between different EEG channels, for example, provides information which is not available from visual assessment of the raw EEG. Nevertheless, the human EEG-er is still required to interpret the findings obtained by the computer. Thus, the situation is that of a fruitful dialog and cooperation, between man and machine.

Before entering our main field of interest, which is the computer-aided analysis of ictal surface and depth-EEG recordings, I should briefly outline the main analysis methods and give some historical flashbacks. I do not intend to present a complete description of the various analysis approaches because Lopes da Silva [11] has recently given an excellent survey on this topic.

Here it should only be pointed to the fact, that a taxonomy of techniques can be done in different ways, depending on the professional background of the investigator. While from a theoretical aspect one can distinguish non-parametric and parametric methods, a quite practical criterion is the difference in whether analog or digital or hybrid computer-systems are used. Moreover, it is well-known that for a function of time there exists an equivalent representation in the frequency domain via Fourier transformation. Consequently, a further important characteristic can be seen in the type of representation, either time domain or frequency domain. Furthermore it can be distinguished between the intended results of an analysis. Particularly whether it is the background activity that has to be described, or transitory patterns, which can be called the foreground. In the case of the background activity, operations in the frequency domain are adequate. The problem of stationarity or finding an appropriate epoch length for applying the Fourier transformation can be solved.

Difficulties arise, however, if very short-lasting transitions are considered, because the transformation has to be carried out with respect to the final epoch length. Therefore, in order to detect time-varying effects, patterns and episodic phenomena, other methods have been successfully developed. The most important are:

Autoregressive Models (Lopes da Silva *et al.* 1975[10])
Iterative Time Domain Analysis (Schenk 1976[18])
Adaptive Segmentation (Bodenstein and Praetorius 1977[2])
Inverse Filtering (Zetterberg 1973[24])
Matched Filtering (Pfurtscheller and Fischer 1978[15]).

Most of these techniques make use of rather sophisticated mathematical paradigms[3].

A last category of analytic approaches is best called "Mimetic Analysis". In contrast to the former ones, "Mimetic Analysis" methods imitate, as close as possible, the decision process as carried out by an human EEG-er[6].

Because of the wide use of the spectral analysis of the EEG, some remarks on its history and rationale should be given:

It is worthwile to remember, that already in 1932, very soon after the first publication of Berger[1] the physicist Dietsch[8] applied Fourier analysis to EEG-recordings. He "digitized" the EEG by measuring manually the enlarged EEG curves. The Fourier transformation was carried out with the help of a mechanical calculator.

Somewhat easier to apply was spectral analysis by means of a set of bandpass filters, pioneered by W. Grey Walter[19] in 1943. Results of this technique were immediately available, whereas in most modern methods this advantage of an analysis in real time has been lost.

With the advent of statistical communication theory Brazier and Casby[3] first applied correlation techniques to the EEG. The discovery of a fast algorithm for the discrete Fourier transform in 1965 by Cooley and Tukey[7] and the increasing availability of fast digital computers made spectral analysis a standard tool in many research centers and even an accepted tool in daily diagnostic practice.

By means of Fourier analysis the EEG is split into a number of sine waves of different frequency. This means, that the EEG, which is a function of time, is transformed into a spectrum which is a function of frequency. Usually, in electroencephalography, the spectrum is displayed as a power spectrum, that is, as power versus frequency, and has the dimension $\mu V^2/Hz$.

The distribution of the power which is common to two EEG channels is the cross-spectrum. Usually the cross-spectrum is normalized and then it is called the coherence-spectrum. The coherence values may be interpreted as correlation coefficients per frequency. The coherence values show the degree of relationship between two EEG-channels in a given frequency range.

An efficient application of spectral analysis methods is almost impossible without digital computers. Processing of the EEG by means of computers requires that the data are digitized. This is done through an analog-to-digital converter. The time difference between two sampling values is called sampling interval and its reciprocal value is called sampling frequency. The analyzed EEG is always only of a certain limited length of the record. The length of the analysis interval determines the frequency spacing in the frequency domain. The half-sampling frequency is the highest possible frequency component which can be represented.

An example, illustrated in Fig. 1 and Table 1 and taken from Rappelsberger[16], should be helpful in explaining the Fourier-transformation: We assume the length of the analysis interval to be 1 sec. The EEG-signal (X_t) of this example (Fig. 1) is the composite of a 2 Hz and 4 Hz sine wave. The 4 Hz sine wave has only half the amplitude of the 2 Hz wave and in addition it is phase shifted, that means the zero-crossings take place at different time. The complex signal X_t is sampled 12 times. The 6 harmonic cosine and sine waves, which are obtained from the 12 sampled points, are shown below. Remember that the highest spectral frequency is given by the half of the sampling frequency. In this example 12 divided by 2, which is 6. Moreover, the basic frequency is 1 because the length of analysis time of our example is 1 sec.

What the computer has to do now performing the Fourier transformation is very simple and shown in Table 1: The components of the sine and cosine waves have to be multiplied with the sampled EEG values at times t_1, t_2 and so on. Then the values obtained this way are added for every given sine and cosine and finally divided by half the sampling value, which is 6 in this example. Now looking to the very right of Table 1 we find only the component of 2 Hz different from zero and the two components of 4 Hz. The phase shift of 45° is indicated by the sum of a sine and cosine component as indicated by both values of these 4 Hz waves.

To calculate the power spectrum, one has to multiply the Fourier coefficient by itself and multiply this value by the analysis time (t). This way a periodogram is

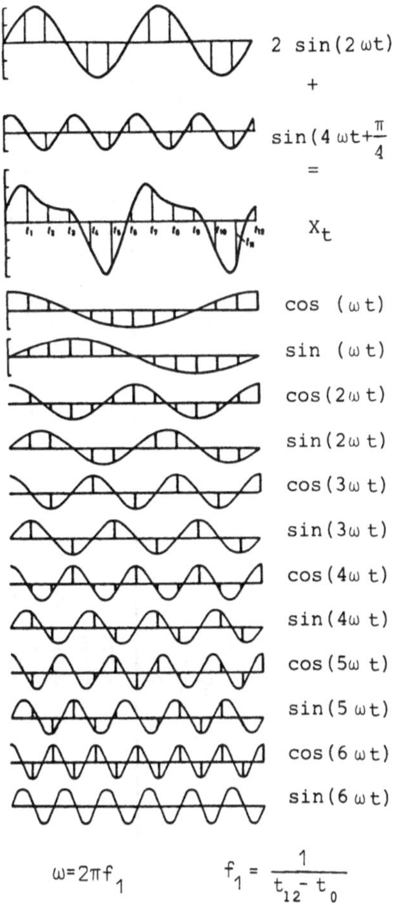

Fig. 1. Illustration of Fourier-transformation: The signal X_t is the sum of both sine waves shown above. It is sampled twelve times ($t_1 \rightarrow t_{12}$). This way six harmonic cosine and sine waves are obtained (from Rappelsberger[16])

obtained (Fig. 2) which in a further step undergoes smoothing. Smoothing is necessary to improve the very bad statistical properties of the periodogram. Smoothing can be done in different ways.

A few practical applications shall illustrate the value of this technique. As already mentioned, spectral analysis is very useful in discribing the background EEG. An example of power spectra from an epileptic patient during the waking state and different sleep stages is given in Fig. 3.

Table 1. *Illustration of Fourier Transformation*. See text (from[16])

		t	t_1	t_2	t_3	t_4	t_5	t_6	t_7	t_8	t_9	t_{10}	t_{11}	t_{12}	
		x_t	1.991	0.766	0.707	-1.473	-2.698	0.707	1.991	0.766	0.707	-1.473	-2.698	0.707	
harmonics	1	cos	0.866	0.5	0	-0.5	-0.866	-1.0	-0.866	-0.5	0	0.5	0.866	1.0	
		sin	0.5	0.866	1.0	0.866	0.5	0	-0.5	-0.866	-1.0	-0.866	-0.5	0	
	2	cos	0.5	-0.5	-1.0	-0.5	0.5	1.0	0.5	-0.5	-1.0	-0.5	0.5	1.0	
		sin	0.866	0.866	0	-0.866	-0.866	0	0.866	0.866	0	-0.866	-0.866	0	
	3	cos	0	-1.0	0	1.0	0	-1.0	0	1.0	0	-1.0	0	1.0	
		sin	1.0	0	-1.0	0	1.0	0	-1.0	0	1.0	0	-1.0	0	
	4	cos	-0.5	-0.5	1.0	-0.5	-0.5	1.0	-0.5	-0.5	1.0	-0.5	-0.5	1.0	
		sin	0.866	-0.866	0	0.866	-0.866	0	0.866	-0.866	0	0.866	-0.866	0	
	5	cos	-0.866	0.5	0	-0.5	0.866	-1.0	0.866	-0.5	0	0.5	-0.866	1.0	
		sin	0.5	-0.866	1.0	-0.866	0.5	0	-0.5	0.866	-1.0	0.866	-0.5	0	
	6	cos	-1.0	1.0	-1.0	1.0	-1.0	1.0	-1.0	1.0	-1.0	1.0	-1.0	1.0	CO(f)
		sin	0	0	0	0	0	0	0	0	0	0	0	0	SI(f)
cross-products	1	cos	1.724	0.383	0	0.737	2.337	-0.707	-1.724	-0.383	0	-0.737	-2.337	0.707	0
		sin	0.996	0.663	0.707	-1.276	-1.349	0	-0.996	-0.663	-0.707	1.276	1.349	0	0
	2	cos	0.996	-0.383	-0.707	0.737	-1.349	0.707	0.996	-0.383	-0.707	0.737	-1.349	0.707	0
		sin	1.724	0.863	0	1.276	2.337	0	1.724	0.663	0	1.276	2.337	0	2.0
	3	cos	0	-0.766	0	-1.473	0	-0.707	0	0.766	0	1.473	0	0.707	0
		sin	1.991	0	-0.707	0	-2.698	0	-1.991	0	0.707	0	2.698	0	0
	4	cos	-0.996	-0.383	0.707	0.737	1.349	0.707	-0.996	-0.383	0.707	0.737	1.349	0.707	0.707
		sin	1.724	-0.663	0	-1.276	2.337	0	1.724	-0.663	0	-1.276	2.337	0	0.707
	5	cos	-1.724	-0.383	0	0.737	-2.337	-0.707	1.724	-0.338	0	-0.737	2.337	0.707	0
		sin	0.996	-0.663	0.707	1.276	-1.349	0	-0.996	0.663	-0.707	-1.276	1.349	0	0
	6	cos	-1.991	0.766	-0.707	-1.473	2.698	0.707	-1.991	0.766	-0.707	-1.473	2.698	0.707	0
		sin	0	0	0	0	0	0	0	0	0	0	0	0	0

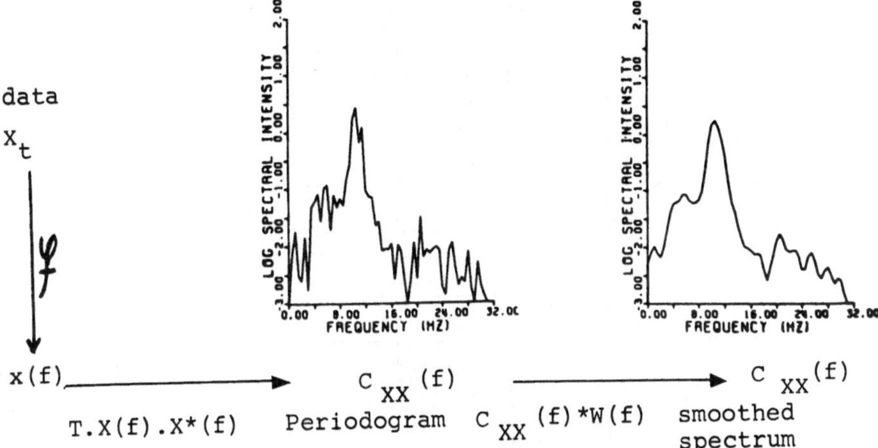

Fig. 2. Arithmetic operations for the calculation of the power spectrum (from[16])

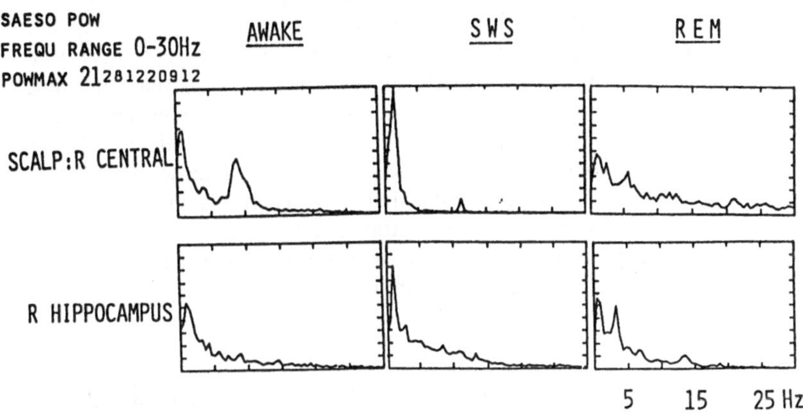

Fig. 3. Power spectra of synchronously recorded EEG from the right central scalp and right hippocampal formation. Note the high alpha-peak in the scalp EEG during waking state and the high delta-peak and a distinct 12/sec sleep spindle-peak during slow-wave-sleep (SWS). During REM a theta peak of about 4/sec emerges in the hippocampus

Similar spectra, now together with coherence and phase spectra are shown in Fig. 4, which is derived from a pain-patient[21,22]. This patient had a stimulating electrode with the target point in the periaqueductal grey matter (PGM) which passed through thalamic nuclei.

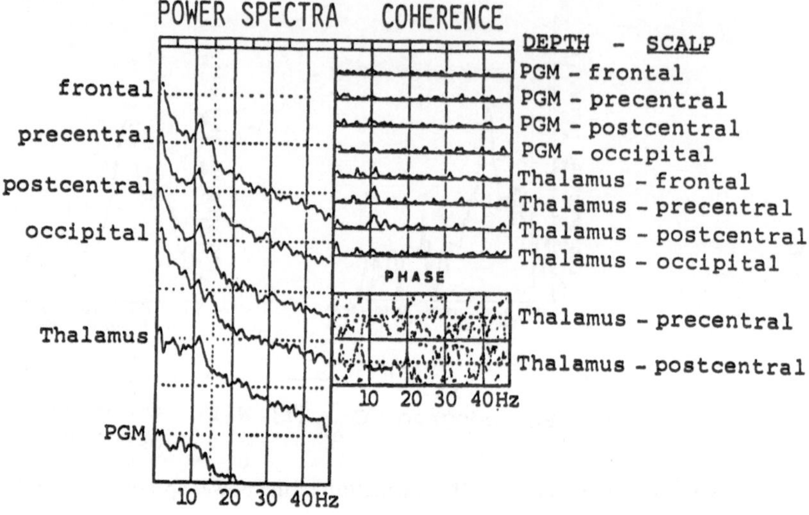

Fig. 4. The power spectra of thalamic and scalp derivations show similar peaks of about 12/sec during spindle sleep. The coherence spectrum shows the degree of relationship between the two EEG channels indicated on the right. As explained, coherence values may be interpreted as correlation coefficients per frequency. The values are between Ø and 1. Ø means no relationship at a given frequency, 1 identical EEGs within this given frequency. As can be seen, the coherence between the thalamic electrode and frontal as well as central scalp electrodes is rather high for this spindle frequency of 12/sec. The phase-spectra indicate a rather stable phase relation, once again only for this frequency. Therefore one can calculate a time-lag between thalamus and postcentral spindle waves of about 8 msec. (A 12 Hz wave has a duration of 83 msec. The indicated phase-lag of about 36 degrees is therefore a tenth of 83 msec.)

We have employed time series of power spectra also for the analysis of ictal depth EEG recordings (Fig. 5). Besides other numerical tabulations[20], we have plotted spectra in a given time interval for all 32 channels. Values are normalized to the maximum power, occurring in all channels in a given interval (Fig. 6). Moreover, spectra were followed in a given channel for all analyzed time intervals (Fig. 7).

The amount of research concerning the analysis of seizure recordings is still very limited. In the analysis of ictal recordings the objective is to determine whether all the seizures of a patient originate in the same area. And if so, where this area is located. This question arises especially for those patients who are candidates for surgical treatment of an otherwise intractable and severe epileptic

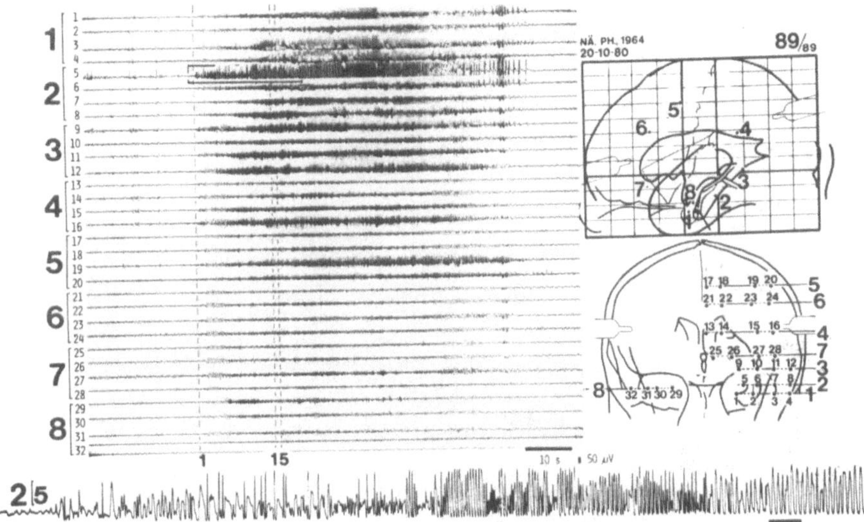

Fig. 5. Depth recorded seizure originating in left hippocampus (electrode 2, recording point 5). Channel *5* is reproduced enlarged at the bottom. Recording is against an inactive common average reference (from Wieser[20])

disorder. Most of these surgical candidates suffer from partial seizures. Propagation and spread of the discharge to other brain areas of one or finally both hemispheres represent severe difficulties, especially if the spread of a seizure is so quick that it cannot be followed by the naked eye and initial clinical features may also escape detection.

Approaches to the analysis of ictal EEG recordings by using computer assisted analysis techniques have started with Mary Brazier's work. Brazier[3–5] applied linear system analysis methods to depth recordings of seizure activity. By estimating coherence and phase between pairs of derivations, she calculated the spread of epileptic discharges within the human brain. Brazier[5] remarked that

> "the detection of a source, that drives the abnormal activity to other parts of the brain ... may have a future in terms of therapeutic procedure. The possibility presents itself that a single coagulation either of the locus itself or of the efferent connections from it might replace the more radical therapy of surgical removal of the temporal lobe".

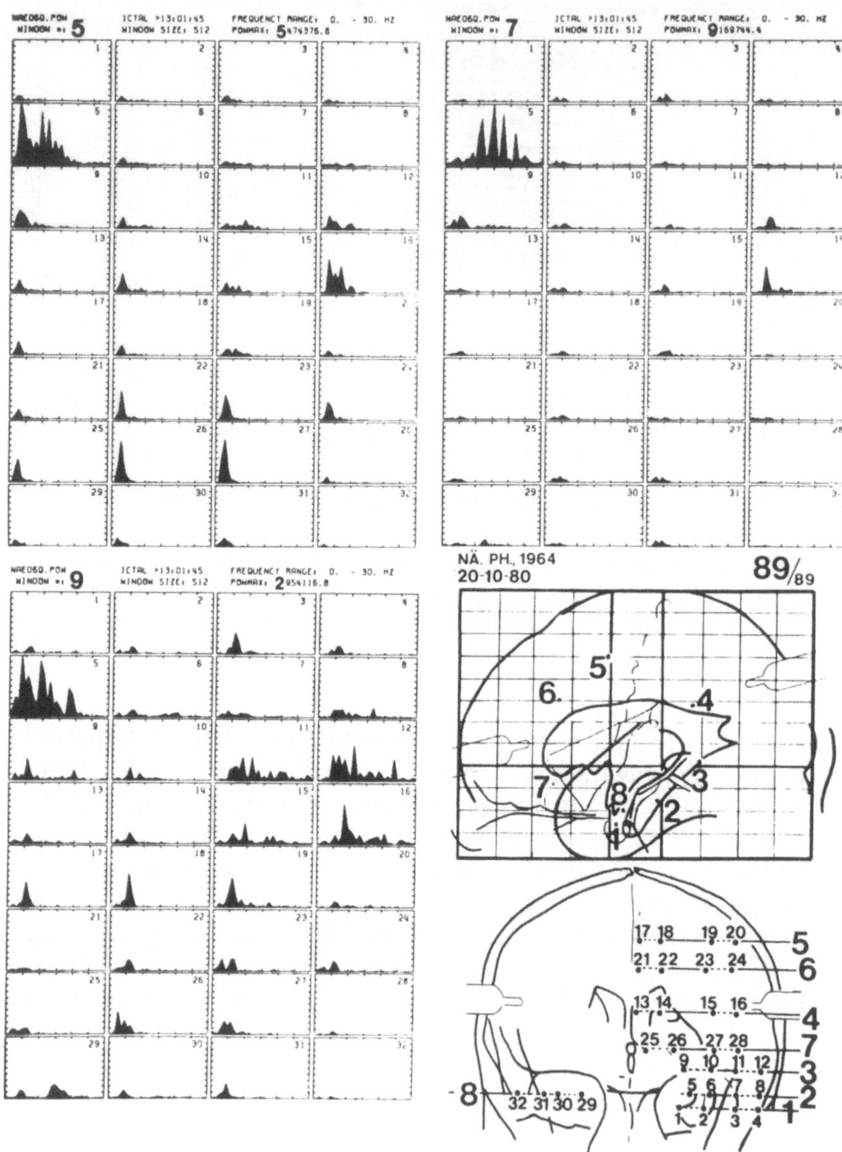

Fig. 6. Power spectra of the 32 channels shown in Fig. 5. Interval numbers (window) *5*, *7* and *9*. Very clearly the channel number *5*, which represents the activity of the left hippocampus, dominates this early seizure stage

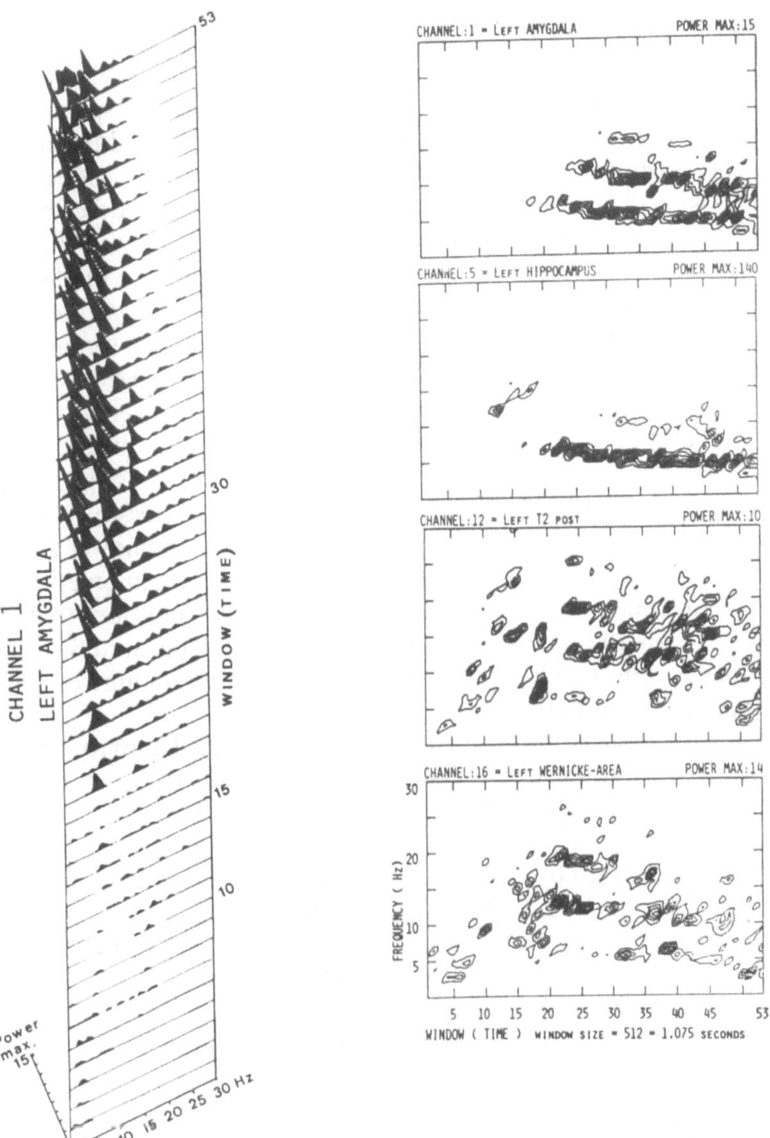

Fig. 7. Compressed spectral array plot (left) of the seizure activity of left amygdala shown in Fig. 5 illustrating the power spectra followed over the analyzed time intervals. Values are normalized to the maximum power occurring in one channel over all intervals. Only those peaks are visible which equal or exceed 10% of the peakpower. On the right another display of the frequency analysis of the same seizure is given. However spectra are now plotted as contour charts to be read like geographical maps. From the top to the bottom are shown: left amygdala, left hippocampus, left second temporal convolution and Wernicke-area. Time is indicated from left to the right, and covers about 1 minute. Maximal power is ten times higher in hippocampus than in the other 3 plots shown here. Note that the spectral array plot of the amygdala on the left is turned now 90 degrees and reproduced in the contour chart at the top

Brazier's delay times derived from the cross power spectra were in agreement with known anatomical pathways. A different and more sophisticated application of linear system analysis is based on the so called "partial coherences" and has been described by Gersch[9] and others in the last ten years. In this method triples of signals are considered. Computing partial coherences implies as a first step elimination from each of the 2 signals of a pair *that part,* that can be considered as being determined by a third signal. If the partial coherence between 2 of the signals partialized on the 3rd signal is very low in a frequency band of high spectral energy, and if only one of the 3 signals has this property, the third signal is considered to drive the 2 others. A single site is sought which appears to drive all other areas by analyzing all possible channel combinations. Computations of the coherences and power spectra is done by the autoregressive model approach. This method of partial coherences, however, requires the assumption that the signal from the causal site is propagated through linear networks to other locations. Coherence measures only the amount of linear dependence of two signals.

Most models for the propagation of neuronal activity contain essential non-linear elements. In Fig. 8 a general model for the generation of 2 EEG signals is shown. In this model the observed signals X and Y, indicated on the right as a function of time, are delayed by amounts Δ_1 and Δ_2 and non-linearly filtered by filters NL_1 and NL_2. The output signals are corrupted by additive noises (n_1) and (n_2).

If only the two observations X and Y are available, the elements of this model cannot be identified. Therefore a simplified model has to be used to describe the relation between 2 EEG signals. It is given in the lower part of Fig. 8.

For non-linear relationships, as exemplified by the EEG, the best analysis method is probably the "Average Amount of Mutual Information" (AAMI) analysis developed by Mars and van Arragon[13]. AAMI is a measure of the predictability of one signal if another is given. In case of Gaussian distributed signal values the AAMI would equal the conventional correlation coefficient.

Because most probably the EEG signals within the brain undergo not only time delays but also non-linear operations, as shown, the correlation coefficient looses its simple interpretation, while the AAMI retains its meaning. Therefore, the main advantage of this AAMI-technique is its very robustness for non-linearities. This technique involves estimating the maximum value

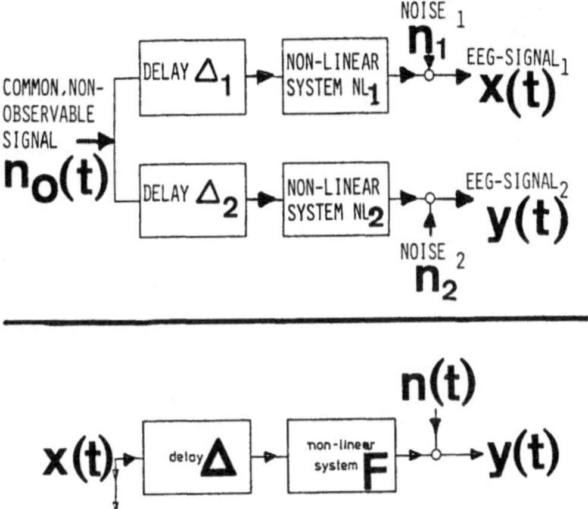

Fig. 8. General model (above) and simplified model (below) for the generation of two EEG signals X and Y. See text (from Mars[12])

of AAMI *and a time lag* at which this maximum occurs. Mars[12] computed AAMI values for lags in the range of — 50 to + 50 msec. He applied this analysis to kindled seizures in the dog and to human depth EEG data. The most important findings of his study are in full agreement with our previously reported studies concerning the coupling of different channels during a seizure. In summary it was found that in focal seizures three periods can be differentiated. The first period is characterized by independence of the local activities in the focus and elsewhere. In the second period there is strong coupling with a consistent time delay between the focus and related areas. In the third period the structures became mutually independently active, that means the coupling disappeared at least between the areas studied. Very important is the finding that during the second period the time delay changed with ongoing seizure time.

In comparison to the method of AAMI, our own approach of measuring functional versus anatomical distances in the brain[14, 23] is mathematically much more simple and has the advantage that results can be visualized directly on TV-screen. An interactive display system permits arbitrary rotation for viewing as well as bidirectional scanning in time.

The objective and method of this analysis methods are[14]: Disregarding EEG signal power and frequency spectrum, we calculated the correlation matrix for 32 intracerebral EEG signals

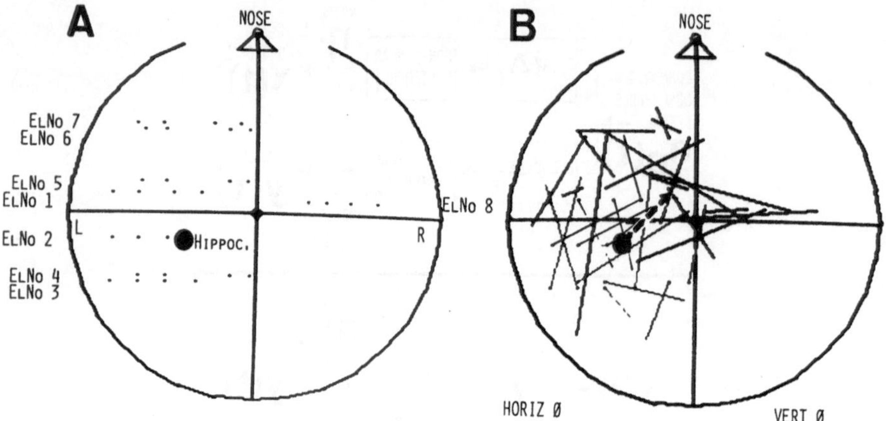

Fig. 9. A) Examples from a movie, illustrating the measurement of functional versus anatomical distances. Dots indicate anatomical locations, as given by the depth probes of the patient, whose seizure is shown in Fig. 5. The left hippocampus is marked by the large dot. B) Essentially coherent activity of most locations during the preictal period, i.e., before the epileptic discharge starts. Note that display of the electrode assemblies are originally identified by colour on the TV-screen. In this figure, the vector of the left hippocampus was subsequently emphasized by dotted lines

for 256 point windows, sampling every channel at 476 c/s. Defining the complexity of these signals as the number of eigenvalues greater than 1, we assumed a visual simplification to a 3 dimensional space to be meaningful and mapped the first three coordinates of the 32 eigenvectors into an idealized unit sphere, representing the skull with the brain (Fig. 9 A). Interpretation is very easy: If the intracerebral signals would be exactly identical, their vectors, indicated by the coloured lines in the TV-display, would all point to one common place (Fig. 9 B). If only one location, *i.e.* one vector, moves off, like in Fig. 10, this location whose activity is unrelated to all others, is a candidate for a seizure originating area. Progressive coupling of other brain areas with such a seizure initiating area showing an aberrant activity-vector, can be interpreted as ictal synchronization. Finally, the anisotropic spread of the seizure discharge to other brain sites can be visualized by this method. If the ends of coloured vector-lines move close together, this indicates ictally active pathways between these structures.

Such an analysis, which is possible in a real time version, brings some practical help and is not restricted to seizures. The

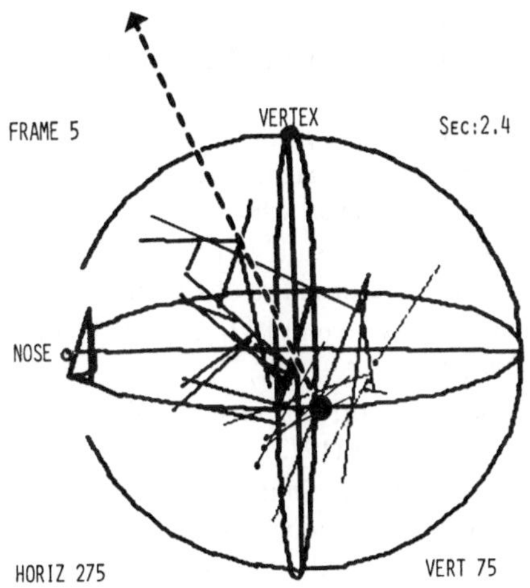

Fig. 10. Strong "individual" activity of the left hippocampus (vector marked by dotted lines) indicates the seizure origin at this location. Same patient and same seizure as in Fig. 5

disadvantage, however, is that time lags between two signals have been disregarded until now. To study these one has to use the AAMI method.

Ictally active pathways have also been studied based on the first 10 seconds and on the entire length of 213 complex partial seizures using multidimensional scaling methods. An unexpected finding was the observation that deep temporal structures—amygdala, hippocampus—were most closely linked to *contra*lateral temporal neocortical association areas[23].

References

1. Berger, H., Über das Elektroenkephalogramm des Menschen. Arch. Psychiat. Nervenkr. *87* (1929), 527—570.
2. Bodenstein, G., Praetorius, H. M., Feature extraction from the encephalogram by adaptive segmentation. Proc. IEEE *65* (1977), 642—652.
3. Brazier, M. A. B., Casby, J. V., Some application of correlation analysis to clinical problems in electroencephalography. Electroencephalography Clin. Neurophysiol. *8* (1956), 325—331.
4. Brazier, M. A. B., Electrical activity recorded simultaneously from the scalp and deep structures of the human brain. J. Nerv. Ment. Dis. *147/1* (1968), 31—39.

5. Brazier, M. A. B., Spread of seizure discharges in epilepsy: anatomical and electrophysiological considerations. Experimental Neurology *36* (1972), 263—272.
6. Burr, W., Computerized pattern analysis of MLE recordings. In: Mobile Long-term EEG Monitoring (Stefan, H., Burr, W., eds.), pp. 275—288. Stuttgart-New York: G. Fischer. 1982.
7. Cooley, J. W., Tukey, J. W., An algorithm for the machine calculation of complex Fourier series. Mathematics of Computation *19* (1965), 267—301.
8. Dietsch, G., Fourier-Analyse von Elektroenzephalogrammen des Menschen. Pflügers Arch. *230* (1932), 106—112.
9. Gersch, W., Causality or driving in electrophysiological signal analysis. Mathematical Biosciences *14* (1972), 177—196.
10. Lopes da Silva, F. H., Dijk, A., Smits, H., Detection of non-stationarities in EEGs using the autoregressive model. An application to EEG of epileptics. In: CEAN Computerized EEG Analysis (Dolce, G., Künkel, H., eds.), pp. 180—199. Stuttgart: G. Fischer. 1975.
11. Lopes da Silva, F. H., Computer-assisted EEG diagnosis: pattern recognition in EEG analysis, feature extraction and classification. In: Electroencephalography (Niedermeyer, E., Lopes da Silva, F. H., eds.), pp. 685—711. Baltimore-München: Schwarzenberg. 1982.
12. Mars, N. J. I., Computer-augmented Analysis of Electroencephalogram in Epilepsy. Proef Schrift, Enschede, Holland, 1983.
13. Mars, N. J. I., Arragon, G. W., van, Time delay estimation in non-linear systems using Average Amount of Mutual Information analysis. Signal Processing *4* (1982), 139—153.
14. Meles, H. P., Wieser, H. G., Computer-generated dynamic presentation of functional versus anatomical distances in the human brain. Appl. Neurophysiol. *45* (1982), 404—405.
15. Pfurtscheller, G., Fischer, G., A new approach to spike detection using a combination of inverse and matched filter techniques. Electroencephalography Clin. Neurophysiol. *44* (1978), 243—247.
16. Rappelsberger, P., Einführung in die EEG-Spektralanalyse. J. Electrophysiol. Technol. *3/1* (1977), 18—38.
17. Rémond, A., Storm van Leeuwen, W., Why analyze, quantify or process routine clinical EEG. In: EEG Informatics: A Didactic Review of Methods and Applications of EEG Data Processing (Rémond, A., ed.), pp. 1—7. Amsterdam: Elsevier, 1977.
18. Schenk, G. K., The pattern-oriented aspect of the EEG quantification. Model and clinical basis of the iterative time-domain approach. In: Quantitative Analytic Studies in Epilepsy (Kellaway, P., Petersén, I., eds.), pp. 431—461. New York: Raven Press. 1976.
19. Walter, W. G., Automatic low frequency analyzer. Electronic Engineering *16* (1943), 9—13.
20. Wieser, H. G., Value of long-term EEG and stereo-EEG in candidates of surgical epilepsy therapy. In: Mobile Long-term EEG Monitoring (Stefan, H., Burr, W., eds.), pp. 121—136. Stuttgart-New York: G. Fischer. 1982.

21. Wieser, H. G., Siegfried, J., Hirnstamm-Ableitungen (Makroelektroden) beim Menschen. 1. Elektrische Befunde im Wachzustand und Ganznachtschlaf. Z. EEG-EMG *10* (1979), 8—19.
22. Wieser, H. G., Siegfried, J., Hirnstamm-Ableitungen (Makroelektroden) beim Menschen. 2. Klinische und elektrische Effekte bei Stimulation im periaquäduktalen Grau (PGM); Augenbewegungs-abhängige Aktivität; visuelle und somatosensorische Reizantworten im PGM. Z. EEG-EMG *10* (1979), 62—69.
23. Wieser, H. G., Electroclinical Features of the Psychomotor Seizure, (242 pp. Stuttgart-New York-London: G. Fischer, Butterworths. 1983.
24. Zetterberg, L. H., Spike detection by computer and by analog equipment. In: Automation of Clinical Electroencephalography (Kellaway, P., Petersén, I., eds.), pp. 227—242. New York: Raven Press. 1973.

Acta Neurochirurgica, Suppl. 33, 35—46 (1984)

Changes of Energy Metabolism and Regional Cerebral Blood Flow Studied by Positron Emission Tomography in the Interictal Phase of Partial Epilepsy

Y. L. Yamamoto[1], R. Ochs[1], W. Ammann[1], E. Meyer[1], A. C. Evans[2], B. Cooke[2], M. Izawa[1], A. Kato[1], P. Gloor[1], W. H. Feindel[1], M. Diksic[1], and C. J. Thompson[1]

With 2 Figures

Summary

We report here results of positron emission tomographic studies on 14 patients with partial epilepsy using fluorine-18 labelled fluorodeoxyglucose for regional cerebral metabolic rate for glucose (rCMRGl) and oxygen-15 for regional cerebral blood flow (rCBF) and regional cerebral metabolic rate for oxygen (rCMRO). Quantitative rCMRGl studies in the interictal phase of partial epilepsy reveal five different patterns of significantly abnormal metabolic changes. These correlate well with EEG findings recorded during the ictal or interictal phase in 12 of 14 cases. However there is no close correlation between rCMRGl and either rCBF or rCMRO findings in the maximum epileptic disturbance during the interictal phase as assessed by electroencephalography.

Keywords: Position emission tomography; partial epilepsy.

Introduction

Epilepsy is a complex sequence of symptoms deriving from a wide variety of causes[10,12]. When neurosurgical treatment of partial epilepsy is anticipated, a delineation of the epileptogenic

[1] Montreal Neurological Institute, McGill University, 3801 University St., Montreal, Quebec, H3A 2B4 Canada.
[2] Atomic Energy of Canada Ltd., Ottawa, Ontario, Canada.

focus in a localized area of the brain is particularly important[14]. At the present time both classification and localization of epilepsy depend heavily on electrophysiological techniques.

Recent positron emission tomographic (PET) studies by a group at UCLA[5a,5b,11] using fluorine-18 labelled fluorodeoxyglucose (FDG) to obtain the regional cerebral glucose metabolic rate (rCMRGl) suggest that the location of the hypometabolic area demonstrated by the FDG scan during the interictal phase in partial epilepsy is closely associated with the epileptogenic focus delineated by interictal and ictal electrophysiological recordings. The UCLA group has also noticed a focal increase of rCMRGl in the ictal or immediate post-ictal state of partial epilepsy[6].

Our findings[7] with respect to regional cerebral blood flow (rCBF) in partial epilepsy, using bolus inhalation of krypton-77 (^{77}Kr PET), indicate that focally increased rCBF occurs not only in the epileptogenic cortical area but also in the supplementary cortical areas during or immediately after ictus. On the other hand, ^{77}Kr PET studies during the interictal phase in 14 partial epilepsy cases reveal no significant changes of rCBF in 7 cases, focal increase of rCBF in 4 cases, and general or focal reduction of rCBF in 3 cases.

We report here our more recent studies using the combined techniques of FDG for rCMRGl and ^{15}O-labelled $^{15}O_2$, $C^{15}O_2$ and $C^{15}O$ for rCBF, regional cerebral metabolic rate for oxygen (rCMRO), and regional cerebral blood volume (rCBV) in the interictal phase of partial epilepsy. We correlated these findings with various electrophysiological measurements in the same patients.

Methods

A. Scanning Procedures

The tomographic device used in most of the following studies was a Therascan 3128, manufactured by Atomic Energy of Canada Limited (AECL). The Therascan system consists of two rings of 64 bismuth germanate (BGO) detectors per ring, with a ring diameter of 43 cm. Both direct and cross slice coincidences are acquired, giving a total of 3 slices simultaneously. Image resolution with a medium resolution collimator used for the present studies is 12 mm FWHM (full width at half maximum). The slice thickness is also a resolution of 12 mm FWHM. The sensitivity of the direct (cross) slice is 55 KHz (98 KHz) per µCi per ml in a 20 cm diameter flood phantom. The camera gantry is aligned with the patient's orbito-meatal line by moving the couch and tilting the gantry. After alignment, the acquisition software controls the indexes of the patient and facilitates scanning of the brain with a slice separation of 6 mm for the temporal region, 10 to 12 mm above the Sylvian level for investigation of partial epilepsy.

Images are reconstructed using the following Therascan software package developed by AECL: 1. automatic correction of random coincidences, 2. normalization of detector sensitivity, 3. attenuation correction using a thresholding method similar in concept to that of Bergstrom *et al.*[1] to avoid the practical difficulties associated with the transmission method, 4. removal of scattered events using a deconvolution procedure similar to that of Bergstrom *et al.*[2], developed independently at AECL, 5. accurate cross calibration between the Therascan system and the well counter. Some of the oxygen-15 studies were performed with our Positome III system, a prototype of Therascan 3128 developed here at the Montreal Neurological Institute[15]. Characteristics of Positome III have been described elsewhere[15,18].

B. Preparation of FDG

FDG is prepared by reacting in situ ^{18}F-acetylhypofluorite (prepared by reacting ^{18}F-F_2 with Na acetate in glacial acetic acid) with triacetyl-D-glucal. After extraction with CH_2Cl_2 and hydrolysis with 2 NHCl, ^{18}F-2-FDG is dissolved in a 1 N phosphate buffer (pH = 7). The specific activity after 30 minutes of irradiation and a 60-minute synthesis is approximately 685 mCi/mmol, with radiochemical purity of about 98%[4].

C. PET Studies

1. FDG Study for rCMRGl

For FDG studies, patients are fasted for 10 hours prior to scanning. 5 mCi of FDG is injected intravenously. Arterialized venous samples are obtained from the vein of the opposite hand heated to 42 °C in a hot-water glove box developed by Phelps *et al.*[13] to arterialize venous blood. For determination of plasma glucose and FDG concentrations, 2 ml of blood are taken every 15 seconds for the first 2 minutes, with sample intervals progressively lengthened. About 40 minutes after injection of FDG, 12 to 16 tomographic images are obtained by the tomograph, starting at the orbitomeatal line. Images are reconstructed and combined with cross calibration factors, glucose concentration, and blood activity measurements to yield the quantitative rCMRGl. The FDG analysis program written by one of us (ACE), is based on the Phelps *et al.*[13] modification of the Sokoloff *et al.*[16] model, including the K 4 rate constant. Values for the rate constants K 1 to K 4 as well as for the lumped constant are those established by Huang *et al.*[9]. A rearrangement of the operational equation, suggested by Brooks[3], has been incorporated. In order to display three-dimensional mapping of rCMRGl, a program has been developed to display sagittal or coronal cuts through the same distribution by recordering and interpolating the existing data.

2. Oxygen-15 Studies

Under local anesthetic, an arterial catheter is placed in a radial artery for blood sampling. The technique consists of three repeated procedures: 1. for measurement of the regional oxygen extraction rate (rOER) the patient breathes oxygen-15 labelled molecular oxygen ($^{15}O_2$) to obtain the steady state, 2. for measurement of rCBF oxygen-15 labelled carbon dioxide ($C^{15}O_2$) is inhaled at the physiological concentration, 3. for measurement of rCBV oxygen-15 labelled carbon monoxide ($C^{15}O$) is inhaled. For the $^{15}O_2$ study, 5 mCi per minute with 65 ml per min flow rate of $^{15}O_2$ are given to the patient through an open plastic mask. After the equilibrium state is reached (in 10 to 12 minutes), PET images are taken at the same planes as the FDG study. For the $C^{15}O_2$ study, 3 mCi per minute with 35 ml per minute flow rate of $C^{15}O_2$ are given to the patient. Following the steady state, which also takes 10 to 12 minutes, PET images are taken at the same planes as the previous studies. The blood samples are withdrawn over a period of 15 seconds to average the respiratory cycles. rCBF, rOER, $rCMRO_2$ and rCBV are quantified with equations developed by Frackowiak *et al.*[8].

3. Data Analysis

PET images are obtained at 6 mm intervals at least 3 to 4 tomographic levels through the temporal region. Each local rCMRGl value is determined using a 12 × 12 × 12 mm voxel size. Two or three areas in each region are measured to calculate the rCMRGl value at the particular plane, then the overall mean rCMRGl value at the particular plane, then the overall mean rCMRGl value is determined from 3 to 4 different tomographic levels in the same region.

D. Electroencephalographic (EEG) Methodology

EEG recordings are made from the scalp by telemetry with and without sphenoidal electrodes during the ictal and interictal phases. Further EEG recordings, using sphenoidal electrodes are made during and after the PET studies. The EEG data is analysed both visually and by computer analysis for epileptiform sharp waves and spikes.

Results

1. Normal Subjects

All subjects reported that they remained awake throughout the study. Light and noise were subdued, but ear plugs or eye patchs were not used. Fig. 1 gives examples of FDG studies in normal subjects, illustrating the symmetry of rCMRGl between the two cerebral hemispheres. Table 1 illustrates the mean values of rCMRGl obtained in 5 normal subjects and rCMRO in 6 normal subjects.

2. Partial Epilepsy

In 14 patients with partial epilepsy, FDG studies were performed during the interictal phase. During and after PET studies, EEG recordings are also taken. In our FDG studies we

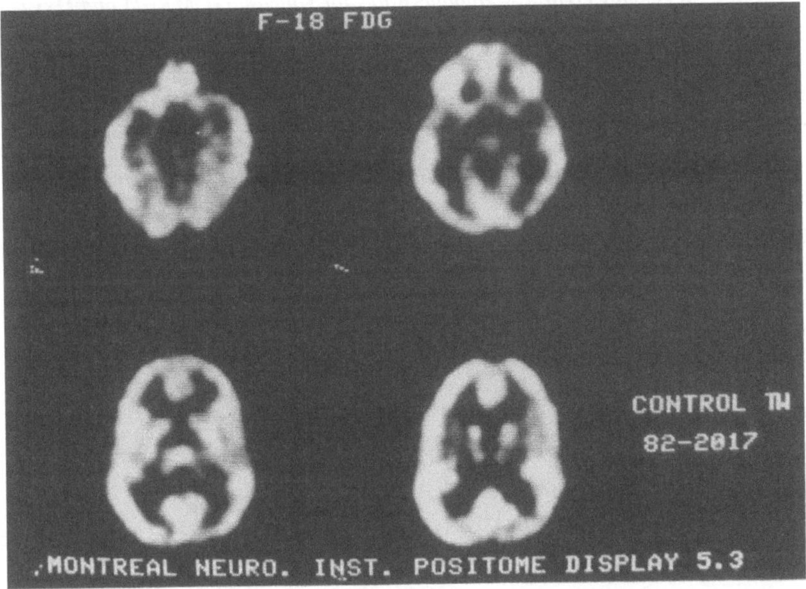

Fig. 1. Four tomographic images for quantitative FDG study in control subjects showing symmetrical rCMRGl in both cerebral hemispheres

observed 5 different patterns of findings during the interictal phase in partial epilepsy, and these are listed in Table 2.

In type I, unilateral focal hypometabolism, 2 cases show 24 to 29% focal reduction of rCMRGl from the control values ($p < 0.005$; < 0.02) which correlate closely with EEG recordings of maximum epileptic discharges during the interictal phase.

In type II, focal hypometabolism with ipsilateral local extension of hypometabolism, the results of 5 cases indicate focal reduction of 28 to 48% of rCMRGl from the control values ($p < 0.001$) in the entire temporal region, with local extension of hypometabolism to the ipsilateral centro-parietal or centro-frontal region. These findings also correlate well with EEG recordings during either ictal or interictal phases in all cases, except one where a porencephalic cyst was found in the area of hypometabolism, while the epileptiform EEG abnormalities predominated contralaterally.

In type III, bilateral focal hypometabolism, 2 cases show a focal reduction of 19 to 24% of rCMRGl from the control values ($p < 0.02$, < 0.005) in the anterior temporal region with left temporal predominance. The interictal epileptiform disturbances in

Table 1. *Regional Cerebral Metabolic Rates for Glucose (rCMRGl) and Oxygen (rCMRO) in Normal Volunteers*

Location	rCMRGl (μmol/100 g/min)	rCMRO (μmol/100 g/min)
Anterior temporal	45 ± 7	227 ± 84
Posterior temporal	46 ± 7	
Parietal	50 ± 9	215 ± 71
Central	47 ± 7	264 ± 136
Frontal	44 ± 8	285 ± 116
Caudate nucleus	43 ± 7	171 ± 43
Thalamus	45 ± 9	190 ± 57
White matter	17 ± 3	81 ± 38
Mean	40 ± 1	165 ± 39

Table 2. *Patterns of FDG Findings in Partial Epilepsy*

Type I	Unilateral focal hypometabolism	2
Type II	Unilateral focal hypometabolism with local extension of hypometabolism	5
Type III	Bilateral focal hypometabolism	2
Type IV	Unilateral focal hypometabolism with contralateral focal hypermetabolism	1
Type V	Diffuse bilateral hypometabolism with maximum unilateral focal hypometabolism	4
	Total	14

the EEG were also bitemporal and showed left temporal predominance.

In type IV, unilateral focal hypometabolism and contralateral focal hypermetabolism, one case shows a focal reduction of 60% of rCMRGl ($p < 0.001$) in the right anterior temporal region with 35% increase of rCMRGl ($p < 0.001$) in the contralateral left anterior temporal region. The main epileptiform EEG abnormalities in this case were on the side of the hypermetabolic zone: the interical epileptiform abnormalities, although bitemporal in location predominated on the left side, and the ictal

EEG abnormalities were localized to the left temporal region. In this case EEG recordings revealed focal epileptic activities in the left midtemporal region during the ictal phase and active epileptogenic abnormalities from the left anterior, mid- and inferior mesial temporal regions with independent spike activities in the right anterior temporal region during the interictal phase.

In type V, bilateral diffuse hypometabolism with unilateral maximum focal hypometabolism, results of 4 cases reveal a diffuse, significant reduction of rCMRGl in both cerebral hemispheres, with maximum focal reduction of 28 to 59% of rCMRGl ($p < 0.001$) in the temporal region. These findings correlate with maximum focal epileptic activities recorded by EEG during either the ictal or interictal phase with a wide variety of diffuse abnormal electrical activities in both cerebral hemispheres.

In spite of various hypometabolic patterns of rCMRGl, the maximum focal hypometabolism matches the maximum epileptic activity recorded during the ictal or interictal phase in 12 of 14 cases with partial epilepsy. In 2 cases, FDG findings disagree with EEG findings (Table 3). Oxygen-15 studies for rCBF, rOEF and rCMRO reveal a wide variety of findings without specific patterns. There is a similar pattern of reduced rCBF, rOEF and rCMRO in most cases but no significant correlation between FDG and rCMRO findings.

Table 3. *Correlation Between EEG and FDG-PET*

Good agreement	10
Fair agreement	2
Disagreement	2
Total	14

Case Presention:

Case 1 (Type II): C.M. a 26-year-old female, has a history of episodes of unresponsiveness with occasional screaming and erratic running around since the age of 6. There is also occasional tonic contraction of the left arm. CT scans showed a moderate diffuse cerebral atrophy in the right cerebral hemisphere. EEG findings, including telemetry and sphenoidal recordings, revealed an epileptic disturbance originating independently from the right temporal area and less often

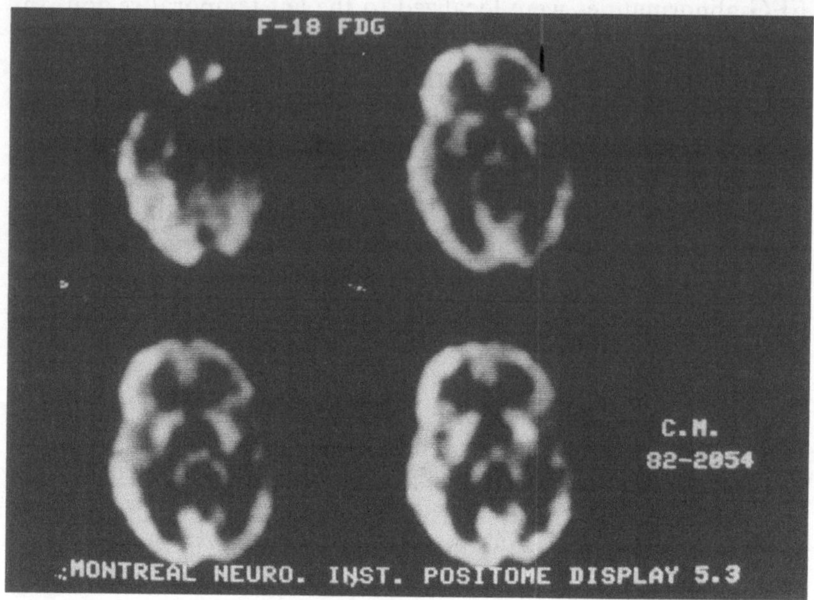

Fig. 2a

Fig. 2. Case 1: C.M.; type 2. a) Four horizontal tomographic images for FDG study, showing marked reduction of rCMRG in the right temporal region associated with moderate reduction of rCMRG in the right parieto-central region. b) Coronal tomographic image for FDG study at the anterior temporal level, showing marked reduction of rCMRGl in the right temporal region. c) Tomographic images for rCBF, rOEF, rCMRO and rCBV at the same level, showing a moderate diffuse reduction of rCBF and rCMRO in the entire right cerebral hemisphere

from the left temporal area during the interictal phase. However, EEG recordings during the ictal phase show an occasional epileptic disturbance originating from the left fronto-temporal areas. Marked atrophy in the right temporal convolution and tough and rubbery cerebral tissue were found during the right temporal craniotomy. Neuropathological examination revealed moderate to marked gliosis in the temporal cerebral tissue and amygdala. FDG findings, illustrated in Fig. 2 for the horizontal (a) and coronal plane (b), show a maximum reduction of 48% (23 ± 6 µmol/100 g/min) from the control values (45 ± 7 µmol/100 g/min) ($p < 0.001$) in the right anterior temporal region, 44% ($p < 0.001$) reduction in the right parietal region, and 23% reduction ($p < 0.05$) in the right central region. Oxygen-15 studies for rCBF, rOEF, $rCMRO_2$ revealed a 49% reduction of rCBF, 12% reduction of rOEF, and 54% reduction of rCMRO in the right anterior temporal region. In the right centroparietal region there was a 26% reduction of rCBF, 11% reduction of rOEF, and 46% reduction of rCMRO.

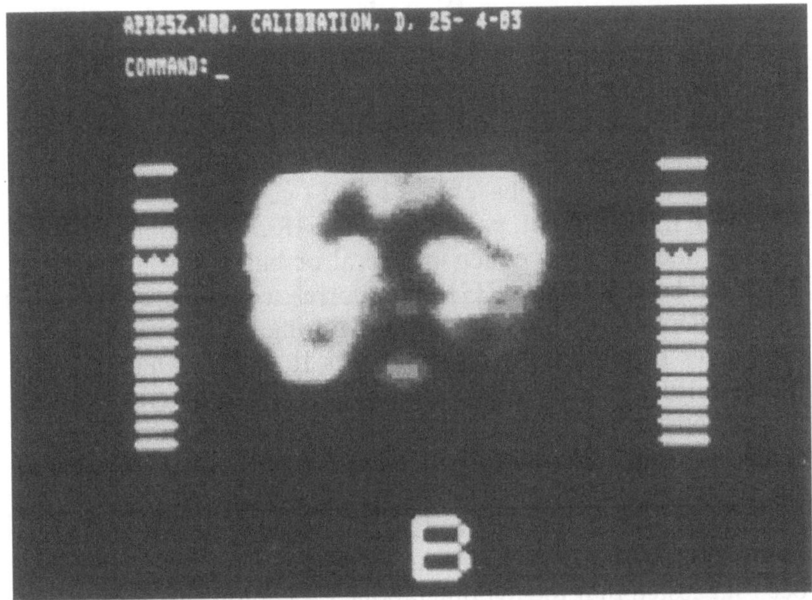
CALIBRATION. D. 25- 4-83
COMMAND:
B

Fig. 2b

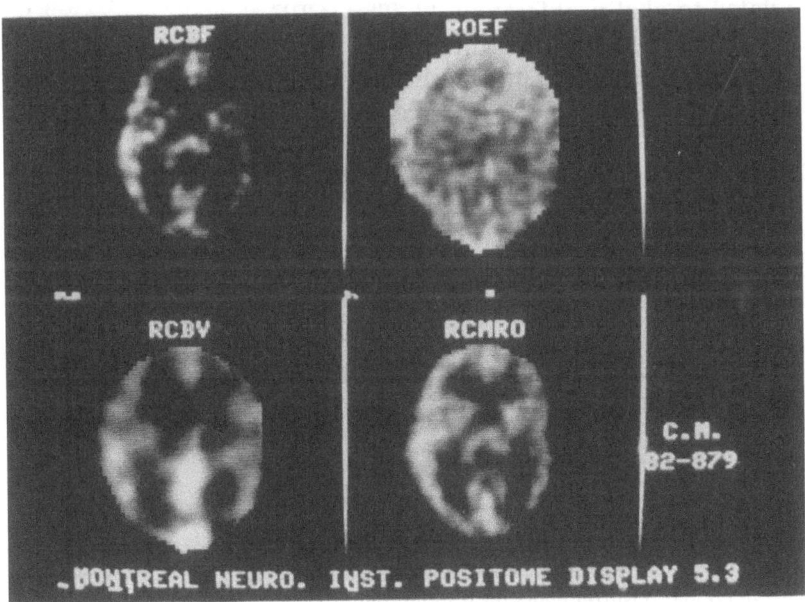
RCBF
ROEF
RCBV
RCMRO
C.M.
82-879
MONTREAL NEURO. INST. POSITOME DISPLAY 5.3

Fig. 2c

Discussion

Quantitative measurements of rCMRGl using the FDG technique in 14 patients with partial epilepsy compared to 5 control subjects indicate significant focal hypometabolism of rCMRGl in the epileptic focus (as delineated by electroencephalograph during the ictal or interictal phase) in 12 of 14 cases. In this study we observed five different patterns of rCMRG1 hypometabolism. Types I and III show either unilateral or bilateral well localized hypometabolism of rCMRGI; these correlate very closely with the focal epileptic abnormality recorded during the interictal phase. The zones of hypometabolism in types II and V, which show a rather diffuse reduction of rCMRG1 in the ipsilateral cerebral hemisphere or in both cerebral hemispheres, are much more extensive than the areas of EEG abnormalities. Localized structural changes such as porencephaly or local cerebral atrophy demonstrated by CT scan correlate closely with the FDG findings, but EEGs often show no significant abnormalities. Although it has been suggested that the hypometabolic zone in the interictal phase of partial epilepsy may represent either functional inhibitory processes or structural changes in cerebral tissue[5a, 5b], the exact mechanism of hypometabolism is still unsettled and may involve much more complex consequences of local abnormal processes related to glial proliferations[17]. The rCBF changes measured by $C^{15}O_2$ technique during interictal partial epilepsy are similar to ^{77}Kr PET results[7]. The significant reduction of rCBF is often associated with a marked reduction of rCMRG1, but the correlation is not significant.

Acknowledgements

The PET program is supported by Grant SP-5 from the Medical Research Council of Canada. The authors would like to express their appreciation to the staff of the Neuroisotope Laboratory and the Medical Cyclotron for their dedicated assistance. Special thanks to Susan Mus for preparing and Dr. Victoria Lees for editing this manuscript.

References

1. Bergstrom, M., Litton, J., Eriksson, L., Bohm, C., Blomquist, G., Determination of object contour from projections for attenuation correction in cranial positron emission tomography. J. Comp. Ass. Tomogr. *6* (1982), 365—372.

2. Bergstrom, M., Eriksson, L., Bohm, C., Blomquist, G., Litton, J., Correction for scattered radiation in a ring detector positron camera by integral transformation of the projections. J. Comp. Ass. Tomogr. *7* (1983), 42—50.
3. Brooks, R. A., Alternative formula for glucose utilization using labeled deoxyglucose. J. Nucl. Med. *23* (1982), 538—539.
4. Diksic, M., Jolly, D., New high-yield synthesis of ^{18}F-labelled 2-deoxy-2-fluoro-D-glucose. Int. J. Appl. Rad. Isotopes (in press). 1983.
5a. Engel, J., jr., Kuhl, D. E., Phelps, M. E., Mazziotta, J. C., Interictal cerebral glucose metabolism in partial epilepsy and its relation to EEG changes. Ann. Neurol. *12* (1982), 510—517.
5b. Engel, J., jr., Kuhl, D. E., Phelps, M. E., Crandall, P. H., Comparative localization of epileptic foci in partial epilepsy by PCT and EEG. Ann. Neurol. *12* (1982), 529—537.
6. Engel, J., jr., Kuhl, D. E., Phelps, M. E., Patterns of ictal and interictal local cerebral metabolic rate studied in man with positron computed tomography. In: Advances in Epileptology: XIIth Epilepsy International Symposium (Akimoto, H., Kazamatsuri, H., Seino, M., Ward, A., eds.), pp. 145—149. New York: Raven Press. 1982.
7. Feindel, W., Gloor, P., Yamamoto, L., Gotman, J., Shimizu, H., Ochs, R., Correlation of EEG and topographic cerebral blood flow in epilepsy by positron emission tomography. In: Advances in Epilepsy: XIIIth Epilepsy International Symposium (Akimoto, H., Kazamatsuri, H., Seino, M., Ward, A., eds.), pp. 151—156. New York: Raven Press. 1982.
8. Frackowiak, R. S., Lenzi, G. L., Jones, T., Heather, J. D., Quantitative measurement of regional cerebral blood flow and oxygen metabolism in man using ^{15}O and positron emission tomography: Theory, procedure and normal values. J. Comp. Ass. Tomogr. *4* (1980), 727—736.
9. Huang, S. C., Phelps, M. E., Hoffman, E. J., Sideris, K., Selin, C., Kuhl, D. E., Noninvasive determination of local cerebral metabolic rate of glucose in man. Amer. J. Physiol. *238* (1980), E69—E82.
10. Jackson, J. H., On the anatomical, physiological and pathological investigation of epilepsies. West Riding Lunatic Asylum Medical Reports *3* (1873), 315. Reprinted in: Selected Writings of John Hughlings Jackson, edited by J. Taylor, *1* (1931), 90—111. London: Hoddler and Stoughton.
11. Kuhl, D. E., Engel, J., jr., Phelps, M. E., Selin, C., Epileptic patterns of local cerebral metabolism and perfusion in humans determined by emission computed tomography of ^{18}FDG and $^{13}NH_3$. Ann. Neurol. *8* (1980), 348—360.
12. McNaughton, F. L., Rasmussen, T., Criteria for selection of patients for neurosurgical treatment. In: Advances in Neurology, Vol. 8 (Purpura, D. P., Penry, J. K., Nalter, R. D., eds.), pp. 1137—1148. New York: Raven Press. 1975.
13. Phelps, M. E., Huang, S. C., Hoffman, E. J., Selin, C. S., Sokoloff, L., Kuhl, D. E., Tomographic measurement of local cerebral glucose metabolic rate in humans with (F-18) 2-fluoro-2-deoxyglucose: validation of method. Ann. Neurol. *6* (1979), 371—388.

14. Rasmussen, T., Cortical resection in the treatment of focal epilepsy. In: Advances in Neurology, Vol. 8 (Purpura, D. P., Penry, J. K., Walter, R. D., eds.), pp. 139—154. New York: Raven Press. 1975.
15. Thompson, C. J., Yamamoto, Y. L., Meyer, E., Positome II: A high efficiency positron imaging device for dynamic brain studies. IEEE Trans. Nucl. Sci. NS-*26* (1979), 583—589.
16. Sokoloff, L., Reivich, M., Kennedy, C., DeRosiers, M. H., Patlak, C. S., Pettigrew, K. D., Sakurada, O., Shinohara, M., The C-14 deoxyglucose method for the measurement of local cerebral glucose utilization: theory, procedure, and normal values in the conscious and anesthetized albino rat. J. Neurochem. *28* (1977), 897—916.
17. Woodbury, D. M., Kemp, J. W., Initiation, propagation and arrest of seizures. In: Pathophysiology of Cerebral Energy Metabolism (Misulja, B. B., Rakic, L. M., Klatzo, I., eds.), pp. 313—351. New York-London: Plenum. 1977.
18. Yamamoto, Y. L., Thompson, C., Meyer, E., Feindel, W., Positron emission tomography for measurement of regional cerebral blood flow. In: Advances in Neurology, Vol. 30 j (Carney, A. L., Anderson, E. M., eds.), pp. 41—53. New York: Raven Press.

Acta Neurochirurgica, Suppl. 33, 47—52 (1984)

C. Communications

Eye Movements and Occipital Seizures in Man

C. Munari[1,2], A. Bonis[1,2], S. Kochen[3], M. Pestre[1], P. Brunet[1], J. Bancaud[1,2], J. P. Chodkiewicz[2], and J. Talairach[2]

With 1 Figure

Summary

49 occipital seizures with an early (first 10 seconds) ocular deviation were recorded during stereo-EEG investigations in 16 patients.

— The ictal discharge usually starts in the medial occipital cortex, below and/or above the calcarine sulcus.

— In most cases (44 seizures, 14 patients), the ocular deviation were "tonic", rapid controlateral to the discharge. Most often (27 seizures, 14 patients), the eye movement was horizontal; in 3 patients (17 seizures) it was upward oblique.

— A "clonic" deviation was rare (4 seizures, 4 patients), but also controlateral to the discharge, horizontal, generally slow.

— Strict relationships exist between the type of the discharge and the modalities of the ocular deviation: a rapid discharge is linked to a "tonic" deviation; slow, pseudorythmic spikes are related to a "clonic" deviation.

Thus, in these patients, the ocular deviation was related to the ictal involvement of the occipital, mainly medial, cortex.

Keywords: Occipital seizures; oculo-motor control; stereo-EEG; clinical neurophysiology.

Introduction

Little is known about the role of the occipital cortex in the control of eye movements in man; most data have been drawn from animal experiments. Moreover the evaluation of this role is hard

[1] Unité 97 de recherches sur l'épilepsie, INSERM, 2ter rue d'Alésia, F-75014 Paris, France.

[2] Service de Neurochirurgie B, Hôpital Sainte Anne, 1 rue Cabanis, F-75014 Paris, France.

[3] Antartida Hospital, Buenos Aires, Argentine.

because of the lack of specific disturbances of oculomotor control in patients with damage of the posterior cortex[5].

On the contrary[8,9], there have been many clinical observations concerning eye movements during the paroxystic desorganisation of the posterior cortex.

Gastaut and Roger[7] showed that the clinical signs of some occipital seizures may be represented only by horizontal "nystagmic jerks", controlateral to the ictal discharge. More recently, Gastaut[6] substituted the term "nystagmus epileptique" with "oculo-clonic seizure". This modification was linked to the hypothesis of a vestibular role in determining ocular deviations[15].

Bancaud[2] and Peschanski[11] showed strict relationships between ocular adversion and a controlateral ictal occipital discharge.

Penfield and Jasper[10] could not obtain any ocular deviation by occipital lobe electrical stimulation; for them, ictal ocular deviation occurred in order to follow visual hallucination moving in the visual field.

The aim of this paper is to describe oculomotor manifestations in relation to ictal disorganization of the visual cortex in man.

Patients and Methods

This study concerns 16 patients admitted to Sainte Anne Hospital (Service de Neurochirurgie B) for severe, drug resistant occipital epilepsy. All these patients underwent a presurgical stereo-EEG exploration (7 to 12 intracerebral multilead electrodes), according to the previously described methodology[1,3,4,12–14]. During stereo-EEG we recorded 49 seizures (at least one in every patient) characterized by an ocular deviation occurring within the first 10 seconds. We chose this relatively short period of time because it allowed for an easier definition of the anatomo-electroclinical correlations. Table 1 shows the position of the 157 electrodes in lateral view. For obvious therapeutic reasons, central and frontal areas were explored by only a few electrodes.

Results

A. Ocular Deviation (Fig. 1)

1. "Tonic" deviation: In most cases (44 seizures, 14 patients), ocular deviation was rapid, abrupt, and extreme; it was rarely slow. The patients, although perfectly aware and conscious, were never able to control this deviation which was always opposite to the side of the ictal discharge. Only one patient, after 4 seizures with a

Table 1. *Early Ocular Deviation (49 occipital seizures in 16 patients)*

	SEIZURES	PATIENTS
TONIC	**44**	**14**
Controlateral	43	14
Homolateral	1	1
Horizontal	27	14
Oblique ↗	17	3
CLONIC	**4**	**4**
Controlateral	4	4
Horizontal	4	4
TONIC-CLONIC	**1**	**1**
Controlateral	1	1
Horizontal	1	1

controlateral deviation, had a fifth seizure with a homolateral deviation. Most often (27 seizures, 14 patients) the eye movement was horizontal; in 3 patients (17 seizures) it was obliquely, upward, never downward.

2. "Clonic" deviation: This type of eye movement is very rare (4 seizures, 4 patients), it is always horizontal, controlateral to the electrical discharge, generally slow and interrupted by a sharp jerk of variable frequency. In the intervals between the jerks, the eyes tend to come back to the midline.

B. Ocular Deviation and Ictal Discharge

1. In every case, the ictal discharge started in an occipital lobe and, specifically, in the medial cortex (43 seizures, 12 patients) above and below the calcarine sulcus. Only the external cortex was primarily affected in one patient (2 seizures); in two patients the discharge simultaneously involves both, medial and external cortex. In 3 patients (9 seizures), the discharge starts above and in 5 patients (16 seizures) below the plane of the calcarine sulcus; in the others, the entire occipital internal cortex is simultaneously affected.

2. No correlation was evident between the initial localization of the discharge inside the medial cortex and the direction (horizontal or oblique) of the ocular deviation.

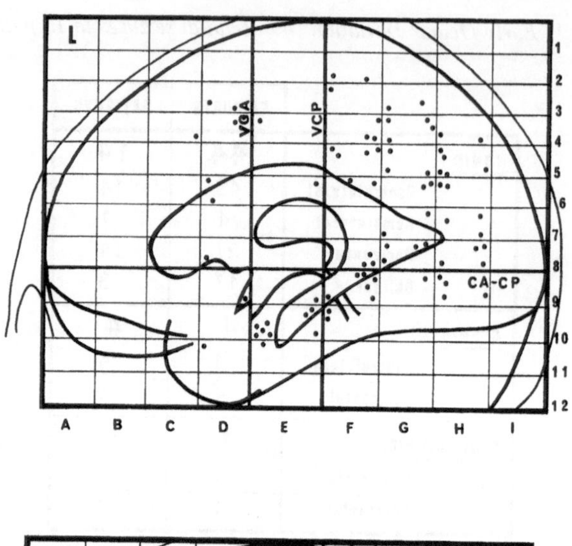

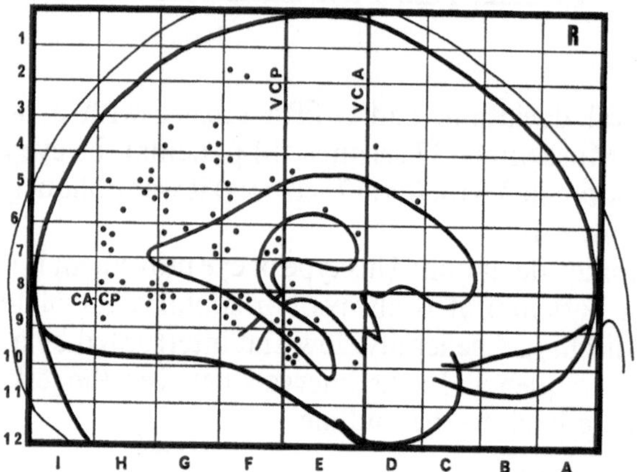

Fig. 1. Lateral projection of 157 electrodes (16 patients). *L* 83, *R* 74

3. There was a strict relationship between the type of the discharge and the modalities of the ocular deviation: when the discharge is fast, the eye movement is rapid and continuous; a discharge of slow, pseudorythmic spikes is related to a brisk, saccadic adversion.

C. Associated Clinical Signs

1. Early: During the first 10 seconds, 10 patients (19 seizures) have bilateral blinking with or without a bilateral mydriasis. Only 3 patients (4 seizures) have visual hallucinations in color in the visual

field opposite the side of the discharge. Two patients had postural modifications of the controlateral upper limb, and an other had chewing activity.

2. Late: Simple and complex visual hallucinations as well as oro-alimentary and simple gestural "automatisms" were more frequent than at the beginning of the seizures. These signs appear to be related to the ictal involvement of other cortical regions (temporo-parietal junction, deep temporal structures, central region). In 4 patients (4 seizures), the ocular deviation, controlateral to the initial deviation, is related to the involvement of the central region, preceding the secondary generalization.

Discussion

Our data seem to show that in patients with occipital seizures, ocular deviation is related to the ictal involvement of the *medial* occipital cortex. Thus, it is understandable why Penfield and Jasper[10] could not obtain ocular deviations by electrical stimulations, to the *lateral* cortex. It also appears that the occipital region responsible for eye movements is more limited in man that in monkeys[16].

The ocular deviation we describe is not related to extra-occipital region discharges, particularly those which occur in the frontal lobe. The deviation is always controlateral to the discharge: in two of the three cases in which it was homolateral, we observed an early involvement of the controlateral occipital lobe.

It is generally admitted[6] that the ocular adversion is always, "clonic" during occipital seizures. This is so also after frontal electrical stimulation in the monkey[17]. In our experience, the most frequent deviations are tonic. The type of deviation seems to us to be strictly linked to the type of discharge: when it is fast, the ocular deviation is "tonic", when it is characterized by rythmic spikes and/or spikes and waves, it is "clonic". Moreover this correlation is confirmed by effects of occipital stimulation in man[2].

References

1. Bancaud, J., Talairach, J., Stereo-electro-encephalography section 1: Macro-stereo-electro-encephalography in epilepsy. In: Handbook of EEG and Clin. Neurophysiol. 10 B (Bancaud, J., ed.), pp. 3—33. Amsterdam: Elsevier Publ. 1975.

2. Bancaud, J., Bonis, A., Kochen, S., Pestre, M., Munari, C., Szikla, G., Chodkiewicz, J. P., Brunet, P., Talairach, J., Aspects du contrôle du cortex visuel sur l'oculomotricité chez l'homme. Revue Neurologique (in press) 1983.
3. Bancaud, J., Talairach, J., Bonis, A., Schaub, C., Szikla, G., Morel, P., Bordas-Ferrer, M., La stéréo-électro-encéphalographie dans l'épilepsie, 321 p. Paris: Masson et Cie ed. 1965.
4. Bancaud, J., Talairach, J., Geier, S., Scarabin, J. M., EEG et SEEG dans les tumeurs cérébrales et l'épilepsie, 351 p. Paris: Edifor ed. 1973.
5. Bender, M. B., The oculomotor system (Bender, M., ed.), 556 p. New York: Harper and Row. 1964.
6. Gastaut, H., Un aspect méconnu des décharges neuroniques occipitales: la crise oculoclonique ou «nystagmus épileptique». In: Alajouanine T., Les grandes activitiés du lobe occipital. 1960, 360 p.
7. Gastaut, H., Roger, A., Une forme inhabituelle de l'épilepsie: le nystagmus épileptique. Rev. Neurol. *90* (1954), 130—132.
8. Herpin, T., Du pronostic et du traitement curatif de l'épilepsie (Baillière, J. B., ed.), 622 p. Paris: 1852.
9. Jackson, J. H., Selected writings, vol. 1. One epilepsy and epileptiform convulsions, 500 p. Londres: Hodder and Stoughton ed. 1931.
10. Penfield, W., Jasper, H., Epilepsy and the functional anatomy of the human brain, 896 p. London: J. A. Churchill ed. 1954.
11. Peschanski, M., A propos des déviations oculaires dans les crises épileptiques à début occipital, 84 p. Paris: Thèse. 1978.
12. Talairach, J., Bancaud, J., Stereotaxic exploration and therapy in epilepsy. In: Handbook of Neurology, vol. XV (1974), 758—782.
13. Talairach, J., Bancaud, J., Bonis, A., Tournoux, P., Szikla, G., Morel, P., Investigations fonctionnelles dans l'épilepsie. Rev. Neurol. *105* (1961), 119—130.
14. Talairach, J., Bancaud, J., Szikla, G., Bonis, A., Geier, S., Vedrenne, C., Approche nouvelle de la neurochirurgie de l'épilepsie. Rev. Neurochir. *20* (1974), Suppl. 20, 240 p.
15. Terzian, H., Sul nistagmo epilettico. Riv. Neurol. *25* (1955), 651—655.
16. Wagman, I. H., Werman, R., Feldman, D. S., The oculomotor effects of cortical and subcortical stimulation in the monkey. J. Neuropath. Exp. Neurol. *1957*, 269—277.
17. Wagman, I. H., Hehler, W. R., Physiology and anatomy of the cortico-oculomotor mechanism. In: Brodal, A., Pompeiano, O., Progress in Brain Research *37* (1972), 619—635.

Acta Neurochirurgica, Suppl. 33, 53—55 (1984)

The Epileptic Seizure with Origin in Frontal Lobe: A Complex Problem for Surgery*

G. Colicchio[1]

Summary

48 epileptic patients underwent SEEG study with a view to surgical treatment. In all cases, among other regions, one or both frontal lobes were explored. 21 patients showed epileptic seizures originating from one or both frontal lobes only. Six different categories of clinical manifestations—at the seizure onset—were established. They included well localized body sensations. It is concluded that the localizing value of clinical manifestations only are unreliable in frontal lobe epilepsy.

Keywords: Epilepsy; frontal lobe; surgery.

The knowledge of the clinical pattern of the epileptic seizures originating from different brain regions represents the starting point for a diagnosis of localization in epilepsy surgery.

Among the different clinical pictures of the epilepsy is it possible to recognize a characteristical feature of the seizures with origin in frontal lobe?

In the attempt to answer this question we reviewed our patients.

Subjects

Forty-eight adult epileptic patients, resistant to pharmacological treatment and candidates for surgery were considered. Several cerebral sites, including the frontal lobes, were explored by stereo-EEG and, in some cases, by electrocorticography, according to indications provided by clinical

---

* Supported by Ministero della Publica Istruzione.

[1] Istituto di Neurochirurgica, Università Cattolica del Sacro Cuore, Largo A. Gemelli, 8, I-00168 Roma, Italy.

neuroradiological and scalp EEG findings. The site of origin of the seizure discharges turned out to be the following:

a) Frontal: 21 cases. The origin of the seizures was from one frontal lobe in 16 patients and from both frontal lobes in 5 patients. It was notable that in 5 cases the causative lesion involved both the frontal and the parietal lobes.

b) Multifocal: 11 cases with independent seizures origin from the frontal lobe and outside of it.

c) Extra-frontal: 10 cases with origin of all seizures outside the frontal lobe.

Twelve of the 21 frontal patients underwent surgery: in the other 9 the epileptogenic zone was either bilateral (5 cases) or involved highly specialized cerebral regions (such as area 4 and left 44 Brodman's areas; 2 cases). Two patients refused surgery. In 7 of the operated patients the excellent results proved that localization of the epileptogenic zone was correct; in 1 case seizures recurred after 3 years; in the remaining 4 the follow-up is still too short.

Clinical Manifestations, at the Onset, of the Seizures with Frontal Origin (21 patients)

These were documented by continuous TV monitoring, simultaneously performed with the electrophysiological study, mainly "chronic" SEEG. 3 to 10 spontaneous seizures were analyzed in each patient. In addition, in some cases, seizures were provoked pharmacologically or by local brain electrical stimulations. The types of the phenomena observed as the first seizure manifestation were the following.

a) Motor: i) tonic (9 cases), mainly adversive head rotation and postural limbs modifications; ipsilateral head turning in 2 cases; ii) clonic (3 cases); iii) complex gesture (2 cases). Loss of consciousness was associated with the i and iii types of motor events.

b) Sensory (3 cases), in the form of a tickle in the armpit, an ache in the knee and a throb in the calf. To be remarked that these sensory phenomena—unaccompanied by movements nor by loss of consciousness—were related to an origin of the ictal discharges from the areas 8 or 6, and that in the 2 patients submitted to areas 8 and 6 corticectomy seizures disappeared.

c) Sensory-motor (2 cases.)

d) Speech arrest (2 cases).

Discussion

The well known variety of functions of the human frontal lobe can easily account for the variety of the clinical patterns of the seizures arising from it. However, some of the clinical events occurring at the onset of the seizures of frontal origin in our patients seem hard to be interpreted. This is particularly true for the pure sensory phenomena.

Several years ago, Penfield stressed the functional unit of the sensory-motor strip[3]. More recently, Bancaud *et al.* reported diffuse, not localized and undefinible sensations as a possible manifestation of ictal discharges from the frontal supplementary motor areas[1,2]. In our cases, however, these sensory manifestations were not associated with motor phenomena and were very well localized in definite parts of the body. For at least 2 of our cases, the frontal origin of the ictal discharge responsable for these sensory phenomena was proven by their disappearance following frontal surgical topectomy.

It appears then that in some cases it is difficult if not impossible that the clinical manifestations of the seizures permits recognition of frontal lobe origin.

Because of this difficulty we suggest that the neurosurgeon, faced with the problem of treating a patient suffering from epilepsy, should remember this aspect of the manifestation of the frontal lobe seizures and check this possibility with any means, clinical, radiological and electrophysiological[4].

References

1. Bancaud, J., Talairach, J., Bonis, A., Schaub, C., Szikla, G., Morel, P., Bordas-Ferrer, M., La stéréoélectroencéphalographie dans l'épilepsie, pp. 321. Paris: Masson. 1965.
2. Geier, S., Bancaud, J., Talairach, J., Bonis, A., Szikla, G., Eujelvin, M., The seizures of frontal lobe epilepsy. Neurology *27* (1977), 951—958.
3. Penfield, W., Jasper, H., Epilepsy and functional anatomy of the human brain, pp. 896. Boston: Little, Brown. 1954.
4. Rossi, G. F., Colicchio, G., Gentilomo, A., Le problème de la recherche de la topographie d'origine de l'épilepsie. Arch. Suisse Neurol. Neurochir. Psych. *115* (1974), 229—270.

Acta Neurochirurgica, Suppl. 33, 57—61 (1984)

Techniques for the Analysis of Spike Trains in the Human Central Nervous System*

F. A. Lenz[1], R. R. Tasker[1], H. C. Kwan[3], J. T. Murphy[2], and H. H. Nguyen-Huu[3]

With 1 Figure

Summary

This paper describes two methods, the cross correlogram and spectral cross correlation techniques, for correlating spike trains and analog signals recorded at operation.

Keywords: Cross correlogram; spectral cross correlation; spike trains.

Introduction

It is often of interest to compare unitary action potentials (spike trains) with other physiologic signals such as the electromyogram (EMG) or electroencephalogram (EEG). These two types of signal differ in their fundamental nature. The spike train is treated as if action potentials are discrete discontinuous events occurring over time (*i.e.* a point process) whereas the other signals vary continuously over time and therefore may be described as analog signals. The relationship between spike trains and analog signals has often been examined by visual assessment of the records.

---

* Supported by the P.S.I. Foundation, Toronto, Canada.

[1] Divisions of Neurosurgery.

[2] Neurology and Clinical Neurophysiology Laboratory, Toronto General Hospital.

[3] Department of Physiology, University of Toronto, Toronto, Canada.

Address correspondence to: R. R. Tasker, Room 7-221, Eaton North Wing, Toronto General Hospital, 101 College Street, Toronto, Canada, M5G 1L7.

However, visual assessment does not allow the relationship between these types of activity to be assessed either quantitatively or statistically. More sophisticated means of assessing the relationship between processes of this type have been developed[1]. The present paper describes the application of these techniques to the analysis of single unit activity recorded in the human central nervous system during stereotactic surgery. As these techniques are described, examples will be drawn from the correlation of spike trains of single thalamic cells with electromyograms (EMG) in parkinsonian tremor.

Methods and Results

Fig. 1 A shows a record of thalamic cell and EMG activity in which there seems visually to be some evidence of correlation between the two signals. Since action potentials in the spike train are represented by discrete points in time, correlation can be established from the average of analog signals time-locked to the occurrence of an action potential, the spike triggered average (STA). The STA shown in Fig. 1 B is characterized by a number of peaks superimposed on a high average level of activity. This type of pattern may indicate correlation between the two signals but may also be seen in the cross correlogram of two uncorrelated signals which occur at similar frequencies. Therefore, the next step is to evaluate the statistical significance of the cross correlation. Statistical evaluation of the cross correlogram is problematic in the analysis of signals which have a large amount of power at similar frequencies[3,4] as in the case of tremor (see Fig. 1 C).

Signals of this type are better analyzed by the technique of spectral analysis. The analog signal, in this case EMG, is digitized and filtered before the Fourier transform is taken. Since the spectra of analog signals are readily calculated on digital computers, the spike train is usually transformed into an analog signal before the Fourier transform is taken[3]. French and Holden[2] have developed a useful technique for generating an analog signal by filtering the spike train with an optimal digital filter. The Fourier transform of this analog equivalent of the spike train is then taken by the same method as employed for the analog signal, EMG, in the current example. Spectra of the individual signals are then used to calculate the auto power spectra of the individual signals and the cross spectrum of the relationship between the two signals. The cross power spectrum is a product of the two individual spectra, which

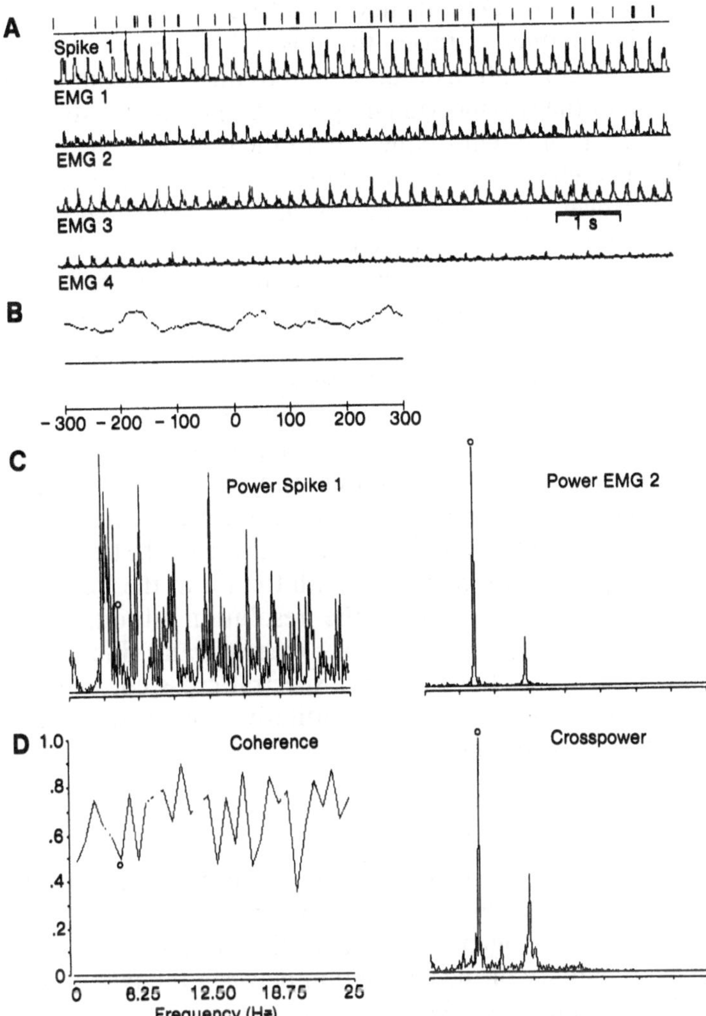

Fig. 1. Example of cross correlation analysis of thalamic tremor cell and EMG in parkinsonian tremor. Fig. 1 A shows a digitized record of four, rectified, filtered EMG channels and one spike channel. Each vertical line in the spike channel indicates the occurrence of an action potential. Fig. 1 B shows the STA for this cell, with the horizontal scale in milliseconds (n = 283). Unsmoothed autopower spectra of spike and EMG signals are shown in Fig. 1 C. Smoothed coherence and unsmoothed cross power spectra are shown in Fig. 1 D. Circles indicate tremor frequency, determined from the EMG record

quantitatively indicates the amount of power shared by the two spectra as a function of frequency. A high degree of shared power at a particular frequency raises the possibility that an important component of correlation occurs at that frequency. In our example, the spectra of the two individual signals, Spike 1 and EMG 2, have major peaks at different frequencies in the tremor frequency band (3–6 Hz). Therefore, cross power at the frequency of tremor must be small. However, there is a small peak in the spike spectrum at exactly tremor frequency, which gives rise to the peak in cross power (Fig. 1 D, right). The significance of this peak can be judged statistically by the evaluation of the coherence function which is computed from the auto power spectra and the cross power spectrum after smoothing of these spectra by averaging eight contiguous spectral estimates. The coherence at the frequency band which includes this small spike peak (0.48, at the circle) is below the significant level because of the power in adjacent components of the unsmoothed spike power spectrum. We can conclude that the spike signal has a substantially different frequency from the tremor signal and is not significantly correlated with tremor at the frequency of maximum cross power, given the resolution of our analysis. Therefore, the peaks in the cross correlogram (Fig. 1 B) are spurious indicators of correlation. Spectral cross correlation has allowed us to understand and quantitatively evaluate a difficult example of cross correlation.

Discussion

The technique of cross correlation by spectral analysis allows quantitative assessment of the amount of periodic activity occurring in each signal, as well as the strength, latency and statistical reliability of the correlation between the two processes. The STA technique is preferable for the analysis of signals without a strong periodic component since it is less involved computationally and it is bandlimited only by the sampling frequency and duration of the averaging interval. The application of power spectral analysis to the study of "tremor cells" in parkinsonian tremor patients has allowed us to measure the properties of cells which may be involved in the generation of tremor. This technique may well be applied to the study of other types of pathology characterized by abnormal periodicity. For instance, correlation of cellular activity with EEG could be used as a quantitative criterion for identifying cells involved in the generation and spread of epileptic activity from one location to another. We believe that this technique is a useful addition to the methods available for the study of single unit activity in the human central nervous system.

References

1. Cox, D. R., Lewis, P. A. W., The Statistical Analysis of Series of Events. London: Chapman and Hall. 1966.
2. French, A. S., Holden, A. V., Alais-free sampling of neuronal spike trains. Kybernetic *8* (1971), 165—171.
3. Glaser, E. M., Ruchkin, D. S., Principles of Neurobiological Signal Analysis. New York: Academic Press. 1976.
4. Jenkins, G. W., Watts, D. G., Spectral Analysis. London: Holden Day. 1969.

Acta Neurochirurgica, Suppl. 33, 63—67 (1984)

Shape Factor Intensity (SFI) Analysis of EEG of Patients Treated Surgically for Epilepsy*

S. H. M. Nyström[1], **P. H. Eskelinen**[1], and **E. R. Heikkinen**[1]

With 2 Figures

Summary

A new method of quantification of EEG has been applied in association with epilepsy surgery. The EEG signal is analyzed in terms of two sets of two parameters, *i.e.*, shape factor and intensity. The method has been used for drug resistant epilepsy treated with stereotactic procedures or lobectomies. Good pictorial interpretability is obtained by the shape factor intensity analysis.

Keywords: Signal processing; EEG quantification; spike detection; epilepsy surgery.

Introduction

Medically refractory epilepsy is a complex problem from the standpoint of its electrophysiological manifestations and treatment. For the electroencephalographer as well as for the neurosurgeon this problem is one of the most challenging ones because successful treatment is generally a laborious and difficult task. Efforts to complete and sharpen human capabilities led early to the implementation of more objective methods in EEG analysis. Since Grass and Gibbs[3] introduced instrumental quantification of

---

* This work was supported by grant no. 7455/304 from the Academy of Finland.

Examinations were carried out in accordance with the Declaration of Helsinki and as research project combined with clinical care.

[1] Department of Neurosurgery, Oulu University Central Hospital, Oulu, Finland.

the electroencephalogram and Walter[6] developed spectral analysis by means of band pass filters, a vast variety of computer techniques has been applied to neurophysiological analysis of epilepsy[1,4] among others. Further very interesting systems have been developed by Gotman and Gloor[2] and Mars[5]. However, some of the computer techniques tend to become complicated for every day clinical use and require an excessive amount of computational arsenal for their implementation. The mathematical methods used, being originally designed for non-biological purposes, does not always provide adequate final results. Delicate, time related alterations involved in ictal brain activity may not be sufficently well transformed to target parameters and thus tend to get lost in the final composition.

A new method of analysis that is easily applicable to minicomputers has been invented by one of us (P.H.E.) and applied by our team to EEG interpretation in connection with surgery for epilepsy at the Department of Neurosurgery of Oulu University Central Hospital. It can produce real-time results during monitoring in the operation unit. Preliminary analyses seem clinically promising. The method has proved useful for us in stereotactic and open procedures. However, our series so far is not extensive.

Methods

All the patients underwent routine investigations involving CT-scan, angiography and extensive preoperative neurophysiological studies including sphenoidal and nasopharyngeal EEG recordings. Medics 6-pole, depth electrodes were used for long duration (24 h) recordings in order to assess origin and spread of seizure activity. The new computer program was utilized for analysis of short duration 1–5 min EEG epochs in various phases of treatment. For peroperative registrations Kaisers 8-pole depth electrodes were used.

Hardware Specification

The computer system consists of a DEC PDP 11/23 computer installed in the operation department in close vicinity of the patient. The computer has 64 KB memory and a floating point unit. The systems mass storage device is a set of two 5 MB RL 01 disks. Auxiliary storage devices include a dual RX02 disk station and an analogue magnetic tape recorder. The results can be displayed on video monitors in two operation theaters. As hard copy output unit we have a Texas SD 422 video printer and an H-P 7225 digital plotter. Programs run under the RT 11 operating system. During the recording the signals are amplified, filtered and transmitted to the computer and digitized on a twelve bits resolution.

Recording on-line and/or off-line can be carried out. Standard sampling frequency is 100 Hz for SFI-analysis.

Software Description

The SFI program is written on Fortran. Signals are visualized as series of positive and negative processes. They are defined by two sets of parameter which are the shape factor (S) and the intensity factor (I). Positive processes of a continous function is defined to exist only if there are consecutive pairs of local extreme values that denote local minimums and maximums. Accordingly, negative processes are defined to exist if consecutive pairs of local extreme values exist. Thus the shape factor is a variable that is dependent on speed, duration and routes of the signal processes. Fast changes usually yield high shape factor values. Intensity is related to signal levels (absolute values as far as 200 microvolts in most cases). The signal is mapped as dots into positive and negative shape-factor intensity planes. The dots are viewed as clusters forming various configurations or they occur outside these as single dots. The method is applicable to all EEG phenomena. It will be published elsewhere in detail.

Clinical Material

The SFI analysis has been applied to normal subjects and in connection with surgically treated patients with medically refractory epilepsy. Temporal lobectomies were performed in 3 patients, hippocampotomy, amygdalotomy and lobectomy in one, amygdalotomy alone in one, amygdalotomy and hippocampotomy in two, fornicotomy in two and scar resections in two. All the patients had extremely severe epilepsy with striking EEG manifestations. Almost seizure-free results were obtained in 3 patients, a clear decrease of frequency and severity of seizures was seen in 6 patients and no results in 2 patients.

Description of a patient treated in this way gives the best impression of the new method used. The first patient to be described is a 29 years old poultry farmer who had suffered from temporal epilepsy since her age of 9. Her working capacity was only sporadic. She had severe and minor fits daily, which defied any kind of antiepileptic drug treatment. CT and angiograms were normal. Registration with surface and depth electrodes using 24 h registrations revealed that her right hippocampus was the main source of epilepsy. To some extent spiking also was generated by her right amygdala. A right hippocampotomy and amygdalotomy was carried out on October 1st 1982. Since then she has had only a few minor fits and her EEG is normalized.

Fig. 1 was obtained by SFI analysis of depth electrode recording in the hippocampal target. The positive and negative processes are

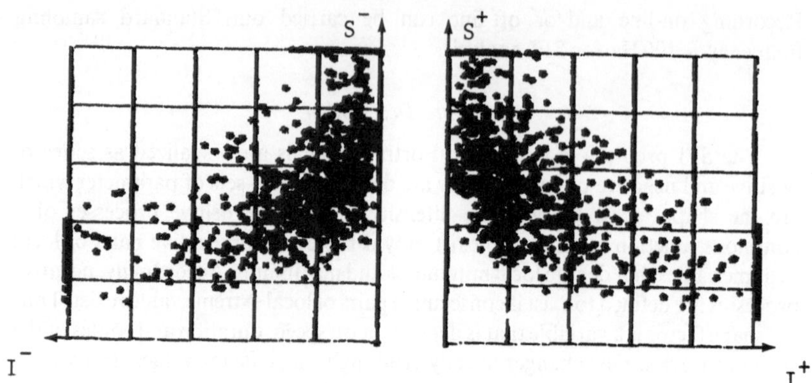

Fig. 1. Shape-factor intensity map of hippocampal EEG prior to hippocampotomy. Quantification of 1-minute epoch. High intensity processes with low shape-factor values are present at lateral margins of map

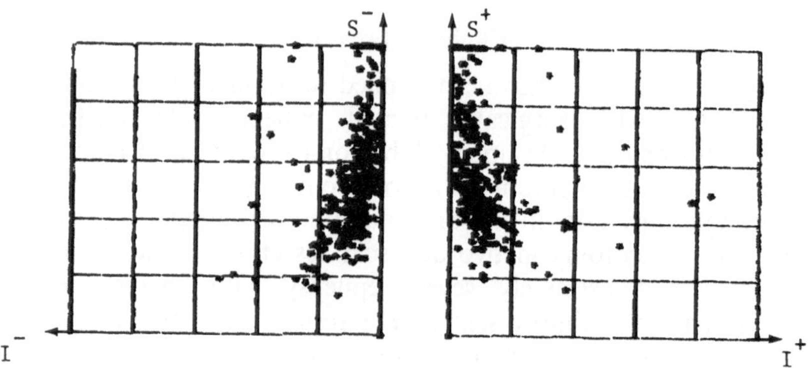

Fig. 2. Shape-factor intensity map of hippocampal EEG following hippocampotomy. Quantification of one minute epoch. Dots are fewer and clustered around hyperbolic structures. Some fast processes are still present at upper margins of map

loosely grouped around a hyperbolic structure of some asymmetry. The cluster map represents an epoch of one minute. S-axis yields speeds and paths of the processes and I-axis signal levels. The dots are largely scattered around the plot with abundant high level slow processes of 0.2–0.4 shape factor values. Also very fast processes above 1 are lined along the upper margine of the plot. Fig. 2 shows the situation after hippocampotomy. Dots are now fewer and clustered much more tightly around the hyperbolic structure.

Discussion

In our opinion the SFI method seems simple and practical. It should save a lot of encephalographers work in subsequent operations when experience with the method has accumulated on large series of patients. The case described is representative of the findings seen in our small series of 11 patients. Our preliminary results suggest that this new method yields good pictorial interpretability. Computationally it is rapid and well accessible. Multifaceted information may be obtained which however still has to be further worked out by computer processing. Thus exploration of the vast information embedded in the various statistical structures will constitute our next efforts. When applied to localization processes of surface or deep epileptic foci the SFI method should be very useful. It reduces data to the essentials but seems to yield very detailed information.

References

1. Brazier, M. A. B., Interactions of deep structures during seizures in man. Synchronization of EEG activity in epilepsies (Petsche, H., Brazier, M. A. B., eds.), pp. 409—427. Wien-New York: Springer. 1971.
2. Gotman, J., Gloor, P., Automatic recognition and quantification of interictal epileptical activity in the human scalp EEG. EEG and Clin. Neurophysiol. *41* (1976), 513—529.
3. Grass, A. M., Gibbs, F. A., Fourier transform of the electroencephalogram. J. Neurophysiol. *1* (1938), 521—526.
4. Lopes da Silva, F. H., Hulten, K. van, Lommen, J. G., Storm van Leeuwen, W., Veelen, C. W. M. van, Vliegenthart, W., Automatic detection and localization of epileptic foci. EEG and Clin. Neurophysiol. *43* (1977), 1—33.
5. Mars, N. J. I., Computer-augmented analysis of electroencephalograms in epilepsy. Thesis. Leiden, The Netherlands. 1982.
6. Walter, W. G., Automatic low frequency analyzer. Electronic engineering *16* (1943), 9—13.

Acta Neurochirurgica, Suppl. 33, 69—73 (1984)

Stability of Interictal Spike Rate as an Index of Local Epileptogenicity. A Study Based on Computer Analysis*

G. F. Rossi[1], P. Pola, and **M. Scerrati**

With 2 Figures

Summary

Automatic analysis of the interictal epileptic potentials recorded with chronically implanted depth electrodes from 7 patients with partial epilepsies was performed. The location of the epileptogenic zone was proven by the disappearance of seizures following its surgical removal. The rate of interictal spikes from the epileptogenic zone showed the highest stability. The relation between local level of epileptogenicity and autonomy of spiking across different physiological and artificially created conditions is stressed.

Keywords: Spike rate stability; stereo-EEG; surgery of epilepsy.

Introduction

Previous personal research based on visual examination of stereo-EEG records[2, 5–7] showed that in certain patients the rate of interictal epileptic potentials recorded from the epileptogenic zone—*i.e.* from the brain zone from which the ictal discharge responsible for the seizure originates—has a peculiar stability or autonomy. The main purpose of the present study was to see whether, by utilizing appropriate automatic elaboration of the stereo-EEG signals, such a phenomenon could be detected in all the epileptic patients.

---

* Supported by the Consiglio Nazionale delle Ricerche and Ministero della Pubblica Istruzione.

[1] Istituto di Neurochirurgia, Università Cattolica del Sacro Cuore, Largo A. Gemelli, 8, I-00168 Roma, Italy.

Material and Method

Seven subjects were analyzed, all of them suffering from severe forms of partial epilepsy. They were selected because:

i) the integration of clinical, neuroradiological, EEG and stereo-EEG findings brought to the identification of an unique epileptogenic zone and of its topographic location[1, 5, 7]; ii) the surgical removal of such a zone was followed by the complete suppression of seizures (shortest follow-up: 1 year), thus proving the correctness of (i) above; (iii) the stereo-EEG recording was protracted for a time long enough to permit the analysis described below and was stored on tape for subsequent elaboration. In 5 cases the epileptogenic zone was in the temporal lobe, in one case it was frontal and in the other one parietal.

The interictal epileptic potentials from most of the explored brain sites (8 to 14 in each patient) were automatically detected according to the method of Lieb *et al.*[3]. The stability, or variability, of the spike rate was evaluated statistically, either by subdividing the mean rate by its standard deviation (conditions 1 and 3 described below), or by the t-Student test (between mean rate of conditions 1 and 2; see Pola and Rossi[4]).

The following conditions were considered: 1. a basic situation of relaxed wakefulness of at least 30 continuative minutes, while the patient was under full pharmacological medication; 2. 30 minutes of wakefulness after some days of marked reduction or suppression of any antiepileptic drug (that was possible in 4 patients only); 3. some hours of night recording, covering wakefulness and all the sleep phases.

Results

1. Basic conditions (relaxed wakefulness). In 6 of the 7 patients the highest stability of interictal spike rate was that of the epileptogenic zone. In the 7th case two cerebral sites showed similar high degree of spike rate stability: one was coincident with the epileptogenic zone (the left Ammon's horn), the other one was very close to it (the left amygdala).

2. Reduction of pharmacological medication. The maximal stability of spike rate—*i.e.* the spike rate less affected by the quantitative variation of the pharmacological antiepileptic treatment—was that of the epileptogenic zone in all the 4 patients available for this type of analysis (Fig. 1).

3. Nocturnal sleep. The high level of stability of interictal discharges recorded from the epileptogenic zone during wakefulness was maintained throughout the night, during all the different phases of sleep (Fig. 2). In 6 patients this level was the highest one; in the remaining patient a level of stability similar to that of the epileptogenic zone (anterior part of the second temporal gyrus) was found in a distant region of the same hemisphere (mesial part of the frontal area 8).

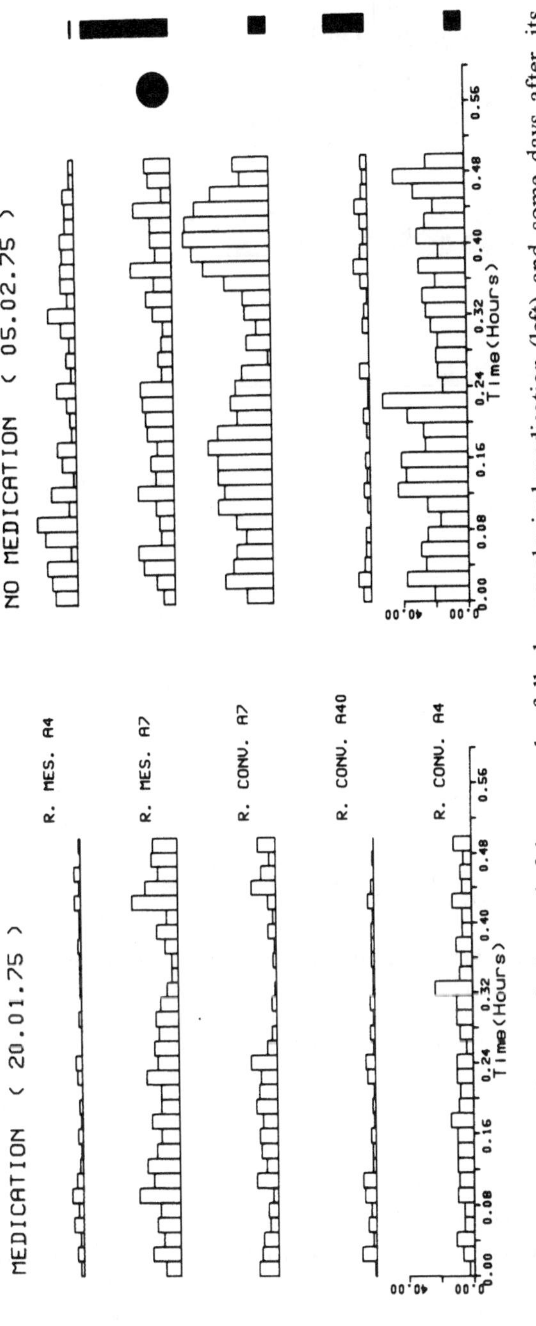

Fig. 1. Interictal spike rate during wakefulness, under full pharmacological medication (left) and some days after its suppression (right). The level of spike rate stability of each structure is indicated by the amplitude of the black vertical bars on the right (t-Student between the mean spike rate of the two conditions examined). In this and in Fig. 2: *A 7*, *A 4*, *A 40* Brodman's areas; *MES* mesial; *CONV* convexity; *R* right; *L* left. The cerebral zone giving origin to the ictal discharges is marked by the black dot

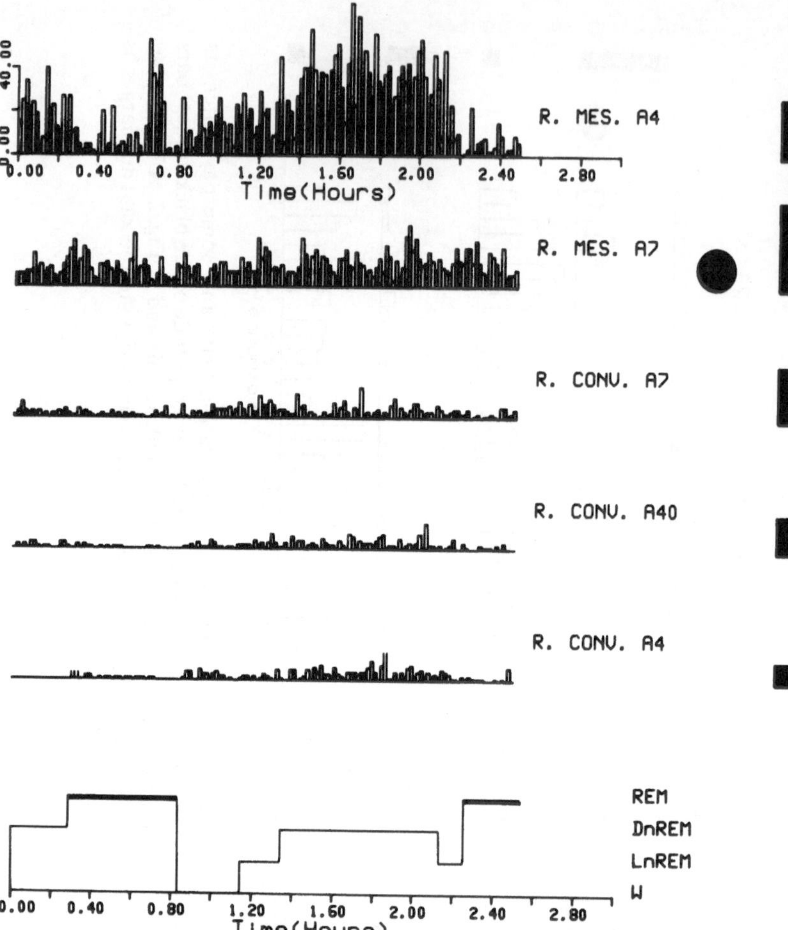

Fig. 2. Interictal spike rate during sleep (same subject of Fig. 1). The level of spike rate stability is indicated as in Fig. 1 (mean rate divided by its standard deviation). The alternation of wakefulness (*W*) and of the sleep phases (*LnREM* phases 1 and 2; *DnREM* phases 3 and 4; *REM* phase REM) is reported on the bottom

Discussion

From the results obtained it appears that the question posed in the introduction can be given a positive answer. The peculiar stability of the rate of the interictal discharges recorded from the cerebral zone giving rise to the ictal activity responsible for the seizures is not an occasional finding; it is a common event in partial epilepsies. This finding was obtained by the use of automatic elaboration.

A relation between local level of epileptogenicity and autonomy of local spiking from internal (*e.g.* sleep) and external (*e.g.* antiepileptic drugs) influences is suggested by the results of our research. Our preliminary observations are thus confirmed[2,5–7]. The phenomenon seems worth of particular consideration for its physiopathological implications and for its possible diagnostic utilization.

References

1. Bancaud, J., Talairach, J., La stéréo-électroencéphalographie dans l'épilepsie, 321 pp. Paris: Masson et Cie. 1965.
2. Gentilomo, A., Colicchio, G., Pola, P., Rossi, G. F., Scerrati, M., Brain depth recording of interictal epileptic potentials during sleep in man. In: Sleep 1974 (Levin, P., Koella, W. P., eds.), pp. 444—446. Basel: S. Karger. 1975.
3. Lieb, J. P., Woods, S. C., Siccardi, A., Crandall, P. H., Walter, R. O., Lake, B., Quantitative analysis of depth spiking in relation to seizure foci in patients with temporal lobe epilepsy. EEG clin. Neurophysiol. *44* (1978), 641—663.
4. Pola, P., Rossi, G. F., Computerized analytic study of stability of interictal spike rate. In: Advances in Stereotactic and Functional Neurosurgery 6 (Gybels, J., *et al.*, eds.), pp. 75—78. Acta Neurochir. (Wien) Suppl. 33. Wien-New York: Springer. 1984.
5. Rossi, G. F., Problems of analysis and interpretation of electrocerebral signals in epilepsy. In: Epilepsy: Its Phenomena in Man (Brazier, M., ed.), pp. 259—285. New York: Academic Press. 1973.
6. Rossi, G. F., Colicchio, G., Gentilomo, A., Pola, P., Scerrati, M., Study of the electrocerebral activity in partial epilepsies. Arch. Ital. Biol. *120* (1982), 160—175.
7. Rossi, G. F., Gentilomo, A., Colicchio, G., Le problème de la recherche de la topographie d'origine de l'épilepsie. Schw. Arch. Neurol. Psychiat. *115* (1974), 229—270.

Acta Neurochirurgica, Suppl. 33, 75—78 (1984)

Computerized Analytic Study of Stability of Interictal Spike Rate*

P. Pola[1] and **G. F. Rossi**

With 2 Figures

Summary

Theoretically there are two methods for the analytic definition of the degree of variability or stability of interictal spike rate, both based on its statistical properties. The first computes the coefficient of variation of the rate of spikes recorded during a particular and well defined functional situation; evaluating the degree of "intrinsic" stability within this situation. The second method computes the ratio between the mean spike rate of the first of two different considered situations and the t-Student between their mean spike rate; it provides information on the "extrinsinc" stability related to the functional variation.

Keywords: Computer analysis; spike rate stability; stereo-EEG.

Introduction

The aim of the present work is to provide an analytical method to study the behaviour of the interictal spike rate in epilepsy. In particular, we wanted to reach a definition of variability or stability. Stability of interictal spikes recorded from a certain zone can be regarded as an expression of the degree of indipendence from any type of external or internal influence[2].

Schematically we can define two types of stability:

1. *"Intrinsic" stability:* the stability of spike rate in a relatively close time during which the functional state of the brain can be

---

* Supported by the Consiglio Nazionale delle Ricerche and Ministero della Pubblica Istruzione.

[1] Istituto di Neurochirurgia, Università Cattolica del Sacro Cuore, Largo A. Gemelli, 8, I-00168 Roma, Italy.

regarded as uniform (*e.g.* a continuous period of relaxed wakefulness).

2. *"Extrinsic" stability:* the stability of spike rate across two different functional situations (*e.g.* a period during which the subject receives full antiepileptic medication and another period of equal duration after suppression of medication).

Methods

The two following methods estimate these two types of stability of interictal spike rate stability.

1. "Intrinsic" stability: mean rate of spikes recorded during the considered uniform functional situation divided by its standard deviation.

2. "Extrinsic" stability: the mean of the rate of spikes recorded during the first one of the two situations divided by the t-Student between the means of spike rate of the two situations.

Results

The results of the application of the proposed methods is shown in Fig. 1 for "intrinsic" stability and in Fig. 2 for "extrinsic" stability. The region with the highest value of "intrinsic" stability (Fig. 1) is usually coincident with the site of origin of the ictal discharge (dark square). For the explored cerebral structures it is possible to define a linear regression between the mean spike rate and "intrinsic" stability of each structure. This can be regarded as a model for the "intrinsic" stability in the examined patient.

Similarly the cerebral area with the highest "extrinsic" stability is coincident with the epileptogenic zone (Fig. 2, dark square). The behaviour of spiking from the cerebral region identified as the most epileptogenic is different as far as "extrinsic" stability is concerned from that of spiking recorded from the other cerebral sites (Fig. 2). A linear regression between the mean spike rate of the first of the two different functional situations and the t-Student, between the means of spike rate of the two situations, is found for all the examined regions but the epileptogenic zone. Also in this case the linear regression may be regarded as a model for the "extrinsic" stability.

Conclusions

The proposed methods seem suited to measure the degree of stability of interictal epileptic spike rate during uniform functional

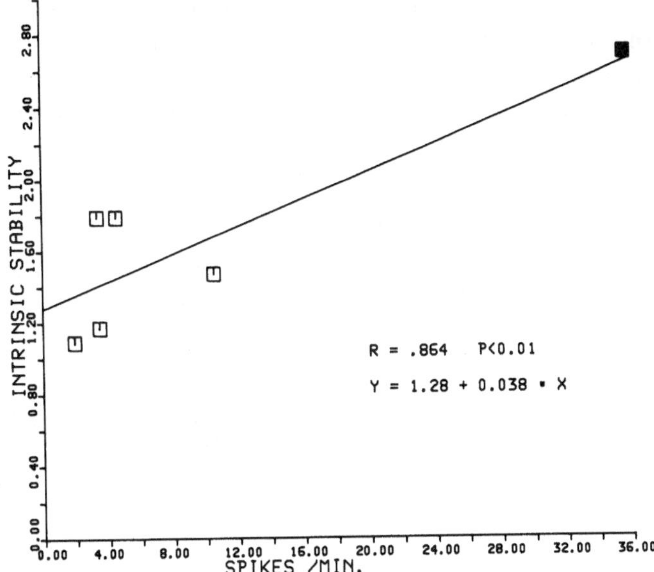

Fig. 1. "Intrinsic" stability during relaxed wakefulness. In this and in Fig. 2 the cerebral zone giving origin to ictal discharge is the dark square

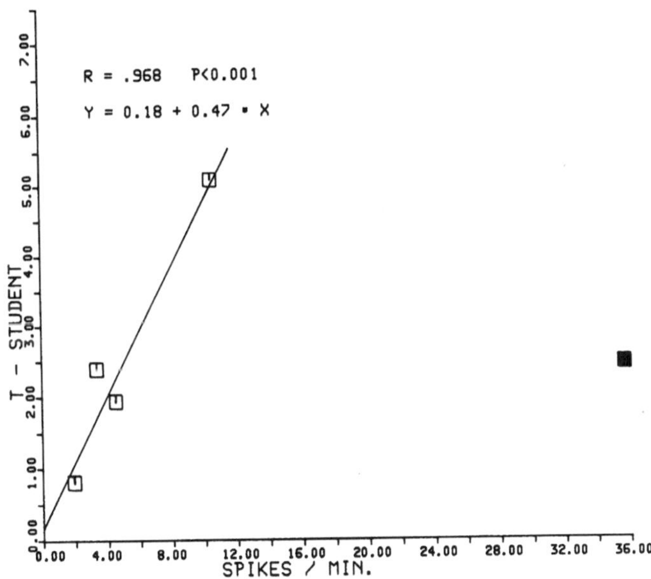

Fig. 2. "Extrinsic" stability across two different situations. The first one is related to a situation in which the patient has a full antiepileptic medication and the second one is after suppression of medication

conditions ("intrinsic" stability) and during different functional situations ("extrinsic" stability). From the applications of the method to epileptic patients it appears that the results of both types of stability are related to the local level of epileptogenicity (see Rossi *et al.* in this issue 1).

References

1. Rossi, G. F., Pola, P., Scerrati, M., Stability of interictal spike rate as an index of local epileptogenicity. A study based on automatic elaboration. In: Advances in Stereotactic and Functional Neurosurgery 6 (Gybels, J., *et al.*, eds.), pp. 69—73. Acta Neurochir. (Wien) Suppl. 33. Wien-New York: Springer. 1984.
2. Rossi, G. F., Problems of analysis and interpretation of electrocerebral signals in epilepsy. In: Epilepsy: Its phenomena in Man (Brazier, M., ed.), pp. 259—285. New York: Academic Press. 1973.

Acta Neurochirurgica, Suppl. 33, 79—83 (1984)

Chronic Burr-Hole ECoG and SEEG in the Assessment of Surgical Treatment for Epilepsy

J. L. Barcia-Salorio[1], **P. Roldán**, **S. Ramos**, **L. López Gómez**, and **J. Broseta**

With 2 Figures

Present day surgical treatment of epilepsy is based on the failure of medical treatment and the localization of epileptic focus. The most accurate technic is stereo-electro-encephalography (SEEG) consisting of chronic implantation of deep electrodes by a stereotactical technique. However the inconvenience of the high cost and risk of cerebral damage due to the introduction of necessarily numerous electrodes must be borne in mind.

To avoid this, the authors followed the method outlined below. In patients who did not respond to any medical treatment, all possible use was made of conventional EEG. This initial study allows the determination of cerebral areas of interest which justify a more detailed study. At a second stage chronic burr-hole corticography (ECoG) is performed (introduction of cortical electrodes)[1], placing the electrodes to complete the data given by the scalp-EEG. From these findings it is possible to deduce which subcortical structures must be explored by deep electrodes to find the exact limits of the trigger focus.

Material and Methods

A group of 10 patients, 6 of which presented epileptic crises unresponsive to all treatment and with numerous daily attacks, and another 4 with psychotic epileptic manifestations were studied by conventional EEG. Evidence of an epileptic focus was found in the majority. In the second phase, ECoG (Fig. 1 a) demonstrated an

[1] Department of Neurosurgery, Hospital Clinico Universitario, Valencia 10, Spain.

epileptic focus not necessarily in the area indicated by the EEG. Electrodes were introduced by the stereotactic technique, with selection of target and positioning of electrodes so that the terminals completely covered the suspected trigger area.

The electrodes have an internal guide allowing rigidity on introduction but flexibility on withdrawal. Although the number of terminals used and the distance between them was variable, the one most frequently used had 7 contacts each, separated by 7 mm covering a distance of 4.5 cm (Fig. 1 b).

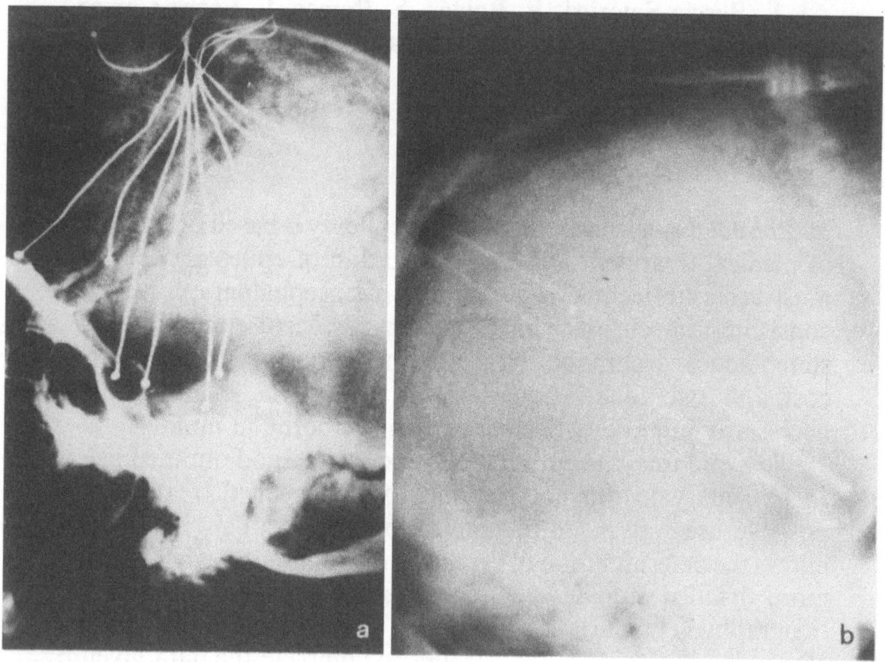

Fig. 1. Lateral X-ray control of electrodes position for (a) ECoG (b) SEEG

Results

The results are summarized in Table 1. It must be noted that EEG findings did not always coincide with those of the ECoG, demonstrating that the latter is much more precise and has a greater power of localization.

On the other hand, SEEG findings coincided generally with those of the ECoG, delimiting the trigger focus with high precission (Fig. 2).

Table 1. *EEG, ECoG and SEEG Findings in Epileptic Patients*. E: Epilepsy. E. Psy.: Epileptic Psychosis. B. D.: Bilateral Discharges. r./l.: right/left. T. F.: Temporal Focus. O. F.: Occipital Focus. No focal: No focalization. L: Lobectomy. Fx: Fornicotomy

Case	Age	Diagnosis	EEG	ECoG	SEEG	Treatment	Radiosurgery	Result	Follow-up
1	45	E	B. D.	l. T. F.	l. T. F.	Fx	—	excellent	7 y.
2	35	E	B. D.	l. T. F.	l. T. F.	L	—	poor	6 y.
3	37	E	B. D.	r. T. F.	r. T. F.	L	—	excellent	6 y.
4	29	E	r. T. F.	r. T. F.	r./l. T. F.	r. T. L.	l. T. F.	good	2 m.
5	31	E	l. O. F.	l. O. F.	l. O. F.	l. O. L.	—	poor	6 m.
6	20	E	B. D.	l./r. T. F.	l./r. T. F.	—	l. T. F.	excellent	6 m.
7	29	E. Psy.	l. T. F.	l. T. F.	l. T. F.	—	l. T. F.	excellent	8 m.
8	25	E. Psy.	B. D.	l. T. F.	No focal	—	—	—	—
9	20	E. Psy.	B. D.	No focal	No focal	—	—	—	—
10	24	E. Psy.	B. D.	l. T. F.	No focal	—	—	—	—

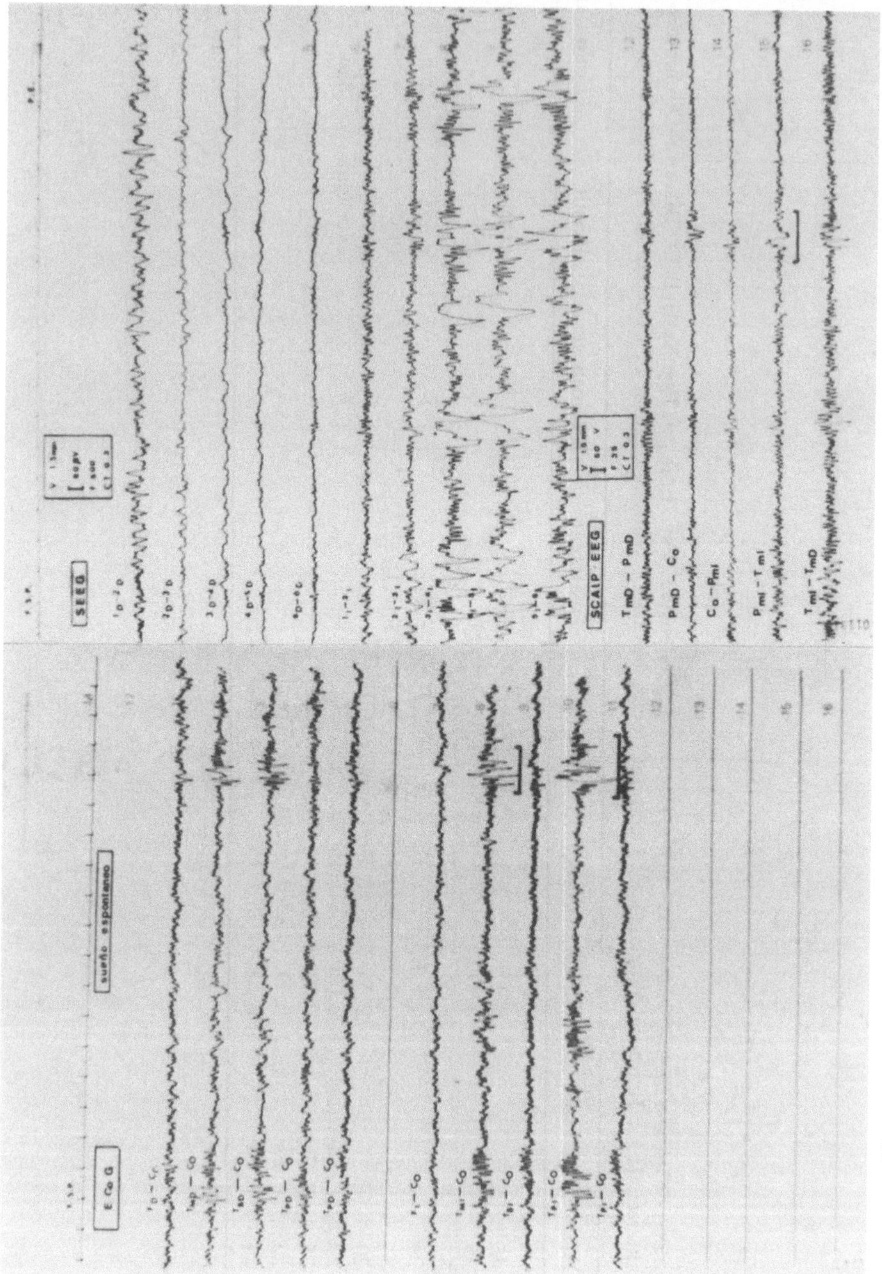

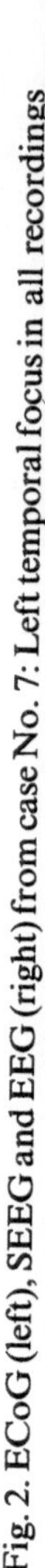

Fig. 2. ECoG (left), SEEG and EEG (right) from case No. 7: Left temporal focus in all recordings

Finally, surgical treatment confirmed ECoG and SEEG findings, and an improvement was seen in the condition of these cases where the focus was extirpated. Extirpation was carried out in 4 cases via lobectomy and peroperative ECoG and SEEG, and in 3 cases of dominant lobe lesions via stereotatic radiosurgery with a dose of 10 Gy and a 10 mm colimator. The short-term results of these cases were favorable although, as yet, the short follow-up does not allow definitive conclusions.

Reference

1. Broseta, J., Barcia-Salorio, J. L., López Gómez, L., Roldán, P., González Darder, J., Barberá, J., Burr-hole electrocorticography. Acta Neurochir. (Wien), Suppl. 30, 91—96 (1980).

Acta Neurochirurgica, Suppl. 33, 85—89 (1984)

Tridimensional Biomagnetic Localization of Epileptic Foci

G. B. Ricci[1], **I. Modena**[2], **S. Barbanera**[2], **F. Campitelli**[3], and **G. L. Romani**[2]

With 3 Figures

Keywords: Magnetoencephalography; focal epilepsies.

The advantages of magnetoencephalography (MEG) with respect to the EEG in localizing intracerebral sources have been confirmed by our study on clinical material, namely focal epilepsies[1,2]. The results obtained by the MEG in studying evoked signals, have also shown the capability of this method to exactly localize 3-dimensionally the sources of such signals. The map of evoked fields on the skull surface, shows two separate areas where the signals are higher and of opposite sign, so called "maxima" or "extrema". Such a pattern suggests a dipolar source, namely a "current dipole" in a spherical conductor medium adopted as model of the head.

If the current dipole model is taken into account, the localization is easily obtained, the source being half-way between the two maxima, at a depth which depends on the distance between the maxima and on the radius of the sphere which best fits the actual shape of the skull[3].

Measurements of evoked fields follows the methodology of the evoked potentials with the difference that the magnetic signal replaces the electric one. The same method applied to spontaneous MEG signals presents difficulties, in that generally a stimulus or

---

[1] Serv. Auton. EEG-Istituto Neurochirurgia, Università "La Sapienza", Roma, Italy.

[2] Istituto di Elettronica dello Stato Solido-CNR, Roma, Italy.

[3] Supported by grant by Elettronica S. p. A.

biological signal cannot be utilized as a trigger. It can be assumed that spontaneous EEG potential, such as sporadic epileptic potentials, also have a dipolar pattern that allows a tridimensional localization. As far as instruments are concerned, the ideal solution is to have a multisensor probe allowing the simultaneous measurements at many points in the area of interest. This is a

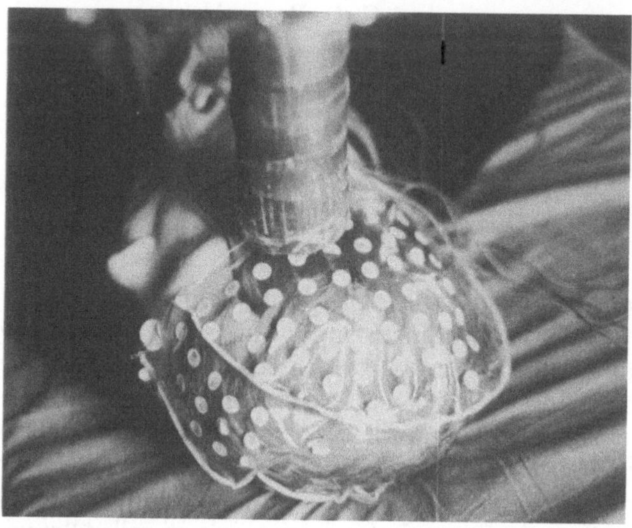

Fig. 1. Grid used for neuromagnetic maps (spacing between point 2 × 2 cm)

technical advance which will be realized in the near future and which will contribute to our knowledge of the MEG in normal and pathological conditions. However, having for now only one sensor available, the alternative is to utilize the EEG signals correlated to the MEG as trigger and to average the MEG on the different locations. This is the way indicated by Barth *et al.*[4] which we have followed in several cases of focal epilepsies in which the EEG showed sustained interictal spiking activity which could be correlated to the corresponding MEG (Figs. 1, 2 a). The case presented is of partial epilepsy with complex psychomotor symptomatology studied in the Institute of Neurosurgery of the Rome University, which showed a sustained interictal spiking activity of high voltage in the right temporal region. The more

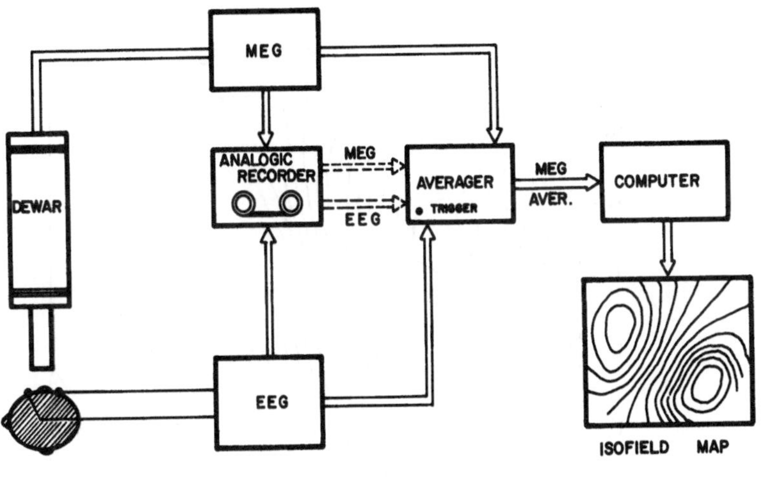

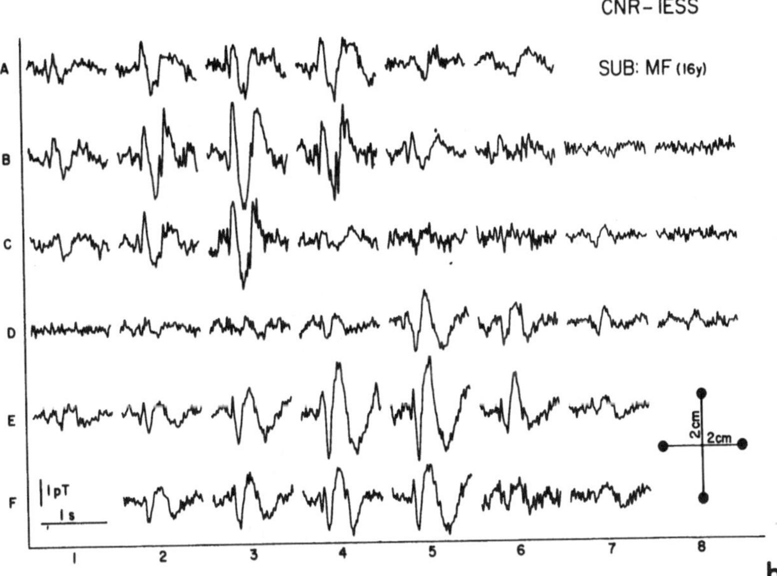

Fig. 2. a) Block diagram of the experimental set-up for simultaneous EEG-MEG measurements. b) Magnetic signals recorded according to the grid of Fig. 1. Every waveform is the result of the average of about 10 samples; the average was obtained using the EEG signal as a trigger

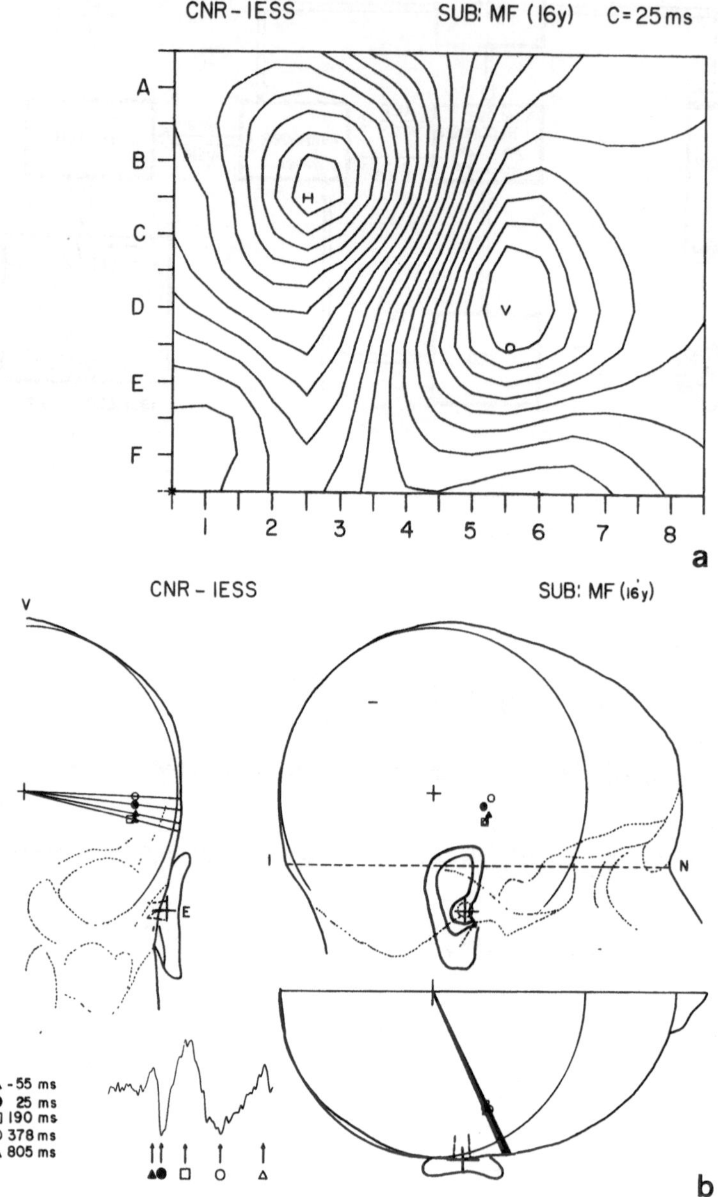

Fig. 3. a) An example of isofield contour-map for a component at a well-defined latency. b) Localization of the possible sources of the five main components of the spiking activity

active EEG derivation was chosen as trigger while the corresponding MEG was averaged (7–12 repetitions) and measured sequentially according to a prearranged matrix (2 cm spacing) that included, in this case, 47 points. The results were plotted as in the case of evoked fields, and the display showed two points of maxima that suggested a temporal lobe localization at the depth of 2.5 cm (Figs. 2 b, 3). Even if in this case a proven anatomical localization did not exist, we can anticipate the suitability of the methodology for a tridimensional MEG localisation in other cases with well-localized lesions (calcifications, paraxytal cyst, etc.). These are extremely important results for clinical application which is presently limited by having only one probe. This limitation makes examination very lengthy, requiring 5 to 6 hours for each case, often repeating the sessions after a few days to check the data. Furthermore a simultaneous display of the MEG in different point is not available and the isofield maps refer only to magnetic signals correlated to electric ones.

Despite these limitations, it is clear that the MEG can give us a static and probably also dynamic tridimensional display of an intracerebral source. This recommends rapid technological implementation of the methodology, where we can already forecast a reconstructive display in the form of slices as in the present CT scanner.

References

1. Modena, I., Ricci, G. B., Barbanera, S., Leoni, R., Romani, G. L., Carelli, P., Electroencephal. Clin. Neurophysiol. *54* (1982), 622—628.
2. Ricci, G. B., Il Nuovo Cimento *2D* (1983), 517—537.
3. Williamson, S. J., Kaufman, L., J. Magn. Mat. *22* (1981), 129—201.
4. Barth, D. S., Sutherling, W., Engel, J., jr., Beatty, J., Science *218* (1982), 891—894.

Acta Neurochirurgica, Suppl. 33, 91—96 (1984)

Stereotactic Methodology in Epileptic Patients with Hemispheric Astrocytoma

C. Munari[1, 2], **A. Bonis**[1, 2], **J. Talairach**[2], **G. Szikla**[1, 2], **J. P. Chodkiewicz**[2], **A. Musolino**[2], and **J. Bancaud**[1, 2]

With 3 Figures

Summary

The usefulness of stereo-EEG investigations in epileptic patients with hemispheric astrocytoma is explored. We will show the results obtained from a 20 year old patient with severe drug resistant epilepsy which began at age 8 years. The stereo-EEG findings (particularly during spontaneous seizures) show that the "epileptogenic" zone widely exceeded the limits of the tumoral lesion shown by CT scan. On the basis of this pre-operative information it is possible not only to remove the tumor, but also to remove the "epileptogenic" area, not necessarily strictly contiguous to the tumor.

Keywords: Epilepsy; astrocytomas; stereo-EEG; epileptic seizures.

Introduction

Recent advances in neurodiagnostic procedures, such as CT scan, permit an earlier detection of small tumours. In epileptic patients the desired result would be to simultaneously treat a tumoral "epileptogenic" lesion as well as the focal epilepsy. The stereo-EEG studies[1, 2, 4] show how variable the topographic relationships may be between a tumor and an "epileptogenic" area.

1 Unité 97 de recherches sur l'épilepsie (J. Bancaud) INSERM, 2ter rue d'Alésia, F-75014 Paris, France.

2 Service de Neurochirurgie B (J. P. Chodkiewicz), Hôpital Sainte Anne, 1 rue Cabanis, F-75014 Paris, France.

Table 1

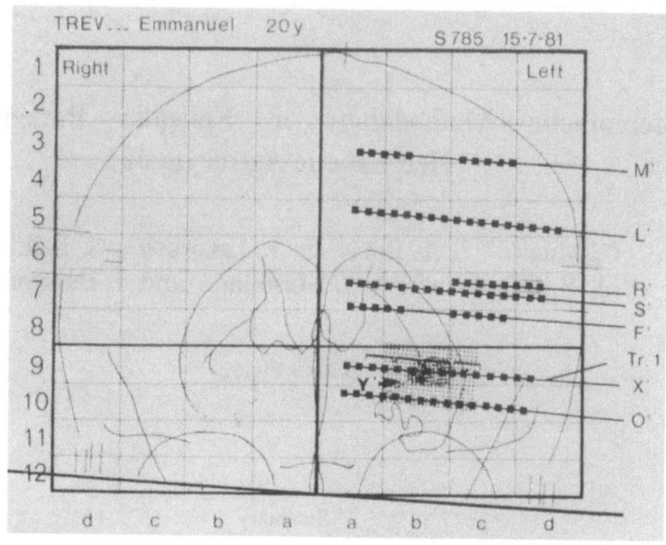
TREV... Emmanuel 20y
S 785 15-7-81
Right
Left
M'
L'
R'
S'
F'
Tr. 1
X'
O'
Y'
d c b a a b c d

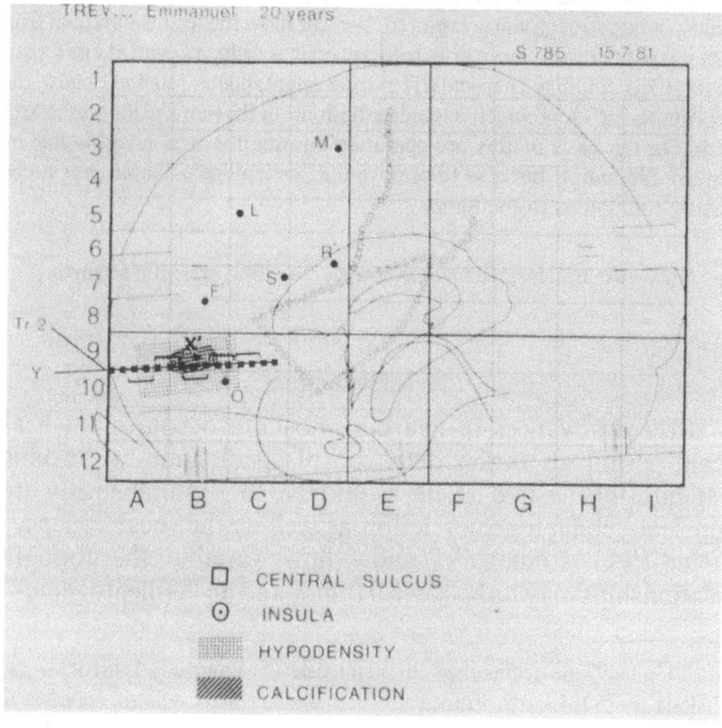
TREV... Emmanuel 20 years
S 785 15-7-81
M'
L'
R'
S'
F'
X'
O'
Tr 2
Y
A B C D E F G H I
CENTRAL SULCUS
INSULA
HYPODENSITY
CALCIFICATION

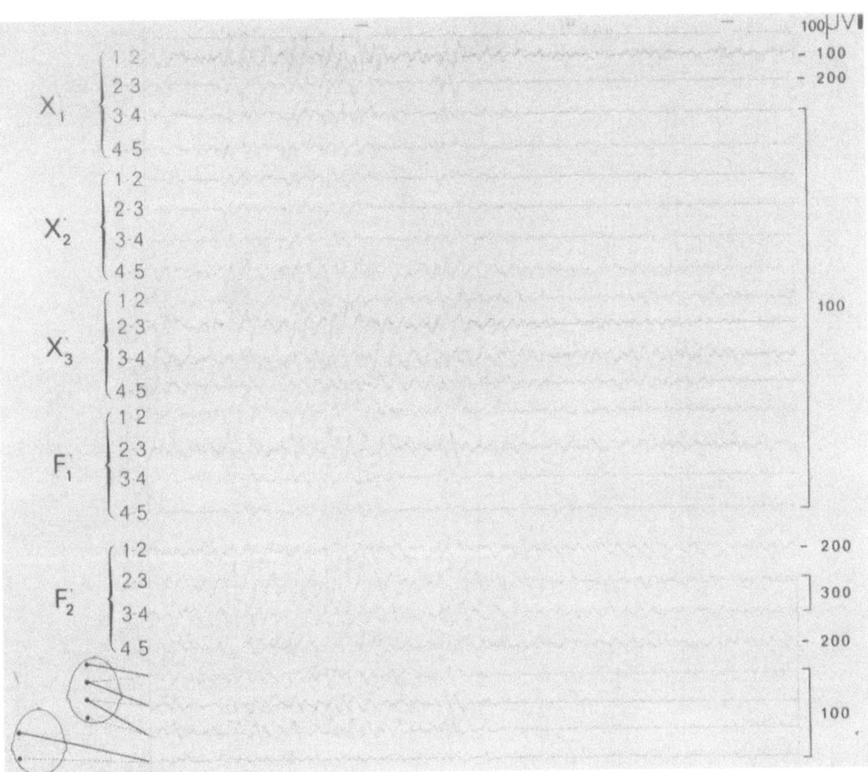

Fig. 1

Patients and Methods

In forty patients with epilepsy and hemispheric astrocytoma, we performed a stereo-EEG exploration with the twofold aim of defining the limits of the tumor and the origin of the seizures. The neurologic, EEG and neuroradiological data characterizing these patients cannot be reported here[3]. We wish only to emphasize that these patients were young adults (10 to 44 years, mean: 25 years) and that epilepsy was, in most of them, the major clinical problem (mean duration of more than 5 years).

Case Report

The patient was a twenty year old man with severe drug-resistant epilepsy which began at age 8 years. This epilepsy had been classified for many years among "primary generalized epilepsies". A schema of ventricular structures, of the tumoral lesion (reconstructed from the CT-scan data), and of the lateral position of the electrodes is represented in Table 1. Figs. 1 and 2 show stereo-EEG findings

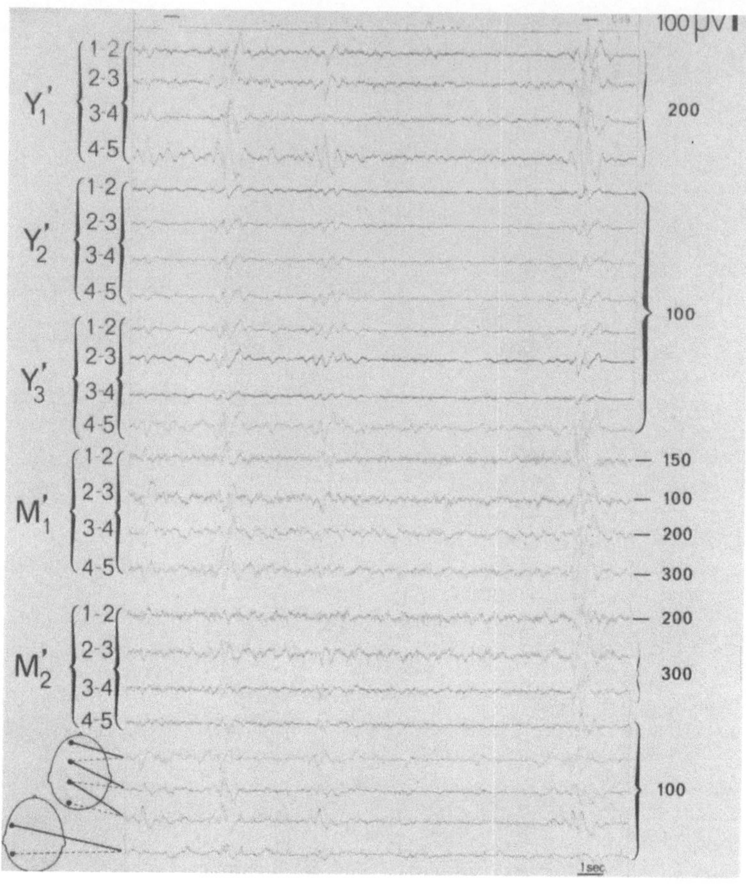

Fig. 2

in the tumor and other cortical regions: areas of very depressed electrical activity (X′1—X′2—Y′2), of slow waves (X′3—F′2) of no altered back-ground activity (M′1—M′2), and of rapid diffused spikes from almost all of the electrodes, including Y′ and X′. Fig. 3 shows a seizure starting on the electrodes Y′ 1—F′ 1—X′ 1—X′ 3—S′ 4—O′ 1—R′ 2. A few seconds later the ictal discharge affects all the electrodes and is visible on the scalp (bilateral spike and waves).

Discussion

The use of stereo-EEG to better define the extent of a small brain tumor is generally admitted[5,6]. In our experience the aid

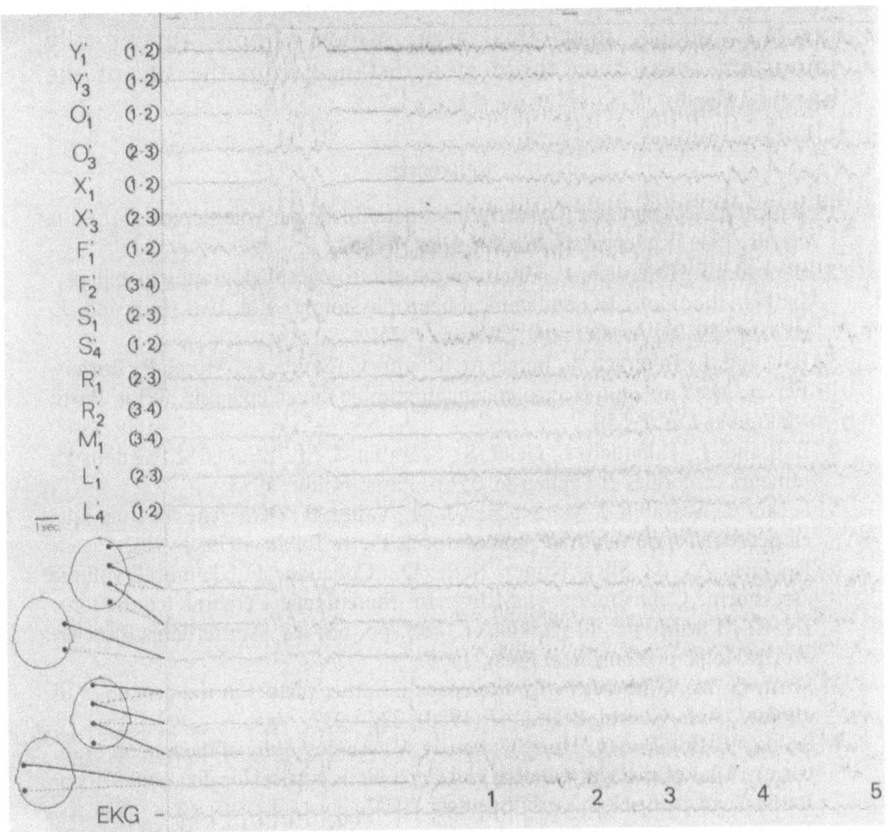

Fig. 3

afforded by this methodological approach is indispensable in patients with epilepsy and slow growing tumors, especially astrocytoma. Some authors claim that epilepsy is a reliable prognostic factor in such patients[7]; a previous stereo-EEG study, however, could improve their prognosis. The neurosurgeon may program his intervention[9], with millimetric precision, before entering the operating theater, knowing: a) the topographic extent of the tumoral lesion and of the epileptogenic area; b) the anatomical modifications induced by the tumor; c) the exact topography of cerebral vessels to be preserved. Using these preoperative information it is possible to achieve: a) as complete a removal of the tumor as possible; b) resection of an epileptogenic area not necessarily contiguous to the tumor; c) preservation of cerebral vessels near this area, which supply functionally important areas even those at a distance from the site of the intervention[8].

References

1. Bancaud, J., Apport de l'exploration fonctionnelle par voie stéréotaxique à la chirurgie de l'épilepsie. Neurochirurgie *5* (1959), 55—112.
2. Bancaud, J., Talairach, J., Macro-stereo-electro-encephalography in epilepsy. In: Handbook of EEG and clinical neurophysiology, Vol. 10 B (Bancaud, J., ed.), pp. 3—33. Amsterdam: Elsevier. 1975.
3. Bancaud, J., Talairach, J., Bonis, A., Schaub, C., Szikla, G., Morel, P., Bordas-Ferrer, M., La stéréo-électro-encéphalographie dans l'épilepsie, 321 p. Paris: Masson et Cie. 1965.
4. Bancaud, J., Talairach, J., Geier, S., Scarabin, J. M., EEG et SEEG dans les tumeurs cérébrales et l'épilepsie, 351 p. Paris: Edifor. 1973.
5. Pecker, J., Scarabin, J. M., Brucker, J. M., Vallee, B., Démarche stéréotaxique en neurochirurgie tumorale. Laboratories Pierre Fabre, 1979, 1—301.
6. Rougier, A., da Silva Nunez Neto, D., Cohadan, F., Tumoral volume assessment: Contribution of SEEG. In: Stereotactic Cerebral Irradiations. INSERM symp. no. 12 (Szikla, G., ed.), pp. 63—68. Amsterdam: Elsevier, North-Holland Biomedical Press. 1979.
7. Scott, G. M., Gibberd, F. B., Epilepsy and other factors in the prognosis of gliomas. Acta Neurol. Scand. *61* (1980), 227—239.
8. Szikla, G., Bouvier, G., Hori, T., Petrov, V., Angiography of the human brain cortex. Atlas of vascular patterns and stereotactic cortical localization, 273 pp. Berlin-Heidelberg-New York: Springer. 1977.
9. Talairach, J., Bancaud, J., Szikla, G., Bonis, A., Geier, S., Vedrenne, C., Approche nouvelle de la neurochirurgie de l'épilepsie. Méthodologie stéréotaxique et résultats thérapeutiques. Neurochirurgie, suppl. 20, (1974), 240 pp.

Acta Neurochirurgica, Suppl. 33, 97—103 (1984)

Depth Recording and Neuropathological Aspects in Symptomatic Tumoral and Non Tumoral Epilepsy

G. Broggi[1], A. Franzini[1], C. Giorgi[1], R. Spreafico[2], and G. Avanzini[2]

With 1 Figure

Summary

Depth EEG recordings have been performed during brain biopsy in 20 epileptic patients with hemispheric deep C.T. scan hypodense lesion. In spite of their epileptic symptomatology, only 3 patients showed "epileptiform" EEG abnormalities at the preoperative scalp EEG recording. In all cases a consistent depression or absence of electrical activity was recorded in correspondence of the "core" of the hypodense lesion. Epileptiform EEG activity was found in 80% of the patients in an area surrounding the electrical silent "core". In no cases this activity reached the surface of the brain (as shown by the scalp EEG recording) except when activation with pentothal was performed.

Keywords: Cerebral tumors; epilepsy; stereo-EEG; stereo-biopsy.

Material and Methods

The present work refers to our experience of deep EEG recording during brain biopsy, on 20 epileptic patients with hypodense lesion in the C.T. scan (Tab. 1). All patients (11 males and 9 females, aged between 12 and 58 years) presented with epileptic seizures as the first and in most cases (14/20) as the only symptom of a brain lesion.

The onset of epileptic symptoms varied from 6 months to 15 years before the C.T. scan demonstrated a hypodense deep lying lesion in one of the brain hemispheres. The site of the lesion was temporal in 8/20 cases, frontal in 2/20, parietal in 2/20, fronto-temporal in 4/20, fronto-parietal and temporo-parietal in

[1] Department of Neurosurgery and [2] Department of Neurophysiology, Istituto Neurologico "C. Besta", Via Celoria N. 11, I-20133 Milano, Italy.

Table 1

No.	Name	Age	Sex	Seizures	Scalp EEG	Neurological deficits
1.	A. G.	41	M	P. C./GEN.	F. S. W.	–
2	A. P.	47	M	P. E.	F. S. W.	–
3	B. G.	48	M	P. C.	A. A.	–
4	B. P. L.	28	M	P. E.	F. S. W.	–
5	C. G.	21	M	GEN.	F. S. W.	right hemiparesis
6	C. M.	45	M	P. C./GEN.	normal	–
7	C. M.	36	F	P. C./GEN.	A. A.	–
8	C. C.	58	M	P. C.	A. A.	–
9	D. C. T.	53	F	P. C./GEN.	A. A.	–
10	F. S.	38	M	P. C.	F. S. W.	–
11	G. E.	42	M	P. C./GEN.	F. S. W.	–
12	M. S.	43	F	P. E.	F. S. W.	right hemiplegia
13	M. A.	16	F	P. E./P. C.	E. A.	right hemiparesis
14	M. L.	40	F	P. C./GEN.	E. A.	–
15	M. G.	13	F	P. E.	F. S. W.	right hemiparesis
16	P. E.	12	F	P. C.	E. A.	–
17	P. T.	18	M	P. E./GEN.	F. S. W.	–
18	P. M.	40	F	P. E.	normal	left hemiparesis
19	R. G.	38	M	GEN.	F. S. W.	–
20	S. A.	53	F	P. E.	F. S. W.	right hemiparesis

P. C. = Partial complex seizures; P. E. = Partial seizures with elementary symptomatology; GEN. = Generalized seizures; A. A. = Aspecific abnorm-

two cases respectively (Tab. 2). In the majority of patients the lesion was in the left hemisphere (15/20).

The preoperative EEG from the scalp was normal in 2 patients, while focal slow waves (theta and/or delta) were found in the majority of patients (11/20). Only 3 patients showed "epileptiform" EEG abnormalities (spikes or sharp waves) while the remaining patients only non specific and diffuse EEG abnormalities were present (Tab. 2).

All the patients had fits, mostly partial (either elementary or with complex symptomatology) with or without secondary generalization. Only two patients had generalized seizures without clinical symptoms of focal onset.

The intra-operative scalp EEG was generally similar to the pre-operative EEG except for the presence of fast activity and slow waves due to the anesthesia. Under general anesthesia the scalp EEG even in 3 patients with epileptic abnormalities on the pre-operative EEG did not show an obvious epileptiform pattern.

Table 1

Site of lesion	Side of lesion	Neuropathology	Anesthesia
T.	L.	P. Encef. Gliosis	AL.
F.-T.	R.	Astrocyt. I–II	AL.
T.	R.	Gliosis	F.
P. POST.	L.	P. Encef. Gliosis	AL. + F.
T.	L.	Astrocyt. I–II	F.
T. P.	L.	Astrocyt. III	AL. + F.
T.	L.	Astrocyt. III	F.
T.	R.	Astrocyt. I–II	local
F.	L.	P. Encef. Gliosis	F.
T.	L.	Astrocyt. I–II	AL.
F.-T.	R.	Astrocyt. III	F.
F.-P.	L.	Astrocyt. I–II	F.
T.-P.	L.	Astrocyt. I–II	F.
F.	L.	Ang. Cav.	F.
T.	L.	Astrocyt. I–II	F.
F.-T.	L.	P. Encef. Gliosis	F.
T.	R.	P. Encef. Gliosis	F.
F.-P.	R.	P. Encef. Gliosis	F.
F.-T.	L.	Astrocyt. Gen. (III)	AL. + F.
P.	L.	Astrocyt. III	local

alities; E. A. = Epileptic abnormalities; F. S. W. = Focal slow waves; T. = Temporal; F = Frontal; P = Parietal; Al. = Althesin; F. = Fluotane.

The stereotactic surgery was performed with a Riechert frame. After a three-dimensional mathematical reconstruction of the C.T. images, the impedance, EEG depth recording and bioptic trajectory were chosen in order to explore the lesion in its major extension[3].

The depth EEG recording was performed by a single multicontact (15 contacts) electrode which was inserted before the biopsy. The later was performed on the same trajectory. The procedure allowed the sampling of brain tissue in the volume corresponding to the defined hypodense areas *i.e.*, particularly, where low or no electrical activity were recorded. The position of recording electrode was also always controlled radiologically. Neuropathological examination of tissue samples demonstrated in 8/20 patients astrocytomas I–II, astrocytomas III in 4 patients (W.H.O. classifiction)[9]. In 6 patients the neuropathological diagnosis was post encephalitis gliosis. In one case an aspecific gliosis was present while in another case a cavernous angioma was found.

Table 2

Site of Lesion

	No.	%
Frontal	2	10 %
Temporal	8	40%
Parietal	2	10 %
Fronto-Temporal	4	20 %
Fronto-Parietal	2	10 %
Temporo-Parietal	2	10 %

Neuropathology

	No.	%
Post-Enc. Glyosis	6	30 %
Astrocytoma I-II	8	40 %
Astrocytoma III	4	20 %
Glyosis	1	5 %
Cavernous Angiom	1	5 %

Fits

	No.	%
Partial-Element.	6	30 %
Partial-Complex	5	25 %
P.C./Gen.	6	30 %
P.S./Gen.	1	5 %
Generalized	2	10 %

Scalp EEG

	No.	%
Normal	2	10 %
Aspecfic Abn.	4	20 %
Focal Slow Waves	11	55 %
Epileptic Abn.	3	15 %

Graphic representations of the series of patients which underwent depth recording and serial stereotactic biopsy. The clinical, neuropathological and EEG features are considered and represented separately. The number and the percentage of patients in different subgroups are indicated within and outside the histograms respectively.

Post-Enc: Postencephalitic.

P. S./Gen: Partial complex seizures with secondary generalization.

P. S./Gen: Partial sensory seizures with secondary generalization.

Abn: abnormalities.

Results

In all the cases consistent depression or absent electrical activity has found during depth EEG recording. Moreover, absence of electric activity was found in most of the hypodense lesions, in which the histopathological examination revealed glial tumors. In patients whose lesion was diagnosed as post-encephalitic gliosis, intra-lesional electric activity was recorded although with very low

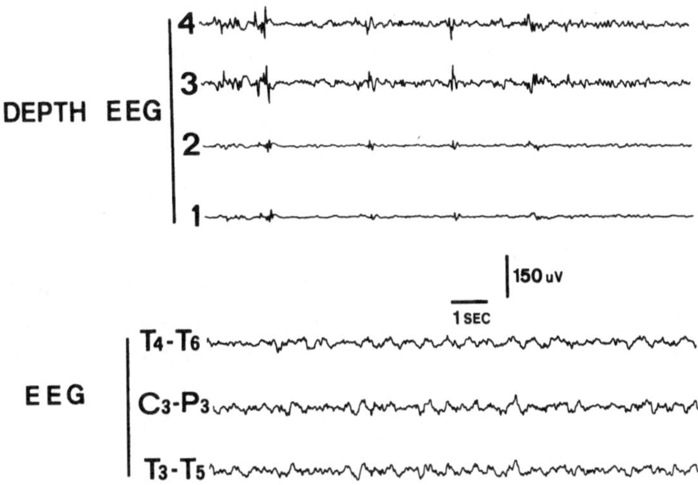

Fig. 1. *1-2-3-4* depth EEG recording. The tip of the electrode (*1* and *2*) is into the "core" of the hypodense lesion, while the other derivations are in the surrounding tissue. Note that spikes of highest voltage are in 3rd contact close to the "core" of low voltage. In the simultaneous scalp EEG recording no epileptiform activity is clearly visible demonstrating that in these conditions the epileptiform discharge did not reach the cortex

voltage as compared to the surrounding tissue. In most cases this reduction or absence of EEG activity was present for no more than 2 contacts (*i.e.* 4–8 mm). This finding is in agreement with previous reports which confirm the utility of depth EEG recording to control the stereotactically estimated target and for most cases for preliminary estimation of the volume and nature of the lesion[2,5,8].

In 80% of patients epileptiform EEG activity was found during depth recording. This activity (predominantly spikes) always had maximum voltage in one of the contacts to the lowest electrical activity (lesional area). Spikes were generally present also in the lesional zone but with lower voltage when compared to the surrounding area, probably due to the spreading of discharge into an "inactive core" (Fig. 1). The presence of maximum voltage epileptiform activity at one point only close to the "inactive core" is explained by the following hypothesis:

1. The entire hypodense lesion detected by C.T. scan cannot be considered the "neoplasm". Only a "core" of proliferative tissue is active and this "core" is generally very small when compared with the radiologically defined lesion.

2. Although this data was not a stereo-EEG-graphy the presence of epileptiform EEG activity in only one side of the lesion and not its opposite area (detected with the other "contact" along the linear trajectory of the electrode) suggests that not all areas "surrounding" the "core" of the lesion can be considered epileptogenic. This epileptogenic area is probably pathologic brain tissue still harbouring neurons able to discharge pathologically.

The epileptiform depth discharge usually did not reach the surface of the cortex, at least during our recordings (Fig. 1) with the exception when "activation" with pentothal was performed[6].

Unidirectional depth recording appears to be advantageous in defining the strategy of biopsy. The mechanism, however, of epileptic discharge diffusion should be studied performing multi-electrode stereo-EEG exploration[1,4,7].

References

1. Bancaud, J., Talairach, J., Geier, S., Scarabin, J. M., EEG et SEEG dans les tumeurs cérébrales et l'épilepsie, pp. 351. Paris: Edifor. 1973.
2. Bancaud, J., Talairach, J., Szikla, G., Stereo-EEG exploration in interstitial irradiation of gliomas. In: Stereotactic Cerebral Irradiations. INSERM symp. no. 12 (Szikla, G., ed.), pp. 57—59. Amsterdam: Elsevier/North-Holland Biomedical Press. 1979.
3. Broggi, G., Franzini, A., Giorgi, C., Servello, D., Spreafico, R., Avanzini, G., Focal C.T. hypodense lesions and epilepsy. Depth-EEG study and stereotactic biopsy. Acta Neurochir. 1984 in press (abstract).
4. Marossero, F., Surgery of epilepsy. Diagnostic importance of SEEG. J. Neurosurg. Sci. *19* (1975), 84—88.
5. Munari, C., Talairach, J., Musolino, A., Szikla, G., Bancaud, J., Chodziewicz, J., Stereotactic methodology of "functional" neurosurgery in tumoral epileptic patients. Ital. J. Neurol. Sci. Suppl. *2* (1983), 69—82.
6. Pampiglione, G., Induced fast activity in the EEG as an aid in the location of cerebral lesions. EEG Clin. Neurophysiol. *4* (1952), 179—182.

7. Rossi, G. F., Problems of analysis and interpretation of electrocerebral signals in epilepsy. A neurosurgeon's view. In: Epilepsy. Its phenomena in man (Brazier, M. A., ed.), pp. 259—285. New York: Academic Press. 1973.
8. Szikla, G., Blond, S., Bilan stéréotaxique des tumeurs cérébrales. Encyclopédie Médico-Chirurgicale 31660 E, 1981.
9. W.H.O., Histological classification of tumors of the nervous system. Geneva 1979.

Acta Neurochirurgica, Suppl. 33, 105—112 (1984)

Positron Emission Tomographic Studies in Focal Epilepsy

B. A. Meyerson[1], L. Widén[2], T. Greitz[3], G. Blomquist[2], and E. Ehrin[4]

With 1 Figure

Summary

Eight patients with various forms of focal epilepsy were examined with positron emission tomography (PET) for the study of cerebral glucose metabolism. A 4-rings (7 slices) positron camera was used. Photosynthetically produced C-11 glucose was employed as a tracer for the analysis of the energy metabolic pattern. All patients underwent X-ray CT examinations. With a specially designed fixation device the head could be aligned in a reproducable position so that identical sections could be studied with PET and CT. Coordinates for stereotactic localization of targets for surgery or electrode implantation could be directly determined on the images obtained from both types of examinations. As a rule, interictal EEG abnormalities corresponded to areas of reduced glucose uptake. In a few cases there was a perfect spatial correspondence between focal EEG changes and the presence of a well localized zone of hypometabolism. Some observations suggest that interictal epileptogenic activity may be associated also with hypermetabolism. Data obtained with PET appear to be particularly useful for the guidance of surgical treatment of epilepsy.

Keywords: Positron emission tomography; epilepsy; glucose metabolism.

Introduction

The possibility of visualizing the regional pattern of biochemical and physiological functions in the live brain with the aid of positron emission tomography (PET) is a great achievement in modern

---

Departments of [1] Neurosurgery, [2] Neurophysiology, [3] Neuroradiology, Karolinska Hospital, [4] Karolinska Pharmacy, S-104 01 Stockholm 60, Sweden.

neuroscience. Hitherto this technique has been applied mainly in basic science-oriented reasearch concerned with the study of cerebral metabolism and blood flow[4,11–13]. One of the few applications of PET which has proven to be of considerable practical value is for the study of epilepsy in patients who may be subjected to surgical treatment. In a series of papers it has been convincingly demonstrated that PET can provide valuable information about the site and extent of regions which may have epileptogenic properties[6–8]. Thus, the PET data may serve to guide subsequent surgical procedures. As a rule, the tactics in epilepsy surgery is based on the clinical characters of the seizures (*e.g.* temporal lobe epilepsy) and on the regional abnormalities of the surface EEG. Exploration of deep structures in an attempt to detect epileptogenic "foci" and other changes correlated to the clinical epileptic manifestations are often done with depth recordings via temporarily implanted electrodes. The selection of targets for implantation is often somewhat arbitrary though generally including certain regions known to have a high likelihood of being epileptogenic, for example the amygdala and the hippocampus. Often, this approach has the feature of "hit or miss". The new imaging techniques such as computerized tomography (CT) has been used in this context for the visualization of morphological pathology which may be of possible significance for the epileptogenic manifestations. For example, the epileptic symtoms may be due to a tumour which is strategically located but too small to give other clinical signs. However, it has been claimed that the chance of detecting a primary epileptotogenic lesion with CT is not more than about 10% compared to almost 100% with the use of PET. Systematic studies of the potentialities of nuclear magnetic resonance (NMR) in this context are not yet available.

In the study of epilepsy, PET has been employed mainly for the demonstration of local changes of glucose metabolism and blood flow, although the method permits the mapping of many other functional characteristics (protein metabolism, distribution of transmittors and other biologically active substances etc.). The relationships between epileptogenic electrical activity recorded both by surface and depth electrodes and the changes of glucose metabolism have been described in detail[6–8]. An important finding seems to be that interictal abnormal activity is consistently associated with hypometabolism whereas seizure activity apparently corresponds to local hypermetabolism[9].

This is a report of our preliminary experiences with the use of

PET in a small number of patients with epilepsy originating from different portions of the brain and with variable clinical characteristics. A method of head fixation enables imaging of identical and reproducable brain sections with PET and CT. Furthermore, both types of tomography are integrated with a stereotactic system so that the coordinates for a surgical target visible on CT or PET images can be directly determined.

Material and Methods

Eight patients have been studied and in six the examination was performed with the aim to provide further information for the decision whether surgical treatment would be advisable. One patient was examined because a routine EEG disclosed focal epileptogenic activity, an other as part of a general neuroradiological study of a cerebral infarction associated with epileptogenic EEG activity. Five of the patients were classified as having temporal lobe epilepsy and one suffered from Grand Mal seizures only.

In all patients the PET-examination was supplemented by a CT-scanning, and in all but one the head was positioned in a glass fiber mould and fixed to the table of the scanner[2].

Three of the patients were examined while their regular antiepileptic medication had been stopped since two or three days. Surface EEG was continuously monitored during the scanning.

The positron camera consists of four detector rings with 96 BGO detectors per ring (details, see[10]). Coincidences are simultaneously recorded withing the rings and between adjacent rings which permit the examination of the activity distribution from seven sections, 13 mm thick. The spatial resolution of the camera is 8 mm.

All the PET-examinations were performed for the study of glucose metabolism using C-11. The isotope was produced by a 16 MeV cyclotrone installed in close proximity to the tomograph. Incorporation of the carbon isotope in glucose was achieved by a photosynthetic process in cultured algae[5].

The examination started at the same time as the 300–600 MBq C-11 glucose activity was injected *i.v.* Eighteen sets of data were sequentially measured, six with a measurement time of 20 seconds, six with 40 seconds and the remaining six with a measurement time of 180 seconds, giving a total examination time of 24 minutes. The reason for the dynamic mode of data recording was to fit the C-11 glucose uptake to a metabolic modell currently being developed. Venous blood samples were drawn during the examination to be used as the input function in the metabolic compartment analysis (in preparation). However, in the present work all data sets were added together, corrected for random and scattered coincidences[1], and reconstructed. In the image reconstruction the absorption correction was obtained with a special edge finding algorithm, described by Bergström *et al.*[3].

A computer program is available for quantitative measurements of the content of glucose and its metabolites in any chosen region of interest.

Results

In all patients the regional pattern of the glucose metabolism differed between the two cerebral hemispheres in at least one or two of the PET images. These differences, which were most conspicuous when displayed in colour, generally appeared as local zones of low activity, interpreted as representing hypometabolism. In a few cases there were signs suggesting focal hypermetabolism. In general, there was some correspondence between the regional PET changes and the characteristics of the surface EEG, but often the EEG abnormalities were more diffusely distributed than would be expected from the relatively well localized areas of hypometabolism. For example, in one patient with a long history of temporal lobe epilepsy the EEG showed widely spread episodes of epileptogenic activity in the right hemisphere being most prominent in the temporal lobe region, and there was also concomitant pathological activity in the left hemisphere. The PET examination demonstrated marked hypometabolism in the right temporal lobe only. The CT-scan in this case was found to be normal.

An other case may illustrate that the relationship between the PET-scans and surface EEG may be much more complex. In that patient, who had temporal lobe epilepsy and occasional Grand Mal seizures, epileptogenic EEG activity was seen in the right fronto-temporal region but was occasionally present also in the left temporal leads. In the CT-scan an area of low attenuation was visible in the left posterior temporal region. PET-examinations were performed twice, five months apart. At the first examination there was a low glucose uptake approximately corresponding to the CT abnormality. On the second occasion this zone of hypometabolism was much less obvious and there was now a similar change seen instead on the right side. Besides, there were indications of hypermetabolism in the right frontal region.

In some other patients the correspondence between the EEG pathology and the presence of hypometabolism was more obvious. The recordings in Fig. 1 were derived from a patient who had had a few episodes of visual blurring and nausea, initially interpreted as migraine attacks. The left occipital lead showed continuous epileptogenic spiking which apparently was confined to this region. The CT-scan was normal but in one section from the PET-examination a small and well circumscribed area of hypometabolism could be detected in the left occipital region (Fig. 1).

Another patient had a long history of Grand Mal seizures and the EEG abnormalities were predominant in the right parietal

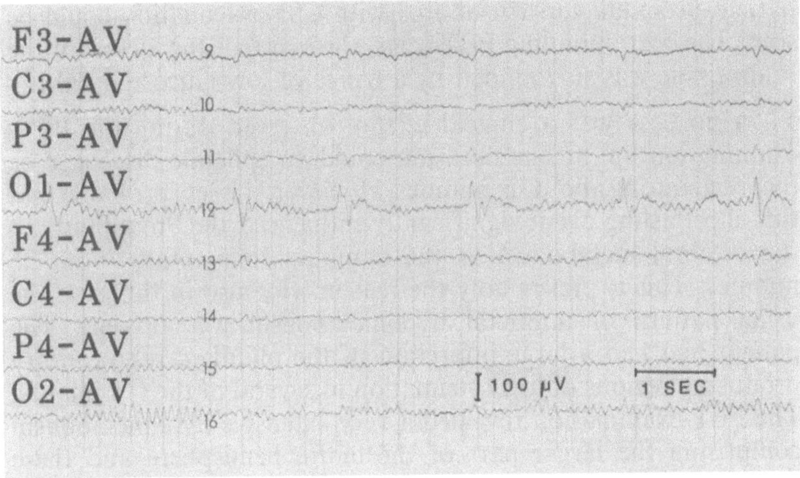

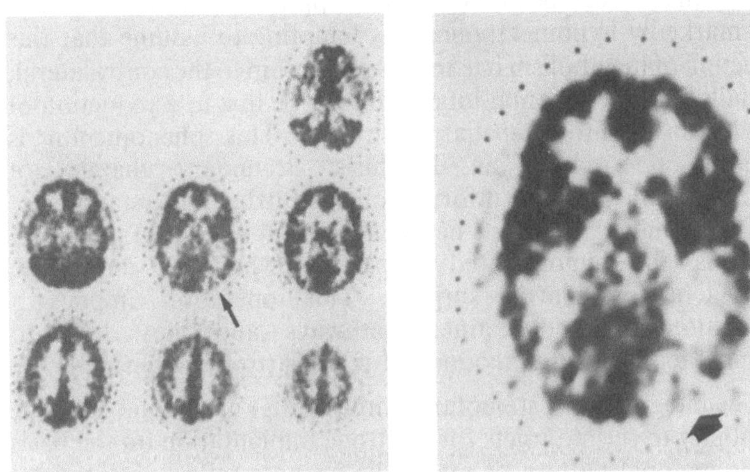

Fig. 1. Above: Surface EEG recorded from a patient with episodes of visual blurring and nausea, initially interpreted as migraine (*AV* average electrode). Below: PET-examination of the same patient showing all the seven sections (left) and (right) a blow-up of the section with a zone of glucose hypometabolism in the left occipital lobe (arrows)

region but present also in the frontal leads. In the CT-images a right parieto-occipital, superficial area with CSF attenuation could be seen. The corresponding PET-scans showed that this defect of the brain tissue was surrounded by a fringe of low glucose uptake.

In no case was a clinical seizure observed during the PET-examination but at one occasion could an epileptic discharge be recorded during about six minutes. However, it is less probable that this shortlasting event significantly influenced the "mapping" of the cerebral metabolism as the scanning time totals about 25 minutes. This is presumably the reason why also in this case the usual pattern of interictal hypometabolism was present. The patient had had a large infarction of the middle cerebral artery producing regions of low attenuation in several of the CT images. The PET-examination revealed a very extensive hypometabolism comprising the larger part of the entire hemisphere and these changes were actually more extensive than what would have been expected from the morphological image obtained from the CT-examination. The PET-images obtained from this patient also showed that the cerebellar hemisphere opposite to the infarcted side was markedly hypometabolic. It is tempting to assume that this reduction of metabolism has some relationship to the contralateral, partially infarcted frontal lobe, and may be due to a reduction of activity in fronto-cerebellar pathways. This phenomenon is generally referred to as diaschisis. Secundary changes of metabolism may provide information and further understanding of the functional relationships between different regions of the brain. This may be demonstrated in patients who have undergone stereotactic psychiatric surgery. This operation implies a destruction of well defined pathways and may lead to hypometabolism in interconnected regions (to be published).

The integration of stereotaxis with the PET-technique gives the possibility to select targets for electrode implantation on the basis of the regional pattern of metabolic changes reflecting interictal epileptogenic foci or zones. It has been claimed that there is a strict correlation between interictal epileptogenesis and hypometabolism but observations on one patient in the present material suggest that also hypermetabolism may occasionally be associated with such activity. In that particular patient who suffered from severe temporal lobe epilepsy the PET-examination revealed the presence of both hypo- and hypermetabolic zones in the temporal lobe. On the basis of these findings electrodes were implanted in both types of regions the locations of which were stereotactically determined directly from the PET-images. It was found that epileptogenic activity could be recorded also from a hypermetabolic region, from where it was later possible at three different occasions to record epileptogenic discharges associated with clinical seizures. Results from an examination of one of the other patients also suggest that epileptogenic interictal activity may exceptionally correspond to a zone with hyper- rather than with hypometabolism. However, these observations warrant further investigations for definite confirmation.

Comments

No doubt, PET has proven to be a most valuable tool in the study of epilepsy since it provides the opportunity to map in detail regional abnormalities of functions which may be closely linked to epileptogenesis. So far, only the metabolism of glucose and cerebral blood flow have been studied in this context but it is conceivable that other aspects of central nervous function may be found to be more specifically related to epilepsy. Of paramount interest is the possibility to use information derived from a physiological and biochemical mapping of the brain as a guide for surgical treatment.

Acknowledgement

This study has been supported by grants from the Swedish Medical Research Council, B 84-17 X-5679-05, Ax-son Johnsons stiftelse, and Torsten and Ragnar Söderbers stiftelser.

References

1. Bergström, M., Eriksson, L., Bohm, C., Blomquist, G., Litton, J., Correction for scattered radiation in a ring detector positron camera by integral transformation of the projections. J. Comput. Assist. Tomogr. *7* (1983), 42—50.
2. Bergström, M., Boëthius, J., Eriksson, L., Greitz, T., Ribbe, T., Widén, L., Head fixation device for reproducible position alignment in transmission CT and positron emission tomography. J. Comput. Assist. Tomogr. *5* (1981), 136—141.
3. Bergström, M., Litton, J., Eriksson, L., Bohm, C., Blomquist, G., Determination of object contour from projections for attenuation correction in cranial positron emission tomography. J. Comput. Assist. Tomogr. *6* (1982), 365—372.
4. Cepeda, C., Menini, Ch., Naquet, R., Mestelan, G., Grouzel, C., Comar, D., Positron emission tomography in a case of experimental focal epilepsy in the baboon. Electroenceph. Clin. Neurophysiol. *54* (1982), 87—90.

5. Ekström, E., Stone-Elander, S., Nilsson, J. L. S., Bergström, M., Blomquist, G., Brismar, T., Eriksson, L., Greitz, T., Jansson, P. E., Litton, J. E., Malmborg, P., af Uggla, M., Widén, L., C-11-labeled glucose and its utilization in positron-emission tomography. J. Nucl. Med. *24* (1983), 326—331.
6. Engel, J., jr., Brown, W. J., Kihl, D. E., Phelps, M. E., Mazziotta, J. C., Crandall, P. H., Pathological findings underlying focal temporal lobe hypometabolism in partial epilepsy. Ann. Neurol. *12* (1982), 518—528.
7. Engel, J., jr., Kuhl, D. E., Phelps, M. E., Crandall, P. H., Comparative localization of epileptic foci in partial epilepsy by PCT and EEG. Ann. Neurol. *12* (1982), 529—537.
8. Engel, J., jr., Kuhl, D. E., Phelps, M. E., Mazziotta, J. C., Interictal cerebral glucose metabolism in partial epilepsy and its relation to EEG changes. Ann. Neurol. *12* (1982), 510—517.
9. Engel, J., jr., Kuhl, D. E., Phelps, M. E., Patterns of human local cerebral glucose metabolism during epileptic seizures. Science *218* (1982), 64—66.
10. Litton, J., Bergström, M., Eriksson, L., Bohm, C., Blomqvist, G., Kesselberg, M., Performance study of the PC-384 positron camera system for emission tomography of the brain. Submitted for publication.
11. Mazziotta, J. C., Phelps, M. E., Carson, R. E., Kuhl, D. E., Tomographic mapping of human cerebral metabolism: Sensory deprivation. Ann. Neurol. *12* (1982), 453—444.
12. Mazziota, J. C., Phelps, M. E., Miller, J., Kuhl, D. E., Tomographic mapping of human cerebral metabolism: Normal unstimulated state. Neurology *31* (1982), 503—516.
13. Phelps, M. E., Mazziotta, J. C., Kuhl, D. E., Nuwer, M., Packwood, J., Metter, J., Engel, J. jr., Tomographic mapping of human cerebral metabolism: Visual stimulation and deprivation. Neurology *31* (1981), 517—529.

Acta Neurochirurgica, Suppl. 33, 113—118 (1984)

Influence of Pregnane Derivates on Metabolism of the Brain and Epileptic Activity in Man

P. Nádvorník[1], M. Lassanova, D. Homerova, T. Turský, and M. Šramka

With 3 Figures

Summary

Clinical and electrophysiological studies show an epileptogenic effect of the pregnan derivates of Althesin in man. The archicortical structures seem the firsts to be affected. Biochemical investigations suggest that the effect is related to the action of the drug on metabolism of glial cells.

Keywords: Epilepsy; pregnan derivates; glial metabolism.

A mixture of pregnandionin and pregnanacetate (3 : 1) is used intravenously as a short-term or pre-anaesthetic drug (Althesin) in dosages up to 100 mg. It differs from other anaesthetics in that pregnan is a physiological chemical component of the human body from which *e.g.* the female sex hormone progesterone and the adrenocortical steroids are derived. It has then a chemical innocuous structure in comparison with toxic anaesthetics.

Electrophysiological Study

In our neurosurgical clinic we began to use Althesin in 1973. During stereotactic surgery for cerebral palsy, we were surprised with Althesin's influence on the electrical activity of the brain. The initial record was unusually changed, reminiscent of epileptic discharges. With further experience with Althesin, we directed attention to these changes in literature[3, 5, 6] and later used a small

[1] Medical School of Comenius University, Bratislava, ČSSR.

quantity of this substance for epileptics. In the EEG record at once a disorder quite characteristic for epilepsy was evoked. Later we made clinical tests also with patients, in whom we introduced chronic electrodes for stimulation therapy of epilepsy. Our aim was to investigate how Althesin influences the activity of deep brain structures before scalp EEG records were affected. Long-term observations were made on 4 patients. Simultaneous EEGs from the scalp, amygdala, hippocampus and the caudatum revealed that small Althesin doses activate pathologic activity of the hippocampus and shortly thereafter of the cerebral cortex. We have confirmed this with another patient. Evidently the archicortical structures of the brain reacts more sensitively than the neocortex.

We introduced electrodes into the oldest paleocortical formations of the brain, fundus striae terminalis, belonging to the septum pellucidum system which is functionally connected to the amygdala. At a dosage of 20 mg, paleocortex was activated immediately and together also the amygdala-hippocampus complex (Fig. 1). When we used a dosage of 70 mg the response was so strong, that a clinical seizure took place. Therefore we used only a dosage of 2 mg, enough to influence the paleocortical system close to the caudate nucleus head (caput nuclei caudati).

We are convinced that we have a very interesting substance. It is common experience, that at puberty or at the menstrual cycle, when the level of sex hormones is rising, epileptic seizures take place often for the first time or they increase.

Biochemical Study

In experiments with slices of cerebral cortex we observed the influence of Althesin on the level of GABA and other amino-acids on the conversion of glucose, acetate and citrate into aminoacids. Glutamic acid, glutamine and GABA and further asparatic acid are produced in the brain from oxidised substrates during the Krebs cycle. The conversion of glucose into these aminoacids takes place especially in the neurones, the conversions of acetate and citrate take place in two compartments of glial cells[1,2]. We also dated the influence of Althesin on the carbondioxide-formation and the incorporation of carbons from the mentioned substrates into proteins and lipids. We used substrate labelled 14 C and express our results in mols of carbon, obtained from glucose, acetate and citrate after 20 minutes of slices incubation.

In the presence of Althesin (43–860 μmols/1) in the incubation media the level of GABA in the slices increased to 130–170%.

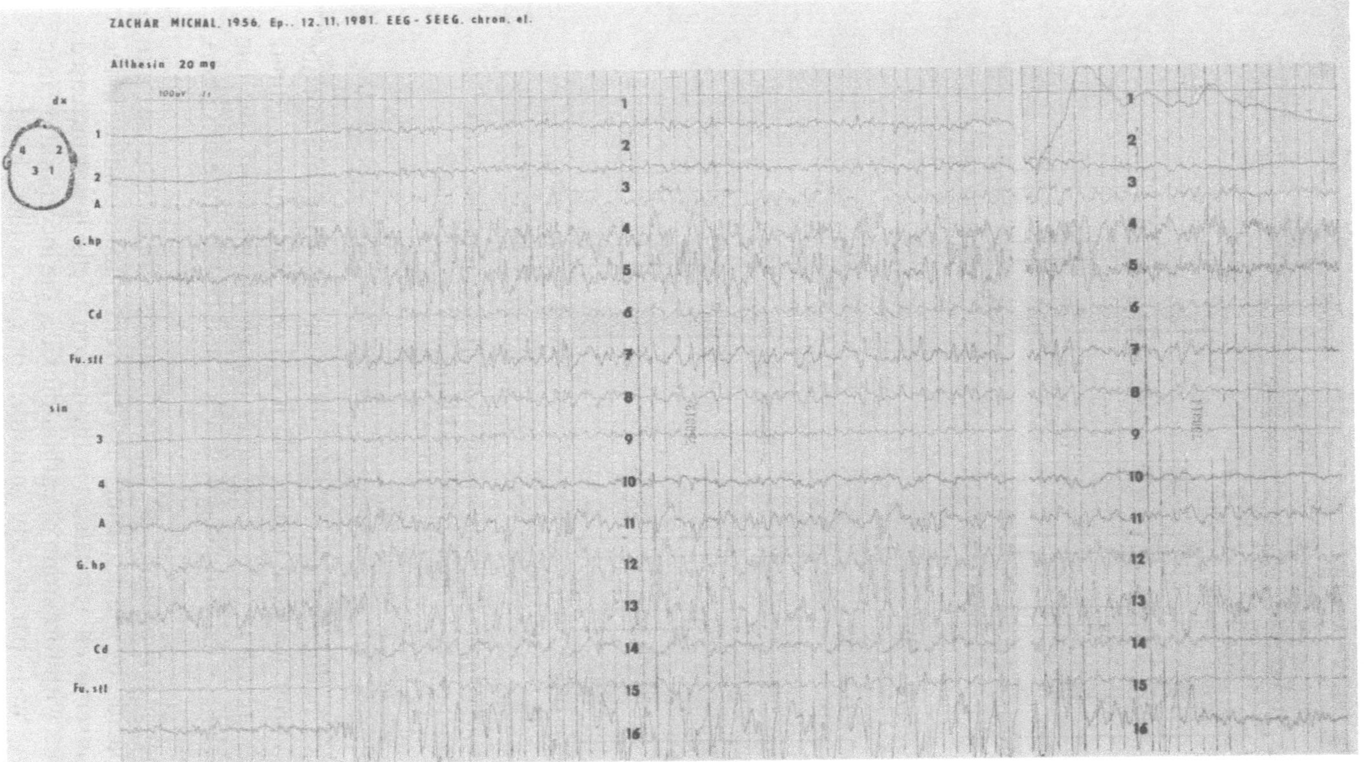

Fig. 1. SEEG record: changes produced by Althesin adminstration (20 mg). *A* amygdala; *Cd* caudatum; *Fu. stt* fundus striae terminalis; *G. hp* gyrus hippocampi

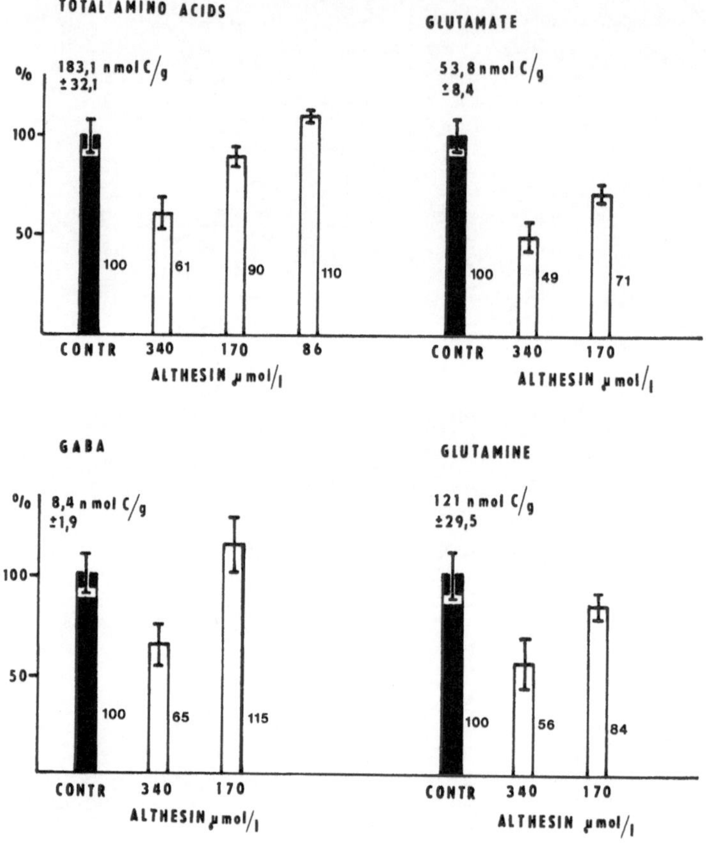

Fig. 2. Glial compartment 1. Incorporation of carbon from the acetate into amino acids. Control = 100% ± SD (n mol C/g wet tissue)

Althesin neither influenced the glutamate decarboxylase nor the GABA transaminase, neither did it influence high or low affinite GABA receptors. In a smaller range it inhibited succinic semialdehyde dehydrogenase, which could be the cause of GABA increase.

The incorporation of carbon atoms from glucose into aminoacids, by which as much as 70 percent glucose oxidised in the brain is removed, is localised in the neuronal cells. It was increased together with formation of carbon-dioxide; the incorporation into GABA was particularly notable; on the other hand, the incorporation into glutamin was reduced, provided that high concentration of Althesin were used (340 μmol/1).

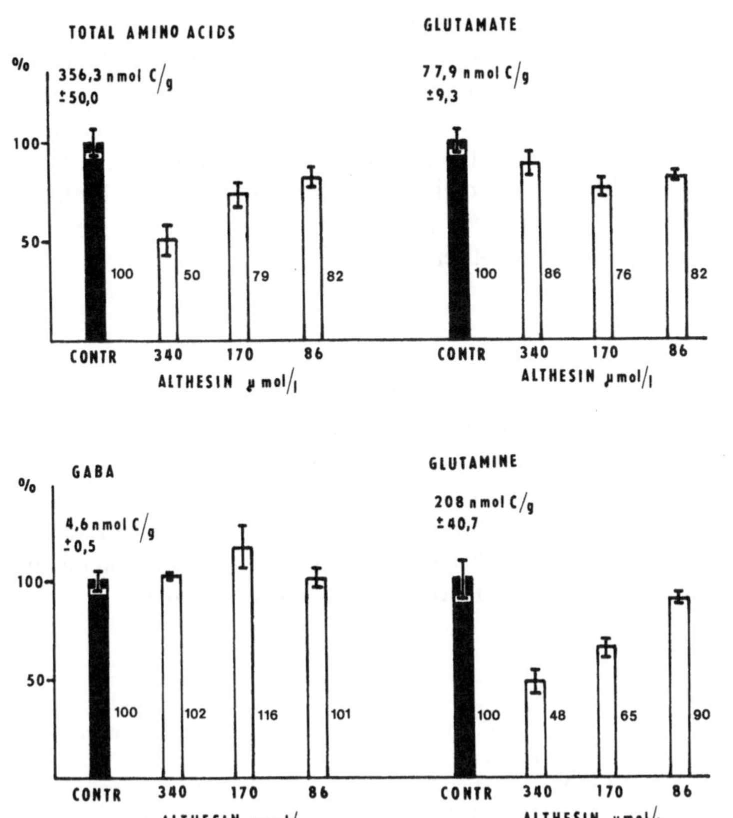

Fig. 3. Glial compartment 2. Incorporation of carbon from the citrate into amino acids. Control = 100% ± SD (n mol C/g wet tissue)

The incorporation of carbon atoms from acetate and citrate into aminoacids takes place in two compartments of the glial cells. Althesin, at concentrations at which it was increasing the conversion of glucose into aminoacids, reduced the conversion of acetate and citrate into aminoacids (Figs. 2 and 3); at the same time the incorporation of carbon atoms into GABA was reduced least. But from carbon atoms incorporated from citrate, GABA gets only 1 percent and 2 percent from acetate, while from carbon atoms, that form aminoacids from glucose, GABA forms 10 percent.

Althesin substantially differs from other anaesthetics. It supports the formation of carbon atoms from oxidised substrates into neuronal and glial aminoacids, in contrast to phenobarbital which slows the formation down[4]. The influence of Althesin on the formation of carbon atoms from glucose, acetate and citrate into proteins and lipids is similarly different.

The formation of all three substrates were reduced with the exception of the lowest concentrations of Althesin. The different action of Althesin, especially on the metabolism of glial cells, which it suppresses, could be a partial explanation of its excitant side effect, in contrast to other anaesthetics.

Conclusions

Pregnan derivates in Althesin produces a remarkable epileptogenic effect. Changes begin in the paleocortical structures of the brain but soon extend into archicortex and neocortex. A biochemical study proved that pregnan derivates interfere with the metabolism of glial cells and neuronal cells. Pregnan derivates limit the entrance of energetic substances into single aminoacids in glial cells upon which the metabolism of neurons depends.

References

1. Balázs, R., Cremer, J. E., eds., Metabolic Compartmentation in the Brain, p. 383. London: Macmillan. 1971.
2. Berl, S., Clarke, D. D., Schneider, D., eds., Metabolic Compartmentation and Neurotransmission, p. 721. New York: Plenum Press. 1975.
3. De Riu, P. L., Susini, G., Ruju, P., Anticonvulsant activity of Althesin on experimental epilepsy. Br. J. Anaesth. *54* (1982), 343—347.
4. Cheng, S.-C., Brunner, E. A., Effects of Anaesthetic agents on Synaptosomal GABA disposal. Anaesthesiology *55* (1981), 34—40.
5. Saady, A., Hicks, R. G., The effects of Althesin on the Electroencephalograph. Anaesth. Intens. Care *8* (1980), 206—210.
6. Šramka, M., Patoprstá, G., Nádvorník, P., Fritz, G., Malatinský, J., Epileptic EEG symptoms and psychic changes following Althesin. Activ. Nerv. Sup. *17* (1975), 287.

Acta Neurochirurgica, Suppl. 33, 119—122 (1984)

Correlations Between rCBF and Computerized EEG in Temporal Lobe Epilepsy

G. Rosadini[1], **G. Rodriguez**[1], **W. G. Sannita**[1], and **F. Arvigo**[1]

With 1 Figure

Summary

Interictal rCBF and quantitative EEG were assessed in 20 epileptic patients with partial seizures with complex symptomatology and a prominent EEG focus of left temporal areas.

1. Hemispheric rCBF values did not differ from controls. 2. An area including 5 probes and corresponding to the scalp projection of the left temporal lobe showed in epileptic patients a significant decrement in rCBF. 3. A consistent asymmetry of the EEG profiles recorded from temporal areas, notably a left predominance in low and fast frequency activities and a right prevalence of alpha activity was also observed.

Keywords: Temporal epilepsy; rCBF; computerized EEG.

Introduction

Regional cerebral blood flow (rCBF) determinations can be useful in the identification of brain regions responsible for, or involved in epileptic seizures. However, the findings reported thus far are comparable only in part[1,2,4].

This paper reports a significant reduction of the rCBF in the temporal lobe of epileptic patients with a prominent EEG focus in the same area.

Material and Method

20 patients with temporal lobe epilepsy (11 males, 9 females; age: 47.1 years ± 16.4) were studied. 13 patients had only partial seizures with complex

[1] Institute of Neurophysiology, University, and Center of Cerebral Neurophysiology, National Council of Research, Genova, Italy.

symptomatology, while generalized convulsions were associated in the others. The average time since onset of seizures was 13.1 years ± 11.2, with frequency of occurrence ranging from 1 per year to 2 per month approximately. Neurological or psychiatric deficits could not be assessed clinically in any patient; neuroradiological findings were indifferent with respect to epilepsy or cerebral circulation (CT in 8 cases). All patients were under treatment, with good control of seizures: 9 were in single-drug; 11 in poly-drug therapy (phenobarbital, 13 cases; carbamazepine 11 cases; diphenylhydantoin, 6 cases). The drug plasma concentration was in all cases within the therapeutic range.

The EEG tracing of one patient was borderline. EEG abnormalities (spikes, slow waves, or combined patterns) were detected in the other patients' tracings upon visual inspection; the amount of abnormalities was always limited. A predominant left temporal focus was identified in all patients; a contralateral temporal focus or multiple foci were associated in 10 cases. The EEG pattern had been steady during the last year in 9 patients, while it had been varying in 11 cases.

Interictal rCBF was assessed by the 133 Xenon inhalation method (32 probes; Harshow Tasc 5 system); patients were normocapnic during the examination. The initial slope index (ISI) was derived for each probe, and values relative to the global hemispheres were computed for each subject[3]. The mean values across subjects were computed for each probe, as well as for the single hemispheres and temporal areas. In addition, each probe was compared with the corresponding mean hemispheric values (intra-hemispheric comparison), as well as with the homologous contralateral probe (inter-hemispheric comparison); only the differences above 10% were considered. Twenty healthy subjects, matched for age, were the controls.

EEG was recorded in standard conditions in concomitance with rCBF and quantified off-line by power spectral analysis (PDP 11/34 A System). For each subject the means were computed for the signal amplitude, its coefficient of variability and the relative power in pre-determined spectral segments (0.5–4.0; 4.5–8.0; 8.5–12.0; 12.5–16.0; 16.5–20.0; above 20.5 Hz).

The left-right differences were computed for each parameter and each patient and averaged across subjects.

Results

1. The epileptic patients did not differ from controls in the across-subject mean rCBF values.

2. One or more probes with rCBF values lower than the homologous contralateral probe were detected in all epileptic patients. The topographic distributions of the probes with reduced rCBF was uneven; the incidence was significantly higher (CHI 2; $p \leqslant 0.01$) in probes 8, 9, 13, 14, 15 of the left hemisphere (Fig. 1). The mean rCBF of the area including these probes was significantly lower in epiletic patients than in the controls (t-test; $p \leqslant 0.01$).

3. Statistically significant asymmetries (Wilcoxon's test; $p \leqslant 0.05$ to $p \leqslant 0.01$) were observed in the patients' EEG power

spectral profiles of the two temporal leads. The power of the low activity (0.5–4.0 Hz) and of the fast frequency components (above 16.5 Hz) and the coefficient of variability were predominant on the left side, while the power on the alpha range was preponderant on the right.

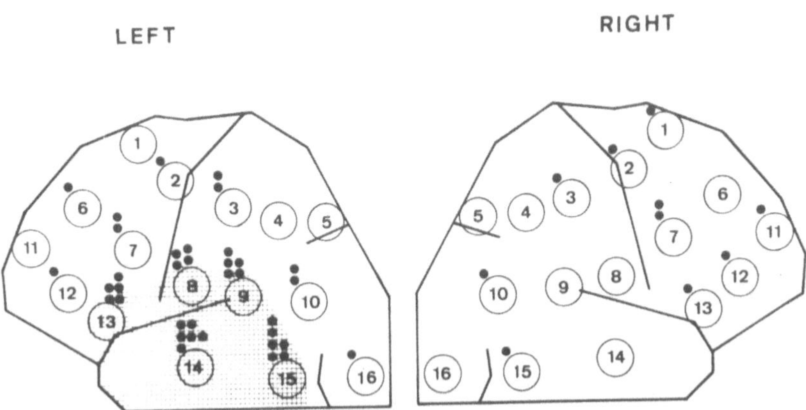

Fig. 1. Inter-hemispheric comparison in epileptics. The black points represent for all the patients the times in which a single probe was reduced more than 10% in comparison with the contralateral one. See also text

Conclusions

1. The antiepileptic compounds administered in this study at therapeutic doses do not affect the hemispheric flow significantly.

2. In interictal periods, a significant reduction in rCBF is evident on the affected temporal area and neighbouring regions of epileptic patients with isolated or predominant, moderately active EEG temporal focus, as compared to healthy controls. An increment in the same area of EEG low and fast frequency activities and a decrement in the alpha activity are associated.

References

1. Ingvar, D. H., Measurements of regional cerebral blood flow and metabolism in psychopathology states. Eur. Neurol. *40* (1981), 294—296.
2. Lavy, S., Melamed, E., Portnoy, Z., Carmon, A., Interictal rCBF in patients with parietal seizures. Neurology *26* (1976), 418—422.

3. Risberg, J., Ali, Z., Wilson, E. M., Wills, E. C., Halsey, J. M., jr., Regional cerebral blood flow by 133 Xenon inhalation. Preliminary evaluation of an initial slope index in patients with unstable flow compartments. Stroke *6* (1975), 142—148.
4. Sakay, F., Meyer, J. S., Naritomi, H., Ming-Chang, H. S. U., rCBF and EEG in patients with epilepsy. Arch. Neurol. *35* (1978), 648—657.

Acta Neurochirurgica, Suppl. 33, 123—126 (1984)

Study of the Role of Defence Mechanisms in Patients with Epilepsy to the Purpose of Neurosurgical Treatment and Rehabilitation

L. Pinkus[1], **L. Provenzano**[1], **A. Bertola**[1], **L. Antinori**[1], and **G. Colicchio**[2]

Keywords: Defence mechanisms; psychology.

Introduction

In the construction of one's identity, the bodily image is the fundamental factor in the passage from non-differentiation of the new-born child to the linked differentiation of his evolution. The epileptic seizures constitute a "lesional" event for the patient's identity, who reacts with the tendency of splitting his sense of identity in: (a) bodily identity, (b) psychic identity[4]. The defence mechanisms that modulate the psychic evolution produce in the epileptic patients a peculiar pattern in order to controle that very tendency toward self-division.

Our study takes into consideration the defence mechanisms of repression and isolation.

Repression: removal from the sphere of consciousness of certain events experienced.

Isolation: tendency to separate the experiences from the emotions that thcy cvoke.

Subjects and Methods

40 patients (20 males, average age 26 years; 20 females average age 26 years; range of age 15 to 40) suffering from partial epileptic seizures with elementary or complex symptomatology, were submitted to tests during a diagnostic procedure with a view to surgical treatment[5].

---

[1] Dipartimento di Psicologia, Università "La Sapienza", Roma, Italy.

[2] Istituto di Neurochirurgica, Università Cattolica del Sacro Cuore, Largo A. Gemelli, 8, I-00168 Roma, Italy.

An homologous control group of healthy subjects was set up. The two groups were submitted to Rorschach's test; the evaluation was made (a) for repression: Rorschach's Index of Repressive Style, R. I. R. S.[3], total R and extent of contents[6]; (b) for isolation: Isolation's Index[1], Form responses (F%) and Accurate form responses (F+%)[6].

Results and Discussion

The epileptic group shows signs of repression more severe than those of the control group (Table 1). We believe that their repression operates to protecte the patient's sense of his own identity from the self division brought on by the seizure.

Table 1. *Repression*

Index	Females	Males
R. I. R. S.	E. G. x = 1.63 C. G. x = 2.32 significant at $P < 0.001$	E. G. x = 1.80 C. G. x = 2.48 not significant
Total R	E. G. x = 13.95 C. G. x = 25.25 significant at $P < 0.001$	E. G. x = 18.5 C. G. x = 20.7 not significant
Extent of contents	E. G. x = 5.5 C. G. x = 10.8 significant at $P < 0.001$	E. G. x = 4.15 C. G. x = 8.35 significant at $P < 0.001$

U (Mann-Withney); E. G. = Epileptic Group; C. G. = Control Group.

In the epileptic group, unlike the control group, the mechanisms of isolation is more often defeated (Table 2). This comes from the patient's need to separate the Ego from the mental image of his own body—an effort which fails.

Therefore the patient:

— loads on the doctor his needs for security and for a confirmation of his self;

— loads on the family group an ambivalent dynamic that shifts between requests for affectionate support and demands for autonomy.

If these defensive mechanisms are too rigid, or if they are badly coordinated with the functioning of the Ego they predispose the patients to reactions patently psychopathological and therefore consitute a counterindication for surgery.

Table 2. *Isolation*

Index	Females	Males
Isolation's index	E. G. x = 0.38 C. G. x = 0.47 not significant	E. G. x = 0.38 C. G. x = 0.47 not significant
F%	E. G. x = 51.34 C. G. x = 58.95 not significant	E. G. x = 55.73 C. G. x = 59.994 not significant
F+%	E. G. x = 57.80 C. G. x = 73.16 significant at $P < 0.001$	E. G. x = 59.59 C. G. x = 63.87 not significant

U (Mann-Withney); E. G. = Epileptic Group; C. G. = Control Group.

In 17 of the 40 epileptic patients considered, surgery was not performed because of the characters of their epilepsy. In the others 23 patients, psychological testing brought to:

i) No counterindication for diagnostic-therapeutic procedure with a view to surgery (8 cases);

ii) No counterindication for surgery provided that the patient should previously receive: supporting psychotherapy (2 cases), therapy finalized in a new family balance (3 cases), psychotropic drug therapy (2 cases) (total 7 cases);

iii) Counterindication for surgery (8 cases).

In the follow-up (1–5 years), the patients treated showed a complete absence of psychopathological reactions and a satisfactory adaptation to life and to human relationships.

In conclusion the value of the interdisciplinary integrated approach seems to be that of a specific psychodynamic intervention bringing into focus the patient's defensive strategies; it has resulted in a complete rehabilitation of the epileptic patient surgically treated[2].

References

1. Bertini, M., Il tratto difensivo dell'isolamento nella sua determinazione dinamica e strutturale, in Atti del XIII Congresso Psicologi Italiani, pp. 71—89, Palermo 1961.
2. Bertola, A., Colicchio, G., Gentilomo, A., Pinkus, L., Provenzano, L., Scerrati, M., Epilessia: un approccio interdisciplinare, pp. 126. Roma: Borla. 1981.
3. Levine, M., Spivack, G., The Rorschach Index of Repressive Style, pp. 164. Springfield, Illinois, U.S.A.: Ch. C Thomas. 1964.
4. Pinkus, L., Die epileptische Erfahrung: Ein Borderlein Syndrom. Dyn. Psychiat. *47* (1977), 425—437.
5. Rossi, G. F., Gentilomo, A., Colicchio, G., Le problème de la recherche de la topographie d'origine de l'épilepsie. Archiv. Suisse Neurol. Neurochir. Psych. *115* (1974), 229—270.
6. Schafer, R., L'interpretazione psicoanalitica del Rorschach, pp. 528. Torino: Boringhieri. 1971.

Section I

Epilepsy

2. Surgical Treatment

Acta Neurochirurgica, Suppl. 33, 129—131 (1984)

A. Introduction

Indications, Advantages and Limits of the Different Rationales of Surgical Treatment of Epilepsy

G. F. Rossi[1]

With 1 Figure

This second part devoted to epilepsy will consider the different surgical approaches proposed so far to treat epileptic patients, and the rationale on which these approaches are based, the indications for each one of them and, finally, their relative advantages and limits.

Let me introduce the subject by presenting you again a scheme which I showed you four years ago, at the Paris meeting[1]. My idea was to synthezise the main basic principles on which surgery can be based. After four years, however, the personal experience of our Institute as well as the experience reported by others, led me to further simplify this scheme.

Today, I think that—schematically—there are two basic principles on which the surgical treatment of epilepsy can be grounded.

1. The first one (Fig. 1 A) aims at the direct and complete removal of the cerebral lesion primarily responsible for epilepsy and of the related primarily epileptic cerebral neurones; the ensemble is called by us the lesional-functional epileptogenic complex. Such a type of surgical treatment is utilizable in unifocal partial epilepsies. It presumes that the location of both the lesional and the functional components of the epileptogenic complex are known in detail and do not involve a brain area of such functional relevance as to prevent its removal. It is the type of surgery which

[1] Istituto di Neurochirurgia, Università Cattolica del Sacro Cuore, Largo A. Gemelli, 8, I-00168 Roma, Italy.

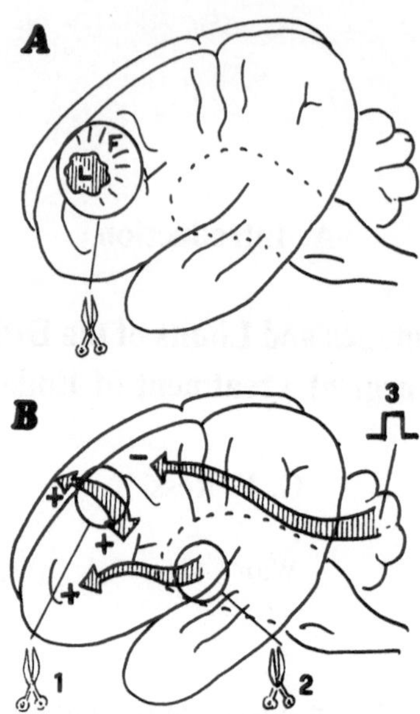

Fig. 1. Schematic representation of the basic surgical approaches to epilepsy. See explanations in the text

seems to offer the best chance of cure, *i.e.* leading to the complete and definitive suppression of seizures.

2. The second type of surgical treatment (Fig. 1 B) aims at reducing the epileptogenicity of the brain and, therefore, the number and the intensity of the seizures. There are several surgical means to reach such a goal.

The most popular of these is interruption of the pathways of propagation of the epileptic discharges from their site of origin to other brain sites (Fig. 1 B *1*). The best example of this type of surgery is provided by the interruption of midline commissures. Such a surgical approach can be used to treat unifocal as well as multifocal partial epilepsies, particularly those with secondary generalization. It presumes knowledge of the topographic organization of the epileptic process, both for the location of the site or sites or origin of the ictal discharges and their main pathways of propagation. It seems likely that the beneficial result on epilepsy is related to the interruption of facilitating reverberating circuits.

A decrease in the level of epileptogenicity is said to be obtained also by making lesions in certain parts of the brain (Fig. 1 B *2*). The amygdaloid nuclear complex and the H-field of Forel are the most popular targets. Amygdaloid lesions are more appropriate when there is a prevalent involvement of the temporal lobe or lobes; H-field lesion would be more suitable in the presence of a prevalent frontal involvement. Whether the effect of these lesions is produced, at least in part, through the interruption of positive feed-back cortico-cortical or cortico-intercortical circuits is hard to prove, but seems likely.

A different way to obtain the same result, *i.e.* a decrease of the level of the brain epileptogenicity would be to artificially provoke or enhance inhibitory influences (Fig. 1 B *3*). This seems possible by stimulating with appropriate electrical parameters certain structures, such as the cerebellum and caudate nucleus.

As said before, it is unlikely that this second group of surgical approaches brings about disappearance of seizures. On the other hand, theoretically at least, it has the advantage of being applicable for almost any type of epileptic syndrome, including those in which the structure of the epileptic process is unrecognizable.

The steadily increasing experience, all over the world, with these different modalities of surgical treatment should permit us to analyze and compare actual data, rather than hypothesis. This is the main purpose of the second part of our meeting on epilepsy.

The evaluation of the correctness of the above schematized different rationales of surgery, as well as their reciprocal advantages and limits, can be based only on analysis of the results obtained by their application. Dealing with epilepsy, we have to take into consideration the effect on the epileptic seizures. I recommend to the speakers that, when reporting their results, a clear distinction be made between disappearance and reduction—even if remarkable—of the seizures. In my opinion, this distinction is very important to compare the validity of the treatment utilized. This is not a theoretical, pragmatic view. It is strictly dependent on the fact that the difference between seizure disappearance and seizure reduction is extremely important for the patient, as all of us know very well.

Reference

1. Rossi, G. F., Why, when and how surgery of epilepsy? Acta Neurochir. (Wien), Suppl. *30* (1980), 7—13.

Acta Neurochirurgica, Suppl. 33, 133—138 (1984)

B. Communications

Temporal Lobectomy for Epilepsy in the Patients with Ipsilateral Extratemporal Brain Lesion

I. I. Ribarić[1] and **N. J. Sekulović**

With 2 Figures

Summary

In a series of 80 patients operated on for epilepsy there were 50 patients with temporal lobe epilepsy. It was found an extratemporal ipsilateral brain lesion in 5 of these patients. It was performed temporal lobectomy for epilepsy in these 5 patients and in the 3 of them the extratemporal brain lesion was extirpated too without resecting the neighbouring cerebral cortex. These 5 patients are seizure free during 1.5 to 5.5 years of the follow up. These cases impose two questions: what surgical strategy should be done in such cases and is there any causative relationship between the extratemporal brain lesion and the epileptogenic features of the ipsilateral temporal structures.

Keywords: Temporal epilepsy; temporal lobectomy; etiology of temporal epilepsy.

Case Reports

Case 1

H. J., age 20, ambidexter girl. She had the tonic-clonic convulsions during the night sleep at the age of 11. One year later she started to have absences and psychomotor attacks preceded by epigastric aura, which were almost everyday.

Neurologically: Without noticeable deficit.

Several *16-channel EEGs* with sphenoidal electrodes and pharmacologically induced sleep showed the active focal epileptic disturbances of the cerebral activity over the left temporal lobe with the phase reversal at the standard position of the electrode Sp 1 and equipotentiality Sp 1 = T 3 and T 3 = F 7.

---

[1] Neurosurgical University Hospital, Višegradska 26, Y-11000 Belgrade, Yugoslavia.

X-Ray examination of the skull and *CT of the brain* showed a small intracerebral calcification in the left frontolateral region. *Left carotid angiography* was normal.

Operation: There was a well circumscribed superficial intracerebral tumor 2.5 cm in diameter, located in front of the Broca speach area. ECoG showed epileptic abnormalities over the inferior part of the sensorimotor cortex and over the Broca speach area. We excised the tumor (histologically: haemangioma) and performed left temporal lobectomy (Fig. 1).

The patient has been seizure free during 3 years of the follow up.

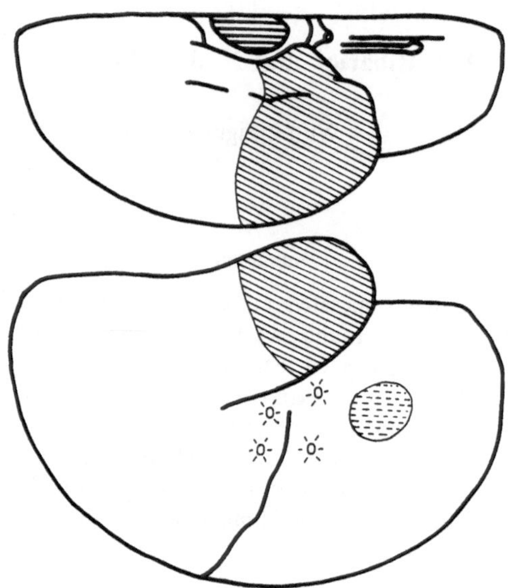

Fig. 1. Operative finding in Case 1 (see text)

Case 2

O. Z., age 18, right handed girl. She had tonic-clonic convulsions during the night sleep at the age of 10. Soon after that she started to have psychomotor attacks with abdominal aura. In the last few years she had psychomotor attacks everyday, often few times daily and generalized tonic-clonic convulsions mainly during the sleep approximately once in two to three months.

Neurologically: Without noticeable deficit.

Several *16-channel EEGs* with sphenoidal electrodes and pharmacologically induced sleep showed the two active focal epileptic disturbances of the cerebral activity: Over the left inferomesial temporal region and over the left midtemporal convexity (phase reversals at the standard position of the electrodes Sp 1 and T 3). *CT of the brain* showed a tumor of very low density in the left frontal brain region. *Left carotid angiography* was normal.

Operation: ECoG showed scant epileptic abnormalities over the anterior part of the temporal convexity. It was performed a cortical resection 2 cm in diameter in front of the Broca speach area and it was extirpated intracerebral frontal teratoma through that approach. The operation was completed by temporal lobectomy. The patient has been seizure free during 1.5 year of the follow up.

Case 3

K. M., age 26, right handed man. He was born in a difficult delivery. He had the tonic-clonic convulsions at the age of 4 and since that time he had had generalized tonic-clonic seizures approximately once a year, always in the night sleep. At the age of 10 he started to have psychomotor attacks with abdominal aura. In the last few years he had psychomotor attacks three to four times weekly. Two years prior to this admission he had been operated on for an intracerebral teratoma in the left occipital region (in an other hospital). This operation had not significant influence to the frequency and type of his epileptic seizures.

Neurologically: Without noticeable deficit.

Several *16-channel EEGs* with sphenoidal electrodes and pharmacologically induced sleep showed the active focal epileptic disturbance of cerebral activity over the left inferomesial temporal brain region.

CT of the brain showed hypodensity and brain shrinkage in the region of the previous operation.

Operation: ECoG showed epileptic abnormalities over the anterior part of temporal convexity. It was performed left temporal lobectomy.

The patient has been seizure free during 1.5 year of the follow up.

Case 4

A. D., age 27, right handed man. He had the head injury at the age of 11. At the age of 16 during the night sleep he had the first epileptic attack in the form of generalized tonic-clonic convulsions. One year later he started to have psychomotor attacks, deja vu, jame vu, olfactory hallucinations and visual illusions. In the last few years he had epileptic attacks once or more times daily.

Neurologically: Without noticeable deficit.

Several *16-channel EEGs* with sphenoidal electrodes and pharmacologically induced sleep showed the active focal epileptic disturbance of cerebral activity over the right inferomesial temporal brain region.

X-ray examination of the skull, right carotid angiography and CT of the brain showed intracerebral calcification in the right temporooccipital brain region (Fig. 2).

Operation: ECoG showed epileptic abnormalities over the anterior part of temporal convexity. It was performed the right temporal lobectomy without touching the region of the calcification. The patient has been seizure free during four years of the follow up. At the repeated CT scans the calcification retained the same size.

Case 5

H. A., age 25, right handed man. At the age of 2 to 5 he had several generalized tonic-clonic convulsions. Two years prior to the admission he started to have psychomotor attacks which were appearing once or more times daily.

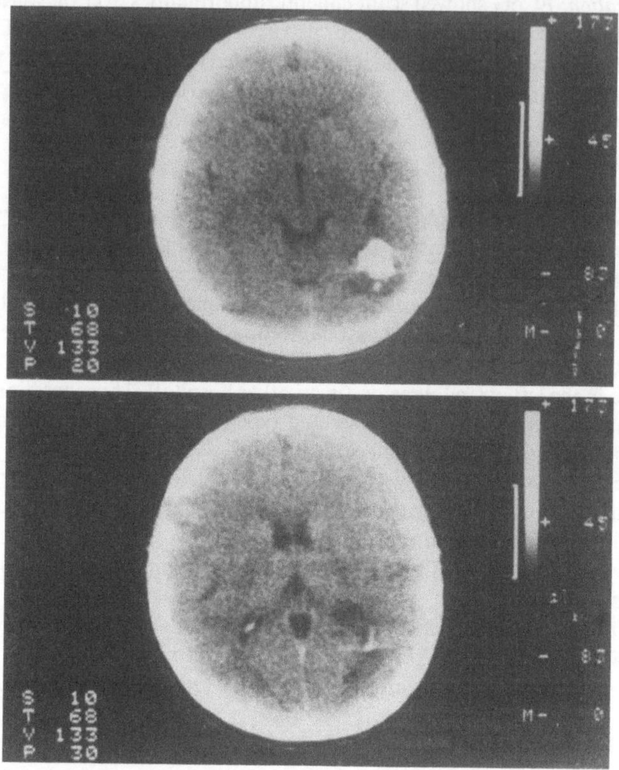

Fig. 2. CT of the brain in Case 4 (see text)

Neurologically: Without noticeable deficit.

In the occipital region he had cranium bifidium with a scalp prominence and an epidural (tissue?) collection.

Several *16-channel EEGs* with sphenoidal electrodes and pharmacologically induced sleep showed the active focal epileptic disturbance of cerebral activity over the right inferomesial temporal brain region, which involved occasionally temporal convexity.

Operation: It was found an anatomic variation in the position of the medial superficial cerebral vein. ECoG showed epileptic abnormalities behind that vein and temporal lobectomy was performed behind the vein.

The patient has been seizure free during 5.5 years of the follow up.

Discussion

In a reported series of 5 patients we performed temporal lobectomy on the basis of clinical epileptic manifestations, repeated EEG findings and ECoG congruence. In Cases 1 and 2 we extirpated the extratemporal brain lesions in addition to the temporal lobectomy because we thought that those lesions were amenable to excision with minimal risk of producing a new neurological deficit. In Case 4 we did not extirpate the intracerebral calcification because there was a great risk of producing contralateral hemianopsie and in the Case 5 the patient refused to be operated on for cranium bifidum.

Varying amounts of hippocampal sclerosis were found in the whole group of 5 patients. The extratemporal brain lesions were obviously congenital except the intracerebral calcification in the Case 4, which was probably calcified intracerebral haematoma. Clinical epileptic manifestations, EEG and ECoG findings showed that the cerebral cortex in the vicinity of the extratemporal lesions did not seem epileptogenic (except in the Case 1 ECoG finding).

Our speculation is that the question concerning the possible causative relationship between the temporal epileptogenic features and the extratemporal (chronic) brain lesion can be answered in the three logical ways:

1. coincidence between the extratemporal brain lesion and the factors that contribute to the development of the mesial temporal sclerosis[2–4, 7];

2. simultaneous congenital malformations in the extratemporal region (proved in the four of five reported cases) and in the mesial temporal region, which perhaps escape our observation.

3. extratemporal brain lesion contributes to the development of the deafferented neurons[8, 9] in the temporal structures causing the development of the epileptogenic focus in the inferomesial temporal region which is well known to have low epileptogenic threshold[1, 6] as well as low threshold for kindling[5].

References

1. Andy, O., Akert, K., Seizure patterns induced by electrical stimulation of hippocampal formation in the cat. J. Neuropathol., exp. Neurol. *14* (1955), 198—202.
2. Earle, K. M., Baldwin, M., Penfield, W., Incisural sclerosis and temporal lobe seizures produced by hippocampal herniation at birth. Arch. Neurol. Psychiat. *69* (1953), 27—42.
3. Falconer, M. A., Genetic and related etiological factors in temporal lobe epilepsy. A review. Epilepsia (Amsterdam) *12* (1971), 13—31.
4. Falconer, M. A., Serafetinides, E. A., Corsellis, J. A., The etiology and pathogenesis of temporal lobe epilepsy. Arch. Neurol. *10* (1964), 233—248.
5. Goddard, G. V., Development of epileptic seizures through brain stimulation at low intensity. Nature (London) *214* (1967), 1020—1021.

6. Kaada, B. R., Somato-motor, autonomic and electrocorticographic responses to electrical stimulation of "rhinencephalic" and other forebrain structures in primates cat and dog. Acta Physiol. Scand. *24* , Suppl. 83 (1951), 1—285.
7. Remillard, G. M., Ethier, R., Andermann, F., Temporal lobe epilepsy and perinatal occlusion of the posterior cerebral artery—a syndrome analogous to infantile hemiplegia and a demonstrable etiology in some patients with temporal lobe epilepsy. Neurology *24* (1974), 1001—1009.
8. Sharples, K. S., Isolated and Deafferented Neurons: Disuse Supersensitivity. In: Basic Mechanisms of the Epilepsies (Jasper, H. H., Ward, A. A., jr., Pope, A., eds.), pp. 329—348. Boston: Little, Brown and Company. 1969.
9. Ward, A. A., jr., The epileptic neurons: Chronic foci in animals and man. In: Basic Mechanisms of the Epilepsies (Jasper, H. H., Ward, A. A., jr., Pope, A., eds.), pp. 263—288. Boston: Little, Brown and Company. 1969.

Acta Neurochirurgica, Suppl. 33, 139—143 (1984)

Surgical Management of Partial Epilepsies: A Critical Evaluation of Electrical, CT Scan, and Pharmacological Studies of the Milan Series

L. Ravagnati[1], **V. A. Sironi, G. Ettorre,** and **F. Marossero**

Summary

From 1959 to 1980, 1,700 patients with non-tumoral epilepsy were admitted at the Institute of Neurosurgery of the University of Milan. In 165 cases surgical procedures have been performed for diagnostic and therapeutic purposes. This paper reports the outcome of 100 cases (mean follow-up: 8 years): 51 patients are seizure-free, or with only occasional seizures; 28 patients had a significant reduction of seizure frequency (from daily seizures preoperatively to a few per year postoperatively); 21 patients were not improved or had a reduction of seizure frequency that was not significant.

The contributions of depth-EEG, CT scan and pharmacological data in surgery for epilepsy are discussed.

Keywords: Partial epilepsy; surgery for epilepsy; depth EEG; antiepileptic drugs; CT scan.

The exact localization of the epileptogenic lesion is one of the necessary conditions for surgical success in epilepsy[2–4]. The difficulty in localizing the lesion by clinical, scalp EEG and traditional radiological investigations has prompted the introduction of sophisticated techniques such as depth-EEG recording. In recent years, computed tomography (CT) has had a great impact in the field of diagnosis and surgical treatment of epilepsy. Moreover, pharmacological investigations, both at plasma and cerebral level, that have become available in the past few years, allow a better understanding about the mechanism of epilepsy[1,5].

---

[1] Istituto di Neurochirurgia, Università di Milano, Via F. Sforza, 35, I-20122 Milano, Italy.

The purpose of this presentation is to critically evaluate the contributions of the electrographic, CT and pharmacological studies for diagnosis and surgical management of partial epilepsy.

Material and Method

Out of 1,700 patients with non-tumoral partial epilepsy admitted at the Institute of Neurosurgery of the University of Milan from 1959 to 1980, 165 were submitted to surgical procedures for diagnostic and therapeutic reasons (Table 1).

Table 1. *Surgery for Epilepsy. Milan Series (1959–1980): 165 Patients*

Surgical procedures	
Lobectomy or topectomy	No. 93
Stereotactic RF lesions	No. 26
Hemispherectomy	No. 17
Depth-EEG only	No. 29

Follow-up of 100 epileptic patients (from 2 to 18 years postoperatively—mean: 8 years)	
Group A (Seizure free or occasional seizure only)	No. 51
Group B (Significant reduction of seizure frequency)	No. 28
Group C (Same frequency or minor reduction of seizure frequency)	No. 21

Surgical outcome according to the localization of the epileptogenic lesion (100 patients)

Epileptogenic lesion	No. of pts	Outcome group A	B	C
Temporal unilateral	41	27	8	6
Temporal bilateral	17	2	8	7
T. P. O.	13	10	2	1
Frontal	19	7	7	5
Hemispherectomy	10	6	2	2

Depth-EEG studies were performed in 114 cases. ECoG was performed in all cases submitted to open surgery. CT-scan is now routinely employed. Plasma level and brain concentrations studies of antiepileptic drugs have been done in 15 cases.

Results

General results. A late follow-up (from 2 to 18 years: mean 8), is available in 100 patients. The results are as follows: 51 patients are seizure free, or have only occasional seizures (less than 2 per year), 28 patients had a significant reduction of seizure frequency (from daily seizures preoperatively, to few per year postoperatively), 21 patients were not improved, or had a reduction of seizure frequency that was not significant (Table 1).

Depth-EEG data. The results of the depth-EEG studies are summarized as follows: a) unilateral temporal EEG foci (30 cases): depth-EEG studies have usually confirmed the unilaterally of the seizure onset in patients who, at scalp EEG, had a clear, well localized, anterior temporal EEG focus, that was constant in different neurophysiological conditions, and positively reactive to drugs. Different temporal structures have been demonstrated to give rise to seizures at depth-EEG (hippocampal formation, amygdala, cortex of the convexity); b) bilateral independent temporal foci (17 cases): depth-EEG has usually confirmed a bilateral, independent origin of spontaneous seizures from both temporal lobes in bitemporal scalp EEG foci. Regarding the results, also when, at depth-EEG, only unilateral seizures have been recorded, surgical outcome has not been favorable; c) temporo-parieto-occipital foci (13 cases): most of the patients with TPO foci were post-traumatic cases, with large anatomical lesions. Depth-EEG has shown the possibility of a multifocal origin of the spontaneous seizures, from different perilesional foci; d) frontal foci (15 cases): depth-EEG has shown an almost simultaneous involvement of the bilateral frontal cortices in about one third of our cases. In post-traumatic cases, the frontal epileptogenic lesion has been found to be large, and, in some cases, beyond the limits of a standard lobectomy; e) miscellaneous (6 cases): depth-EEG has been able to show a clear-cut epileptogenic lesion (2 temporal unilateral, 4 frontal) in a small number of patients in whom scalp EEG, radiological and clinical studies were unconclusive. On the contrary, in 29 patients, depth-EEG recordings have shown complicated lesions (bilateral, multiple, or unclear foci) not amenable to surgery.

Pharmacological data. Besides allowing a better selection of candidates for surgery, pharmacological studies, carried out during depth-EEG recordings, have demonstrated the hierarchical organization of the epileptogenic lesions and the functional complexity of partial epilepsy. In multifocal epilepsy, epileptogenic foci that used to give rise only rarely to full electroclinical seizures, were seen to became more active and fully independent when plasma levels of anticonvulsant drugs were reduced. At zero level, areas that were silent at steady-state level, have been observed to become active, and give rise to spontaneous seizures.

CT-scan data. The incidence of cerebral lesions in epilepsy, after CT-scan introduction, has been found to be higher than previously suspected or documented. Out of 20 surgical cases with CT, 11 had localized lesions. In 7 cases, in whom CT has shown a small localized lesion and in whom clinical and EEG data were coincident with those of CT, surgery has been successfully performed without prior depth-EEG study. ECoG alone has given the operative indications regarding the epileptogenic areas to be removed.

Discussion

The validity of surgery for epilepsy has been confirmed by the results of our series, which, in agreement with the literature, shows fairly good results in about 3/4 of the treated patients. Our experience confirms also the validity of depth-EEG, that has given in many cases precise operative indications.

However, in the future management of our patients, we are going limit in the use of depth-EEG.

In cases with a clear-cut epileptogenic lesion in areas amenable to radical excision, as in the anterior temporal lobe, when there is a coincidence of clinical, scalp-EEG and CT data, surgery, in our opinion, can be successfully performed without prior depth-EEG studies.

On the other hand, we have lowered the expectations in complicated clinical and scalp EEG cases since depth-EEG has often demonstrated the presence of bilateral, or multiple foci and has not given definitive operative indications.

References

1. Baruzzi, A., Cabrini, G. P., Gerna, M., Sironi, V. A., Morselli, P. L., Anticonvulsant plasma level monitoring in epileptic patients undergoing Stereo-EEG. In: Antiepileptic Drug Monitoring (Gardner-Thorpe, C., Janz, D., Meinardi, H., Pippenger, C. E., eds.), pp. 317—334. Kent: Pitman Medical. 1977.
2. Marossero, F., Ettorre, G., Ravagnati, L., Miserocchi, G., Franzini, A., Sironi, V. A., Cabrini, G. P., Chirurgia delle epilessie parziali: ruolo della Stereo-EEG e risultati operatori. Riv. Ital. EEG Neurofisiol. Clin. *2* (1979), 611—620.
3. Marossero, F., Ravagnati, L., Sironi, V. A., Miserocchi, G., Franzini, A., Ettorre, G., Cabrini, G. P., Late results of stereotactic radiofrequency lesions in epilepsy. Acta Neurochir. (Wien), Suppl. *30* (1980), 145—149.

4. Purpura, D. P., Penry, J. K., Walter, R. D., Advances in neurology, vol. 8: Neurosurgical management of the epilepsies. New York: Raven Press. 1975.
5. Sironi, V. A., Cabrini, G. P., Porro, M. G., Ravagnati, L., Marossero, F., Antiepileptic drug distribution in cerebral cortex, Ammon's horn and amygdala in man. J. Neurosurg. *52* (1980), 686—692.

Acta Neurochirurgica, Suppl. 33, 145—148 (1984)

Excision of Two and Three Independent and Separate Ipsilateral Potentially Epileptogenic Cortical Areas

I. I. Ribarić[1]

With 1 Figure

Summary

In the series of 80 patients operated on for epilepsy, in 2 cases we excised, respectively, two and three separate ipsilateral epileptogenic cortical areas. The indication to surgery was based on the clinical epileptic manifestations, EEG and ECoG findings. The patients are seizure feee since 4 and 1.5 years, respectively. We suggest that the same criteria for excision of a single cortical resection can also be applied to each individual separate ipsilateral focus.

Keywords: Cortical excision for epilepsy; multifocal epilepsy.

Cortical excision in the treatment of partial (focal) epilepsy is based on the assumption that the epileptic discharge responsible for the seizure originates from a circumscribed cortical area[1–5]. Two or more independent and separate epileptogenic cortical areas amenable to surgical excision are identified. The question can be raised of the justifiability of simultaneous multiple cortical excisions.

Material

In the series of 80 patients operated on for epilepsy, in 2 cases we excised, respectively, two and three independent and separate ipsilateral potentially epileptogenic cortical areas.

[1] Neurosurgical University Hospital, Višegradska 26, Y-11000 Belgrade, Yugoslavia.

Case 1. S. G., age 14, right handed girl. She had generalised convulsions at age 3 to 8 months. At the age of 9 years she started to have three types of seizures: 1. sudden laughter which was disagreeable to her, lasting 2 to 3 minutes and occasionally followed by loss of consciousness, head turning to the left and generalised tonic-clonic convulsions; in the last years these attacks appeared a few times daily; 2. sudden loss of contact, senseless talking, psychomotor movements; these occurred 2 to 3 times a day; 3. sudden loss of consciousness, falling down with tonic-clonic convulsions; she had these attacks approximately once a month. The patient had behavioural abnormalities with temper tantrums, emotional instability and difficulties in coping with home and school situations. No neurological deficits were noted.

Several 16-channel EEGs with sphenoidal electrodes and pharmacologically induced sleep showed two independent focal epileptic disturbances: the most active one over the right fronto-lateral region and the less active one over the right parieto-occipital region.

X-ray examination of the skull, right carotid angiography and vertebral angiography showed intracerebral calcifications in both parieto-occipital regions, more pronounced on the right side.

The appearance of these calcifications suggested Sturge-Weber Syndrome (without facial nevus). CAT of the brain showed the same calcifications.

Operation: In the right parieto-occipital brain region there was an area of gyral shrinkage which corresponded to the calcifications. ECoG showed two independent cortical areas with frequent spikes: over the anterior edge of the shrunken cortex and over the frontal premotor convexity. We excised the two cortical areas.

The patient is seizure free 4 years after surgery and her behaviour has been considerably improved.

Case 2. B. A., age 18, right handed girl. At the age of 10 she started to have four types of epileptic attacks: 1. sudden staring and subsequent tonic contraction of all muscles during 1–2 seconds; 2. absence, pale face followed by senseless talking; occasionally deja vu or jame vu; 3. strange feeling in the left arm associated with feeling of sweating and subsequent spread of the same feeling into the whole body; 4. sudden inability to talk followed by loss of consciousness and tonic-clonic convulsions. She had epileptic attacks almost every day. No neurological symptoms.

Several 16-channel EEGs with sphenoidal electrodes and pharmacologically induced sleep showed two independent active focal epileptic disturbances of cerebral activity: over the right infero-medial temporal region and over the right fronto-lateral region.

X-ray examination of the skull and CAT of the brain were normal.

Operation: The brain was macroscopically normal. ECoG showed frequent epileptic abnormalities over two separate cortical areas: the temporal convexity and the inferior half of postcentral gyrus. Over the frontal cortex epileptic abnormalities were scant. Three separate cortical excisions were performed as shown in Fig. 1.

The patient is seizure free 1.5 years after surgery.

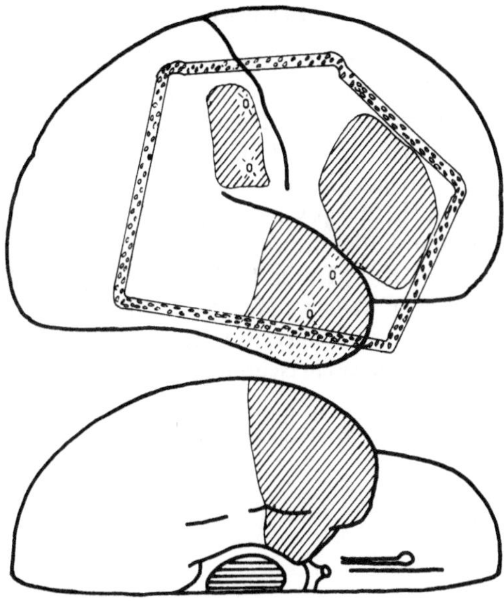

Fig. 1. B. A. scheme of the operative finding: the hatched fields—the excised cortical areas; 0—the maximum of the epileptic abnormalities in the ECoG

Discussion

The rationale for double cortical resection in Case 1 was as follows: in favour of the right parieto-occipital area excision were EEG and ECoG findings and the fact that this active electrographic epileptic focus was quite close to an obvious brain lesion; in favour of the frontal area excision were the clinical types of seizures, EEG and ECoG findings.

The rationale for triple cortical resection in Case 2 is as follows: in favour of the temporal lobectomy were the clinical epileptic manifestations, EEG and ECoG; the frontal lobectomy was mainly suggested by the repetitive EEG findings and by the clinical epileptic manifestations (and a scant ECoG confirmation).

The ultimate decision concerning the cortical resection for epilepsy can be made by integrating our present knowledge of the localising values of the clinical seizure manifestations, of EEG and ECoG signals, of brain pathology and of the amenability to excision of the specific cortical areas. If the diagnostic findings indicate that the epileptic syndrome is related to two or more separate ipsilateral cortical areas their excisions seem to us justified.

References

1. Jasper, H. H., Ward, A. A., jr., Pope, A. (eds.), Basic Mechanisms of the Epilepsies, p. 835. Boston: Little, Brown and Co. 1969.
2. Magnus, O., Lorentz de Haas, A. M. (eds.), The Epilepsies. In: Handbook of Clinical Neurology, Vol. 15 (Vinken, J. P., Bruyn, G. W., eds.), p. 860. Amsterdam: North Holland Publ. Co. 1974.
3. Penfield, W., Jasper, H., Epilepsy and the Functional Anatomy of the Human Brain, p. 896. Boston: Little, Brown and Co. 1954.
4. Purpura, D. P., Penry, K. J., Tower, D., Woodbury, M. D., Walter, R. (eds.), Experimental Models of Epilepsy. New York: Raven Press. 1972.
5. Purpura, D. P., Penry, J. K., Walter, R. D. (eds.), Neurosurgical Management of the Epilepsies, In: Advances in Neurology, Vol. 8, p. 356. New York: Raven Press. 1975.

Acta Neurochirurgica, Suppl. 33, 149—154 (1984)

Additional New Approach in Treatment of Temporal Lobe Epilepsy

J. A. Ganglberger[1]

With 3 Figures

Summary

Based on electrophysiological and anatomical evidence stereotactic interruption of the amygdalo—mediothalamic pathway, has been added to the different conventional targets commonly used in the stereotactic treatment of temporal lobe epilepsy. This pathway has a most important rôle in the break-through of limbic seizures to other structures of the brain. In 9 cases the interruption has been performed at the oro-ventral pole of Nc. medialis (dorsomedialis) thalami and in one case at the border of prothalamus and hypothalamus latero-occipital to the columna fornicis in the intercommissural plane. This later intervention can be combined with fornico- and anterior commissurotomy in an one stage operation, using an insulated stylet or string electrode.

Keywords: Amydalo; mediothalamic pathway interruption.

Introduction

Because of the multitude of pathway connections in the limbic system several target structures are approached in the course of stereotactic treatment of temporal lobe epilepsy in order to interrupt the traffic of abnormal discharges to other parts of the brain.

The author initially prefers interuption of the crossing of the of fornix and anterior commissure (Umbach). Since 1965 special care has been taken to section the stria medullaris thalami and the stria terminalis as well[6]. Some prefer medial

[1] Department of Functional Neurosurgery and Clinical Neurophysiology, Neurosurgical Clinic, University of Vienna, Alser Strasse 4, A-1090 Wien, Austria.

amygdalotomy at the first stage[11]. After 1961 (in Freiburg) fornix and anterior commissure was occasionally combined with medial amygdalotomy. Later (in Berlin) this combination was used as a routine first stage operation[2] and changed in 1970 to combination with baso-lateral amygdalotomy[9]. Bouchard[1] combined fornicotomy with a stylet electrode lesion in the anterior pole of the thalamus. An additional target was introduced in 1971. The interruption of the amygdalo-mediothalamic pathway at the oro-ventral pole of the Nc. medialis (dorsomedialis) thalami[7] and the site for this interruption changed to a few millimeters latero-occipitally to the columna fornicis in the intercommissural plane in 1981. The physiological and anatomical reasoning for the interruption of this important pathway will be discussed later.

Material and Methods

41 patients with temporal lobe epilepsy and grand mal seizures had unsatisfactory results from previous fornico- and anterior commissurotomy. In 9 patients the amygdalo-mediothalamic pathway was interrupted at the oro-ventral pole of the Nc. medialis thalami in a second stage operation, and in one case a third stage operation (after medial amygdalotomy in the second stage).

In a further case after incomplete dissection of the fornix in the first stage operation this pathway was interrupted after re-fornicotomy in November 1981 at the border of prothalamus and hypothalamus where it still runs with the inferior thalamic peduncle, using an insulated laterally drive-out electrode. The incomplete dissection of the columna fornicis was caused by a shift of the brain due to loss of C.S.F. through the stereotactic trephine hole in combination with cortical atrophy.

In all cases pharmacological treatment was continued, drug reduction being considered at the earliest after 3 years of complete freedom of seizures.

Results

Of these 10 cases four are now free of attacks (including temporal auras). The first case operated upon in October 1971 remained free of seizures until February 1983 when occasional short seizures of a different type commenced, hardly noticeable by an observer, accompanied in the EEG by short groups of 2.5 seconds Spikes and Waves pronounced over the operated hemisphere. The case with the three stage operations showed no improvement. The rest were considerably improved, the psychomotor attacks now of rare occurance and of much shorter duration quite often without complete amnesia, the patients hearing what is said to them but being unable to respond.

Discussion

In 1970 Ganglberger *et al.* found distant cortical responses and distant extinction (originally known as a local phenomenon[4]) over prefrontal cortex while stimulating the ipsilateral amygdala. The latencies (onset of deflection) of 16–18 milliseconds clearly suggested a polysynaptic transmission, explained by a detour via the Nc. medialis (dorsomedialis) thalami, being the specific projecting nuclear mass to the prefrontal cortex. When Brazier at a Vienna Symposium in September 1971 reported that in more than 50 cases of temporal lobe epilepsy with chronically implanted electrodes the break-through of limbic seizures to other parts of the brain invariably happened in the Nc. medialis thalami, the literature was searched for anatomical evidence. The first description of an amygdalo-mediothalamic connection in animals[5], was later confirmed. In man this pathway has been impressively demonstrated[10]. Originating from the baso-lateral amygdala the pathway traverses the internal capsule and runs, partially extracapsular, with the peduculus thalami inferior following it through the hypothalamus, before turning to and inserting into the Nc. medialis thalami at its oro-ventral pole.

A fortnight after the presentation of Brazier's important paper the first patient had been operated upon successfully. The lesion was placed at the oro-ventral pole of the medial nuclear mass, where the pathway is still quite compact.

With an additional new approach at the inferior thalamic peduncle at the border of prothalamus and hypothalamus (see Fig.) so far one case has been operated in November 1981. This male patient has now only very rare short attacks without amnesia. During such attacks he hears and comprehends what is said to him but is unable to react for 10 to 15 seconds.

It is a fact that some patients can be completely freed of seizures by a single interruption of pathways leading away from the hippocampal-amygdaloid activator of seizure discharges. The actual epileptogenic lesion may be elsewhere in the anterior temporal lobe or in some cases even paratemporal. The first case with fornico- and anterior commissurotomy operated on in the spring of 1965 is now completely free of seizures and without drugs, working as a fully trained medical orderly. Before operation he suffered from up to 8, sometimes even up to 10 psychomotor attacks per day and three to four seizures of the grand mal type per month.

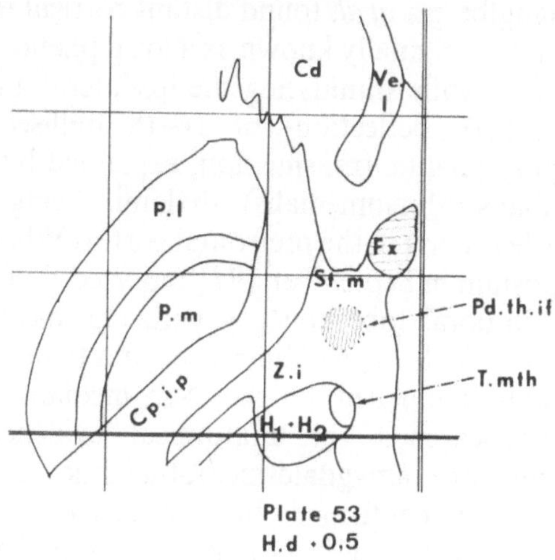

Fig. 1. Horizontal section

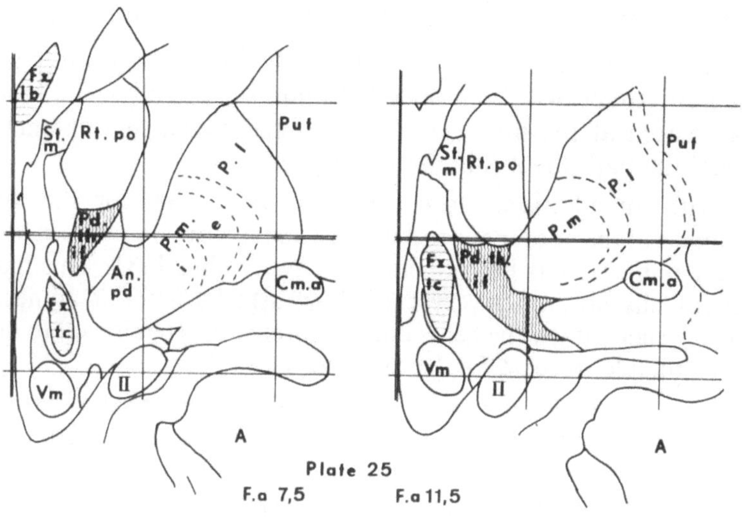

Fig. 2. Frontal section

Cm. a commissura anterior, *Fx. lb* pars libera columnae fornicis, *Fx. tc* pars tecta columnae fornicis, *Pd. th. if* pedunculus thalami inferior, *St. m* Stria medullaris thalami

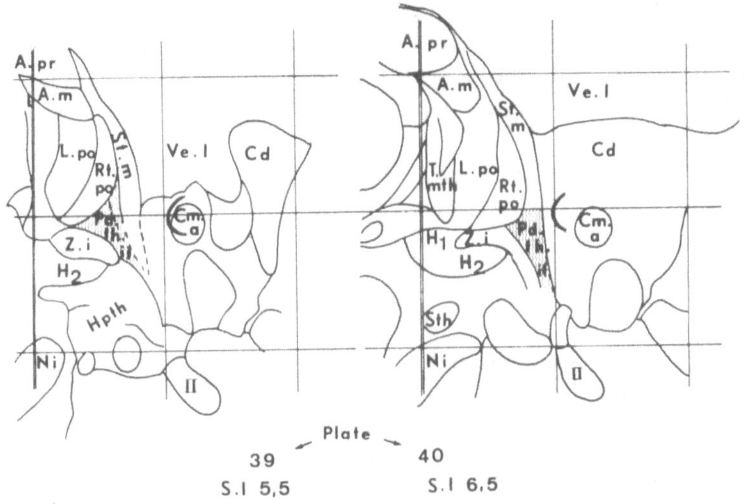

Fig. 3. Parasagittal section

Seizures of the grand mal type are abolished in more than 90% of the cases after fornico- and anterior commissurotomy, combined with interruption of stria medullaris thalami and stria terminalis. In the optimal cases limbic seizures are also abolished, in the others at least considerably reduced in frequency and duration although after years of freedom of seizures they may reoccur.

Patients without substantial improvement by the first operation may want further improvement. The author now recommends interruption of the amygdalo-mediothalamic pathway for this second stage procedure. It seems a great pity that this most important pathway is still widely ignored. It is not even mentioned in the otherwise excellent chapter on the limbic system in the new textbook on stereotaxy of the human brain[13].

It should be considered whether interruption of this pathway on the border of prothalamus and hypothalamus should be performed in combination with fornico- and anterior commissurotomy (including stria medullaris thalami and stria terminalis) in a single first stage intervention, using the laterally drive-out stylet electrode, requiring only insertion of a single electrode shaft, thus restricting brain damage. It has to be emphasized that extreme care has to be taken not to damage the A. polaris (a branch of the A. comm. post.) and its ramifications. Recording of the depth EEG with the insulated stylet electrode in situ, using a time constant of 1.2

seconds indicates the eventual nearness of an artery by pulse artifacts. By retraction or further protrusion of the laterally drive-out stylet electrode the nearness of an artery can be deliminated more accurately (a method which has been proved useful to us since 1967).

The figures taken from the atlas of Schaltenbrand and Wahren[12] show the relation of the inferior thalamic peduncle to columna fornicis and anterior commissure.

References

1. Bouchard, G., Basic targets and the different epilepsies. Acta Neurochir. (Wien), Suppl. *23* (1976), 193—199.
2. Bouchard, G., Umbach, W., Langzeitergebnisse der stereotaktischen Therapie bei psychomotorischer Epilepsie (Heppner, F., ed.), Limbisches System und Epilepsie, pp. 90—93. Bern-Stuttgart-Wien: H. Huber. 1973.
3. Brazier, M. A. B., Interaction of deep structures during seizures in man, pp. 409—424 (Petsche, H., Brazier, M. A. B., eds.), Synchronization of EEG activity in epilepsies. Wien-New York: Springer. 1972.
4. Dusser de Barenne, J. G., McCulloch, W. S., Local stimulatory inactivation within the cerebral cortex, the factor for extinction. Amer. J. Physiol. *118*, (1937), 510—524.
5. Fox, C. A., Amygdalo-thalamic connections in Macaca mulatta, Anat. *103* (1949), 537—538.
6. Ganglberger, J. A., Stereotaktische Fornikotomie (Heppner, F., ed.), Limbisches System und Epilepsie, pp. 100—105. Bern-Stuttgart-Wien: H. Huber. 1973.
7. Ganglberger, J. A., New possibilities of stereotactic treatment of temporal lobe epilepsy (TLE). Acta Neurochir. (Wien), Suppl. *23* (1976), 211—214.
8. Ganglberger, J. A., Groll-Knapp, E., Haider, M., Computer analysis of electrophysiological phenomena during stereotaxic fornico- and amygdalotomy, pp. 149—155 (Umbach, W., ed.), Special topics in stereotaxis. Stuttgart: Hippokrates-Verlag. 1971.
9. Kim, Y. K., Effects of basolateral amygdalotomy, pp. 69—78 (Umbach, W., ed.), Special topics in stereotaxis. Stuttgart: Hippokrates-Verlag. 1971.
10. Klingler, J., Gloor, P., The connections of the amygdala and of the anterior temporal cortex in the human brain. J. Comp. Neurol. *115,* 3 (1960), 333—369.
11. Narabayashi, H., Stereotaxic amygdalotomy (Its long term results). Excerpta Medica, Intern. Congr. Series *193* (1969), 8.
12. Schaltenbrand, G., Wahren, W., Atlas for stereotaxy of the human brain, 2nd ed. Stuttgart: G. Thieme. 1977.
13. Schaltenbrand, G., Walker, A. E., Stereotaxy of the human brain, anatomical, physiological and clinical applications. Stuttgart: G. Thieme. 1982.

Acta Neurochirurgica, Suppl. 33, 155—159 (1984)

Caudate Nucleus Stimulation During Epilepsy Treatment

V. Drličkova[1], M. Šramka, and P. Nádvorník

Summary

Experience with the standard stimulation program (10 and 100 Hz, 1 msec, 10 V, 10 min, once a day) in the treatment of epilepsy by means of caudate nucleus stimulation was evaluated on 13 patients after an interval of three years. The favourable influence of stimulation on grand mal turned out to be temporary. With mixed forms of epilepsy a gradual reduction of seizures, and sometimes their total disappearance, was attained; three patients were able to work again. The inhibitory influence of the caudate nucleus with bilateral stimulation was revealed whilst measuring action potentials from other brain depth structures.

Keywords: Epilepsy; caudate nucleus stimulation.

Introduction

Ablation of the caudate nucleus under experimental conditions suggested that its function is connected with motion reactions, especially defensive ones[6]. Later electrophysiological research brought into evidence a moderating influence on the cerebral cortex motor cells[4,5]. Stimulation of the caudate nucleus evokes a transitional period of silence. At the same time, special spindles in subcortical structures can be noted, especially in the thalamus, similar to some synchronous waves in epilepsy[1]. Further observation showed that the caudate nucleus inhibits the spreading of epileptic discharges and joins in its extra-rhinencephalic control[7]. The caudate nucleus has connections with the nucleus amygdalae and through its outlet pathway stria terminalis with the oldest cortical structures of the brain at septum pellucidum.

[1] Research Laboratory of Clinical Stereotaxy, Research Institute of Medical Bionics (Director Doc. Dzurik R., M.D., Dr.Sc.), Bratislava, Czechoslovakia.

Therefore Cooper's[3] experience with cerebellar stimulation for epilepsy encouraged us to stimulate the caudate nucleus. We described our first experiences with caudate nucleus stimulation in treatment of epilepsy in 1976.

Method

Since 1980 we have performed stimulation treatment in caput nuclei caudati with 13 patients; today we can evaluate the results after a three year interval. We inserted chronic electrodes bilaterally and symmetrically into the caudate nucleus, nucleus amygdalae and hippocampus and, in same patients, into the thalamus reticular nucleus. The study of the clinical effects of caudate nucleus stimulation was integrated with the study of the effect on the electrical activity of these deep brain sites.

The chronic electrodes were externalized and the caudate nucleus stimulation was usually performed on both sides at the same time. Our stimulation program utilized electric impulses with a frequency of 10 and 100 Hz lasting 0.5 and 1 msec up to 10 V. We stimulated once a day for ten minutes at a certain time in the morning or irregularly during the day. Therapy stimulation was performed with patients who had daily epileptic seizures refractory to drug treatment. The type of epileptic seizures, the duration of the stimulation treatment and the results obtained are summarized in Table 1. The optimal duration of stimulation therapy was about one month. If stimulation lasts longer, there is danger of epileptic activity returning.

Results (see Table 1)

The grand mal type of epilepsy respond to stimulation by temporary disappearance of seizures. The seizures reappear after 2 to 4 weeks, but with lower frequency. Mixed type of epilepsy with psychomotor seizure prevalence gradually reduces during caudate nucleus stimulation and can even disappear completely; drug treatment, however, has to be maintained; three of the patients of this group returned to work. Only a short and transitional effect on caudate nucleus stimulation was found with a patient who, according to EEG examination, suffered from centrencephalic epilepsy. Psychologic examination did not show significant changes caused by stimulation.

From the analysis of repeated electrophysiological observations, it was clear that a favourable clinical result from caudate nucleus stimulation can be expected when epileptic activity in SEEG record is reduced. Epileptic activity appeared in caudate nucleus only once. Spontaneous registration of electric activity from caudate nucleus shows the tendency to a slow rhythm, which is not essentially changed by stimulation.

Table 1

	Patient	Onset and type of seizures	Stimulation therapy	Effect on seizures
1.	D. A. f., 1951	17 y., GM	17. 9. 1974—6 d	Suppression 4 weeks
2.	Č. V. m., 1953	17 y., GM	24. 1. 1975—4 d	Suppression 4 weeks, reduction
3.	K. T. f., 1955	7 y., temp.	17. 6. 1976—14 d	Reduction
4.	T. A. f., 1948	16 y., temp.	17. 6. 1977—70 d	Suppression 2 weeks, reduction, recurrence
5.	H. L. f., 1967	11 y., temp.	30. 6. 1977—21 d	Short reduction
6.	S. M. f., 1953	6 y., GM—temp.	13. 10. 1977—30 d	Progressive reduction then suppression
7.	Z. R. m., 1959	14 y., GM—temp.	14. 10. 1977—14 d	Progressive reduction
8.	K. K. m., 1951	4 y., GM—temp.	2. 3. 1978—40 d	Progressive reduction
9.	H. J. m., 1956	14 y., GM	3. 3. 1978—7 d	Suppression 4 weeks, reduction
10.	M. V. m., 1939	31 y., GM—posttraum.	30. 2. 1978—19 d	Suppression (subsequent hypothalamotomy)
11.	T. J. m., 1968	3 y., centrenceph. EEG	15. 5. 1979—30 d	Reduction 2 weeks
12.	L. O. m., 1956	3 y., GM—temp.	14. 1. 1980—65 d	Progressive reduction
13.	R. O. f., 1936	7 y., GM	27. 5. 1980—60 d	Suppression 4 weeks, reduction

Discussion

Systematic observation of caudate nucleus stimulation to influence epileptic seizures is not often reported. Therefore, every new piece of knowledge is a contribution to the recognition of the new therapy process effect and to the better understanding of the disease substance[8]. Our own experience is to a certain extent the same as that of Cchenkeli[2]. Low frequencies are probably more effective. Stimulation was carried out only once a day, therefore it is reasonable to except that further modification of the treatment program will show further possibilities. Probably neither the duration nor the distribution of stimulation during the day are substantial.

The results confirm the experimental experience that the caudate nucleus has inhibitory influence on movement manifestations of epileptic seizures. Stimulation probably intensifies this inhibitory action. But under clinical conditions we did not attain caudate spindles in the brain depth structure. The proper electric activity of the caudate nucleus does not change according to stimulation. Sporadic observations of specific epileptic activity in the caudate nucleus may be explained by the stimulation electrode lying near the fundus striae terminalis touching the head of the caudate nucleus and possibly participating in the transmission of epileptic discharges in the brain.

References

1. Buchwald, N. A., Wyers, E. J., Okuma, T., Heuser, G., The "caudate spindle". Electrophysiological properties. Electroenceph. clin. Neurophysiol. *13* (1961), 509—518.
2. Cchenkeli, S. A., Lordkipanidze, G. S., Chirurgičeskoe lečenije epilepsii, p. 80. Tbilisi: Mecnierva. 1980.
3. Cooper, I. S., Reversibility of chronic neurologic deficits. Some effects of electrical stimulation of the thalamus and internal capsule in man. Appl. Neurophysiol. *43* (1980), 244—258.
4. Davis, G. D., Caudate lesions and spontaneous locomotion in the monkey. Neurology *8* (1958), 135—139.
5. Dean, W. H., Davis, G. D., Behavior changes following caudate lesions in rhesus monkey. J. Neurophysiol. *22* (1959), 524—537.
6. Klosovskij, B. N., Volžina, N. S., O funkčním významu nucleus caudatus. Vopr. nejrochirurgii *21* (1957), 8—12.
7. La Grutta, V., Amato, G., Zagami, M. T., The importance of the caudate nucleus in the control of convulsive activity in the amygdaloid complex and the temporal cortex of the cat. Electroenceph. clin. Neurophysiol. *31* (1971), 57—69.

8. Mundinger, F., Indication and long-term results of stereotactic operations in therapy-resistant epilepsy. Arch. Psychiatr. Nervenkr. *231* (1981), 1—11.
9. Šramka, M., Fritz, G., Galanda, M., Nádvorník, P., Some observations in treatment stimulation of epilepsy. Acta Neurochir. (Wien), Suppl. *23* (1976), 257—262.

Acta Neurochirurgica, Suppl. 33, 161—167 (1984)

The Reduction of Seizures in Cerebral Palsy and Epileptic Patients Using Chronic Cerebellar Stimulation

R. Davis[1], **E. Gray**[1], **H. Engle**[2], and **A. Dusnak**[1]

Summary

With the use of chronic cerebellar stimulation (CCS) for the reduction of spasticity and improvements of performance in our clinic since 1974, 329 spastic patients (89% cerebral palsy) were implanted and studied. Ninety-five (29%) had had a history of seizures prior to the implantation. Group 1 comprised 65 patients (20%) who had no seizures in the 3 years prior to implantation, none had had a seizure during the CCS period (average 4.3 year/patient). Group 2 comprised 30 patients (9%) who were having seizures although under medical care during the 3 years prior to implantation; of the 19 having grand mal seizures 15 stopped and 3 were reduced, of the 8 having petit mal 4 stopped and 2 were reduced, of 5 having myoclonic episodes 1 stopped and 3 were reduced. Overall CCS effects on the 27 patients followed in Group 2 for an average of 4.3 year/patient showed 17 (63%) stopped seizuring, 7 (25%) reduced and 3 (12%) no effect.

Of 6 epileptic patients implanted, 5 were followed and underwent CCS for an average of 4.6 year/patient. Of 4 patients having grand mal seizures, 2 stopped, 1 reduced and 1 unchanged. Petit mal occurred in 1 patient whose seizures were reduced with CCS. Of 2 patients having 50+ psychomotor seizures per day, 1 stopped.

Overall of the 32 patients having intractable seizures, CCS stopped 18 (57%) of the patients seizuring, reduced a further 9 (28%) with no effect in 5 patients (15%). The most successful equipment involved fully implanted pulse stimulators using hermetic sealing, lithium batteries and constant current output (1–2 μC/sqcm/ph), rate was not a factor.

Keywords: Cerebellar Stimulation; cerebral palsy; epilepsy; seizures.

Introduction

Overall there have now been 55 patients with intractable seizures treated with chronic cerebellar stimulation (CCS) reported[1,3–6], 34 patients (62%) have benefitted (Table 1).

[1] Department of Neurological Surgery and [2] Department of Pediatrics, Mt. Sinai Medical Center, Miami Beach, FL 33140, U.S.A.

Table 1. *Seizures—CCS Clinical Series*

Report	Patients	Benefitted
Cooper (1978)	32	18 (56%)
Gilman (1977)	6	5 (83%)
VanBuren (1978)	5	0 (0%)
Heath (1983)	9	8 (89%)
Madrazo (1983)	3	3 (100%)
SubTotal	55	34 (62%)
Davis	32	27 (84%)
Total	87	61 (70%)

The following report presents 32 new cases of intractable seizures treated with CCS, 27 have spastic disabling condition (23 patients—cerebral palsy) and 8 patients with intractable epilepsy.

Methods

Clinical Series: From February, 1974 to June of 1982, 329 spastic patients (cerebral palsy: 89%) and 6 patients with intractable epilepsy underwent the implantation of cerebellar stimulating systems[2]. Of the 329 spastic patients, 95 (29%) had a history of having of at least 1 seizure during their lifetime.

Group 1: Comprised 65 patients (20%) who had a history of seizures from birth up to 3 years prior to the implantation.

Group 2: Comprised 30 patients (9%) who had seizures occurring during a period 3 years prior to implantation and had been under medical treatment. The age distribution of the 95 patients showed in the 4–10 year age group: 46 patients; in the 11–20 year age group: 27 patients; and in the 21–42 year age group: 22 patients. The prime reason for the spastic patients to undergo CCS was to reduce spasticity[2], however, the 6 patients with the intractable epilepsy aged 4 to 25 years (Table 3) underwent CCS specifically to reduce their seizure activity. The cerebellar stimulators used during this study have been described previously[2]. In summary of the 95 spastic patients, 68 were implanted from February 1974 to November 1978 with the Avery Radio Frequency System (I 108 receiver, 0.5 mamps, 0.5 msec, 180 pps, 7 min ON/OFF). From May 1979, 27 patients had a combination of the Avery Twin Pad Electrodes connected with the totally implantable Lithium powered constant current pulse generator (Neurolith 601, Pacesetters Systems, Inc., Sylmar, CA), producing 1.0 mamps (601-A) or 1.4 mamps (601-B), 150 pps, 4 min ON/OFF. The charge density for both the Avery and the Neurolith systems was 1.0–1.8 μC/sqcm/ph. In the epileptic group, 3 patients had the combination of the Avery cerebellar leads connected to the Cordis 900 series fully implantable programmable stimulator (1–2 μC/sqcm/ph, 10–30 pps, continuous).

Results

Spastic Patients with Seizure History: Group 1: Of the 65 patients, 2 were lost to follow-up and 1 had died in 1980 (CCS: 3 years); all were cerebral palsy patients, 53 had had a history of grand mal seizures, 6 had had petit mal, and 3 had had a combination of different types of seizures (myolonic, psychomotor). As was stated above, none of these 62 patients had a seizure during the 3 years prior to implantation; none had had seizures since undergoing CCS for the reduction of spasticity for an average of 4.3 year/patient (range 6–84 mos).

Group 2: Of the 30 spastic patients who were having seizures during the 3 years prior to CCS, 27 were evaluated and 3 were lost to contact. CCS had been applied for an average of 4.5 year/patient (12–84 mos). Table 2 shows the results of CCS in 19 spastic patients having grand mal seizures and 8 patients having petit mal attacks.

Grand mal seizures were present in 19 of the spastic patients followed, 2 patients were having more than 1 seizure a week, 3 patient were having 2–20 per day. Two patients were having more

Table 2. *CCS*

Grand mal seizures

	SCP	EP	Total	%
Stopped	15	2	17	74
Reduced	3	1	4	17
No effect	1	1	2	9
Patient	19	4	23	100

Petit mal seizures

	SCP	EP	Total	%
Stopped	4		4	44
Reduced	2	1	3	33
No effect	2		2	22
Patient	8	1	9	100

Table 3. *Epilepsy—CCS*

Case Age/Sex	Duration Implantation	Equipment (Date)	QD/Rate	Seizures	CCS	Behavior	CCS
1. E. C. 25/F	—	A (7/74)	—	GM 10–15/ day	—	aggressive	—
2. L. L. 21/F	80 mos	AI 108 (10/75) C 900 (11/1979) C 900 (1/1980)	? 1.0/10 0.8/10 1.1/30	GM 15–40/ day	none	slow ataxic institution	more alert learning more home more often
3. B. C. 15/M	67 mos	C 199 (11/1976) C 900 (2/1979) C 900 (1/1981)	0.8/10 1.0/10 1.3/10	psychomotor 50–100/day	none	very aggressive non-trainable supervision	calm working
4. C. B. 4/M	63 mos	AI 108 (3/1977) AI 110 (1/1979)	0.8/10 1.0/10	GM 2–10/ day myoclonic 30/day	2–3/day 5–30/day	slow untrainable	no change

5. R. L. 12/F	34 mos	C 900 (8/1979)	1.0/10	GM 5/day PM continu.	none minimal	slow untrainable self-stim.	alert learning stop self-stim.
6. J. M. 19/M	30 mos	E (1/1980)	1.1/10	GM 3–5/ day psychom. 50+/day	3–5/day 50+/day	slow	no change

GM = grand mal.
PM = petit mal.
A = Avery.
C = Cordis.
E = Epilith.
QD = charge density (μC/sqcm/ph).
Rate = pulses per sec.

than 1 seizure a month, 6 were having more than 1–2 seizures a year, and 6 patients were having more than 1 seizure every 3 years. With CCS, medication generally continued unchanged except 4 stopped, 1 needed more and 1 started.

Epilepsy Per Se: Of the 6 patients that underwent CCS for intractable epilepsy 5 were followed for over an average of 4½ years per patient. Table 3 shows the details of the 6 patients.

In summary, of the 4 patients having grand mal seizures, 2 (Case 2, 5) have been controlled and both cases have the Cordis 900 stimulator. The other patient (Case 3) had the psychomotor controlled with CCS using the Cordis stimulators for 7 years. All 3 patients have had marked improvement in their behavorial problems.

Discussion

CCS (0.8–2.0 μC/sqcm/ph, 10–180 pps cycled or continuous) has been safe and efficacious for the reduction of intractable seizures in 27 (84%) of the 32 patients over a 7 year period (Table 1). The seizures stopped in 18 patients (57%) while 9 (28%) had their seizures reduced, and 5 (15%) were unaffected. The results appeared not to be dependent on the stimulation rate (10–180 pps) whether continuous or intermittent.

Including these 32 patients with the 55 already reported[1,3–6], CCS has produced benefits by reducing or completely stopping seizures in 61 patients (70%, Table 1). Fully implantable stimulators, have been an improvement not only in reliability but in results especially in cases[2,3,5] of the epileptic series.

References

1. Cooper, I. S., Riklan, M., Amin, I., Cullinan, T., A long-term follow-up study of cerebellar stimulation for the control of epilepsy. In: Cerebellar Stimulation in Man (Cooper, I. S., ed.), pp. 19—39. New York: Raven Press. 1978.
2. Davis, R., Engle, H., Kudzma, J., Gray, E., Ryan, T., Dusnak, A., Update of chronic cerebellar stimulation for spasticity and epilepsy. Appl. Neurophysiol. *45* (1982), 44—50.
3. Gilman, S., Dauth, G. W., Tennyson, V. S., Kremzner, L. T., Defendini, R., Correll, J. W., Clinical, morphological, biochemical, and physiological effects of cerebellar stimulation. In: Functional Electrical Stimulation (Hambrecht, F. T., Reswick, J. B., eds.), pp. 191—223. New York: Dekker. 1977.
4. Heath, R. G., Cerebellar vermis stimulation: long-term response in intractable behavioral disorders and epilepsy. In: Cerebellar Stimulation for Spasticity and Seizures, in press (Davis, R., Bloedel, J., eds.). Boca Raton: CRC Press. 1983.

5. Madrazo, I., Rosas, V. H., Chronic cerebellar stimulation for reduction of grave behavioral changes and seizures in psychiatric patients. In: Cerebellar Stimulation for Spasticity and Seizures, in press (Davis, R., Bloedel, J., eds.). Boca Raton: CRC Press. 1983.
6. VanBuren, J. M., Wood, J. H., Oakley, J., Hambrecht, F., Preliminary evaluation of cerebellar stimulation by double-blind and stimulation and biological criteria in the treatment of epilepsy. J. Neurosurg. *48* (1978), 407—416.

Section II

Cerebral Tumours

Acta Neurochirurgica, Suppl. 33, 171—181 (1984)

Introductory Lecture

Morphologic Evaluation of Stereotactic Brain Tumour Biopsies

P. Kleihues[1], **B. Volk, J. Anagnostopoulos,** and **M. Kiessling**

With 2 Figures

Summary

The validity of morphologic diagnosis of stereotactic brain tumour biopsies was evaluated in a series of 600 patients treated since 1977 at the University Hospital, Freiburg. Combined cytological (smear preparations) and histological examination of paraffin-embedded samples revealed the tumour type and approximate grading in 492 (82%) of cases. In 66 patients a clinically suspected neoplasm could be ruled out. In the remaining 42 cases (7%), the presence of a tumour was confirmed but the available samples did not allow an unequivocal classification of the neoplasm. Inaccurate diagnoses were most frequently due to sampling errors in non-homogeneous tumours, *i.e.* biopsies taken from sites not representative for the entire neoplasm (tumour necroses, infiltration zone). In the future, the use of immunohistochemical methods for the identification of tumour markers and cytoskeleton proteins may partially compensate for the limited size of stereotactic biopsy samples.

Introduction

In recent years stereotactic biopsy has been increasingly used to identify the nature of intracranial lesions[6,8,9,12]. With the advancement of computed tomography (CT), very small tumours (less than 1 cm diameter) can now be precisely located and a

---

[1] Abteilung Neuropathologie, Pathologisches Institut der Universität Freiburg, Albertstrasse 19, D-7800 Freiburg im Breisgau, Federal Republic of Germany.

Address for correspondence: Dr. P. Kleihues, Abteilung Neuropathologie, Institut für Pathologie, Universitätsspital, CH-8091 Zürich, Switzerland.

stereotactic probe taken from sites inaccessible to open surgery. However, the volume and number of stereotactic biopsy samples are limited and require a specialized histopathological approach.

In this report the following questions are addressed:

— Is stereotactic brain tumour biopsy, from the pathologist's point of view, a reliable method?

— Which are the diagnostic problems and limitations and how can they be reduced?

To answer these questions we have reviewed the histopathology of 600 consecutive cases operated in the Division of Stereotactic and Functional Neurosurgery at the University of Freiburg in the years since 1977.

Sample Processing

Depending on the size and location of the lesion 2 to 10 biopsies were taken stepwise at distances of 3 to 10 mm along the puncture tract with a specially designed biopsy forceps[6,8]. The diameter of the stereotactic forceps is 0.8 mm and the volume of tissue removed approximately 1 mm^3 per biopsy site. In all cases of this series the final neuropathological diagnosis was the result of two different diagnostic procedures: Rapid intraoperative diagnosis by cytological analysis of smear preparations[1,4], followed by histological examination of serial sections from additional paraffin-embedded material. More recently we have also used plastic embedding (Araldite) for semi-thin sections (Figs. 1 and 2) and electron microscopy. For smear preparations, biopsy material was placed on glass slides, gently spread out with needles, stained with methylene-blue and slightly pressed with a coverslip.

Tumour Classification and Grading

Histological classification of CNS tumours was carried out according to the guidelines published by the WHO[13]. In our view, this scheme has proven to be very useful and assisted considerably to unify the terminology of CNS tumours. This is particularly important when results of various therapeutic measures are compared in multi-center studies. However, the WHO classification needs constant revision to include tumour entities more recently recognized, *e.g.* primitive neuroectodermal tumours (PNET, see Table 2). Similarly, we have applied the grading proposed in the WHO classification, since the estimated biology is usually the rationale for the selection of adjuvant radiation

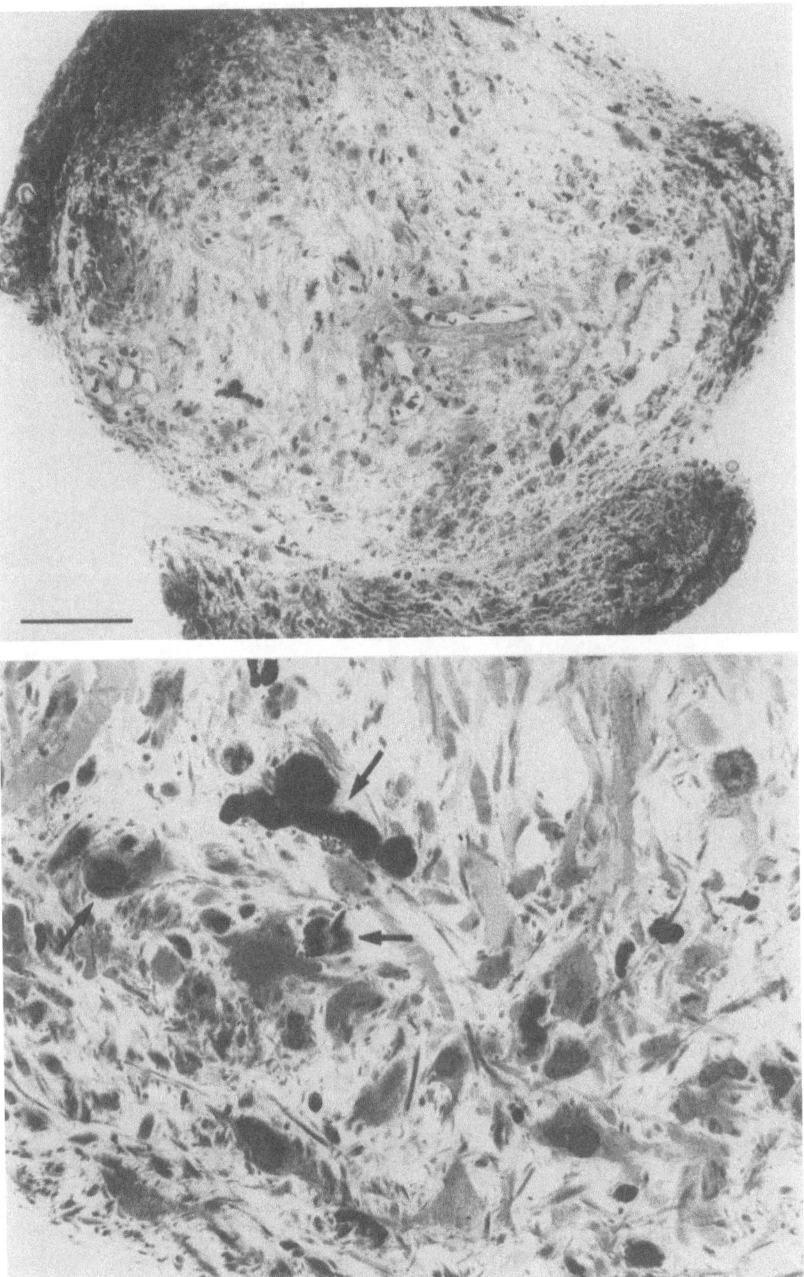

Fig. 1. Araldite-embedded semi-thin section of a stereotactic biopsy from a pilocytic astrocytoma. The horizontal bar in the upper photograph corresponds to 0.1 mm. Higher magnification (lower) shows irregularly shaped tumour cells in a dense fibrillary network with occasional Rosenthal fibres (arrows). (Toluidine blue, × 175 and × 715)

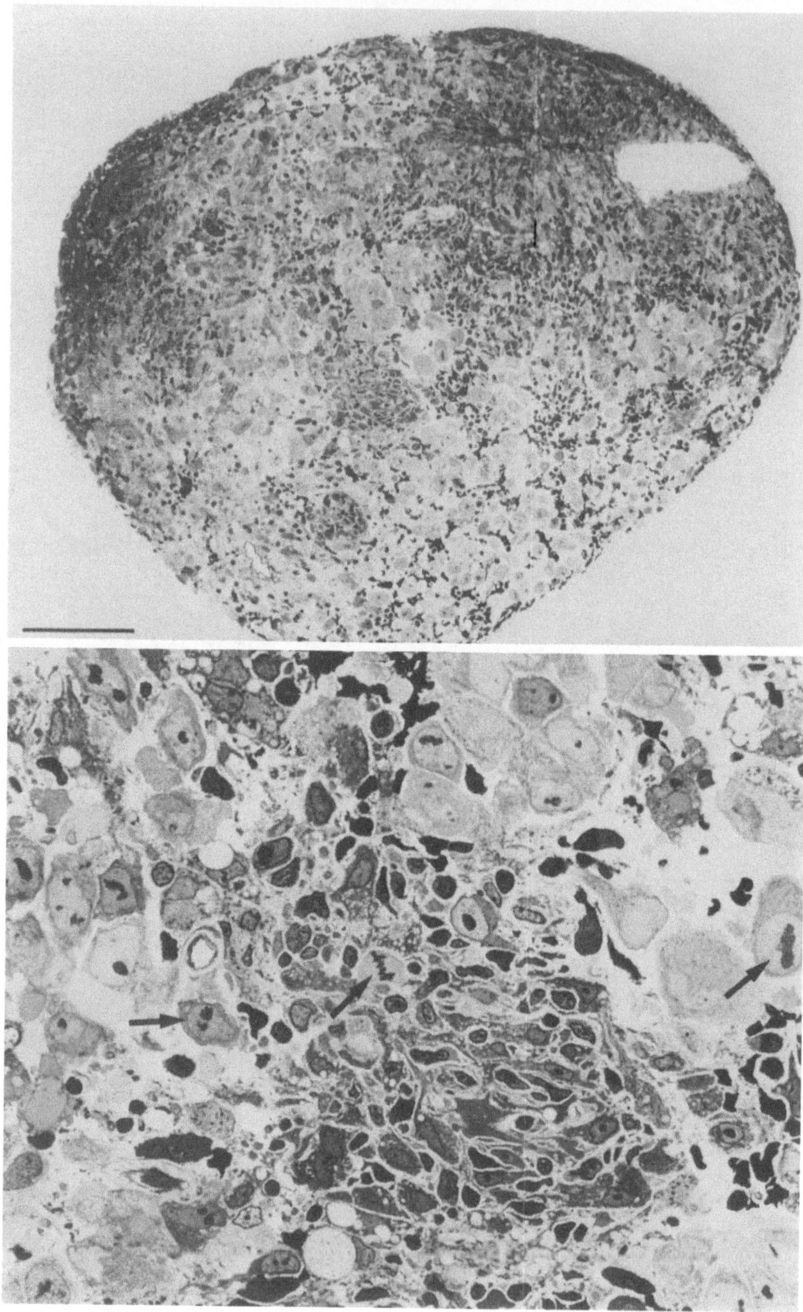

Fig. 2. Semi-thin section of a stereotactic biopsy from a germinoma of the pineal region. The horizontal bar (upper) corresponds to 0.1 mm. At higher magnification (lower) the "two cell type" nature of the neoplasm is clearly recognizable with small hyperchromatic lymphoid cells (center), and large polygonal cells with central pale nuclei, prominent nucleoli and numerous mitoses (arrows). (Toluidine blue, × 175 and × 715)

therapy. Interstitial radiotherapy is being carried out in both benign and malignant neoplasms whereas external radiation is usually restricted to grade III and IV tumours.

Location and Nature of Biopsied Lesions

The age distribution of stereotactically operated patients was very similar to that reported earlier[5]. When compared to open surgery, patients were generally younger, with an early peak in the first and second decade. This was mainly due to the high percentage of deep-seated low grade astrocytomas in children and younger individuals.

The majority of biopsied lesions was located supratentorially (Table 1). The cerebral hemispheres were the site most frequently

Table 1. *Localization of Biopsied Lesions (600 cases)*

Supratentorial		84%
Hemispheres	46%	
Basal ganglia	20%	
Diencephalon	11%	
Ventricles	4%	
Base of skull	3%	

Infratentorial		16%
Midbrain-Pineal region	8.5%	
Pons-Medulla	6.0%	
Cerebellum	1.0%	
Ventricle	0.25%	
Base of skull	0.25%	

involved (46%), with a marked predilection for functionally important hemispheric regions such as the central region and the speech area. Second in frequency were locations close to midline structures such as basal ganglia and hypothalamus (20% and 11% respectively) followed by the midbrain-pineal region (8.5%) and pons-medulla (6%). Rarely encountered were intraventricular tumours and extracerebral lesions at the base of the skull.

Table 2. *Tumour Types (600 Stereotactic Biopsies)*

Tumour type	n (%)
Astrocytic tumours	297 (49.5%)
Pilocytic astrocytoma	86 (14.5%)
Astrocytoma	122 (20.5%)
Anaplastic astrocytoma	68 (11.5%)
Subependymal giant cell astrocytoma	1 (0.5%)
Glioblastoma	81 (13.5%)
Metastatic tumours	27 (4.5%)
Oligodendroglial tumours	25 (4%)
Oligodendroglioma	21 (3.5%)
Anaplastic oligodendroglioma	2 (0.5%)
Mixed oligo-astrocytoma	2 (0.5%)
Germinoma	15 (2.5%)
Craniopharyngioma	15 (2.5%)
Ependymoma	10 (1.5%)
Meningeoma	10 (1.5%)
Plexus papilloma	6 (1%)
PNET	4 (0.5%)
Medulloblastoma	4 (0.5%)
Teratoma	3 (0.5%)
Pituitary adenoma	3 (0.5%)
Pineoblastoma	2 (0.5%)
Lymphoma	2 (0.5%)
Pineocytoma	1 (0.5%)
Chordoma	1 (0.5%)
Unclassified tumours	14 (2.5%)

Histopathological diagnoses obtained in the present series of 600 cases are given in Table 2. There was a marked prevalence of astroglial tumours (50%). This was particularly true for pilocytic and grade II astrocytomas which occurred approximately 3 times more frequently than in a comparable series of patients treated by open surgery[5]. There was also a relatively high incidence of pineal germinomas whereas meningeomas and neurinomas were rare due to their easily accessible extracranial location.

Diagnostic Potential and Accuracy of Stereotactic Brain Tumour Biopsies

After combined cytological and histological examination a definite tumour diagnosis including tumour type and approximate grading was made in 492 (82%) out of 600 stereotactic biopsies (Table 3). In additional 66 cases (11%) a clinically suspected

Table 3. *Diagnostic Potential of Stereotactic Brain Tumour Biopsies (Smear Preparation + Paraffin-embedded Sections)*

Tumour + tumour type + approximate grading	82%
Tumour clinically suspected, but not confirmed	11%
Glioma without grading	4.5%
Tumour (unclassified)	2.5%

neoplastic lesion was definitely ruled out by the combination of both procedures. In 27 cases (4.5%), a glioma was diagnosed but precise grading was not possible. In the remaining 15 cases (2.5%) the presence of a tumour was confirmed, but tissue samples available were insufficient for histopathological classification.

Data on the accuracy and reliability of stereotactic diagnoses as verified by clinical follow-up or autopsy (87 cases) are summarized in Table 4. Stereotactic diagnoses were confirmed by subsequent therapeutic craniotomy, additional biopsies of recurrent tumours or autopsy in 67 cases. In 9 cases radiation necroses were found following interstitial radiotherapy of previously diagnosed neoplastic lesions. Diagnostic discrepancies were encountered in 11

Table 4. *Accuracy of Stereotactic Diagnosis*

Clinical follow-up	Confirmation	Radiation necrosis	Discrepancy
Subsequent open surgery	20	1	4[a]
Recurrency (additional open surgery)	7	1	2[b]
Recurrency (additional stereotactic biopsy)	23	5	3[c]
Autopsy	17	2	2[d]

[a] Necrotic tissue/anaplastic ependymoma; astrocytoma II/astrocytoma III–IV; gliosis, no tumour/craniopharyngioma; oligodendroglioma II/astrocytoma II.

[b] Necrotic tissue/astrocytoma III–IV; astrocytoma II/astrocytoma III–IV.

[c] Necrotic tissue / astrocytoma III; astrocytoma II / astrocytoma III; germinoma/gliosis (1st diagnosis was correct).

[d] Pilocytic astrocytoma/cystic necrosis with reactive gliosis and Rosenthal fibres (old hemorrhage); astrocytoma III/metastatic hemangiosarcoma.

cases. Of these, 5 were obviously due to sampling errors, *i.e.* the initial or subsequent stereotactic biopsy had only shown gliosis or necrotic tissue. In 3 cases the clinical follow-up revealed a higher grade of malignancy but it is difficult to decide whether this was due to a sampling error or to tumour progression with increasing dedifferentiation and anaplasia. In the remainder 3 cases the discrepancy was due to a diagnostic error mainly based on the small sample size.

Smear Preparation versus Tissue Embedding

To estimate the diagnostic relevance of cytological analysis the correlation of diagnoses obtained from smear preparations and paraffin-embedded sections was evaluated (Table 5). Results

Table 5. *Correlation of Diagnoses Obtained from Smear Preparations and Paraffin Sections*

Smear diagnosis confirmed		77%
Tumour type and grading	60%	
No tumour	10%	
Tumour type only	4.5%	
Tumour only	2.5%	
Lack of correlation		10.5%
Difference in tumour type	5%	
Difference in grading	4%	
Presence of tumour	1.5%	
No discrepancy, no confirmation (sampling error, border zone, necrosis)		12.5%
Diagnosis from smear preparation only	11.5%	
Diagnosis from paraffin section only	1%	

showed a confirmation of the cytological diagnosis by subsequent histological examination of additional samples in 462 cases (77%). The cytological diagnosis had to be substantially changed in 63 cases (10.5%), with discrepancies related to tumour type or grading in 54 (9%) cases. A diagnostic error in smear preparations concerning the presence of tumour tissue occurred in 9 cases (1.5%). In 75 cases (12.5%) the verification by one procedure alone was not possible. This was predominantly due to sampling errors:

the biopsy material of one of the two methods employed contained a border zone of the lesion or consisted only of necrotic or hemorrhagic areas. In these cases, the final diagnosis was usually based on the intraoperative smear preparation.

Major Problems in the Histological Evaluation of Stereotactic Biopsies

Sample size. In neoplasms with a homogeneous tissue architecture, *e.g.* pilocytic astrocytomas, grade II astrocytomas and oligodendrogliomas, the sample volume of 1 mm^3 proved to be sufficient for diagnostic evaluation. However, in tumours with varying tissue components, *e.g.* anaplastic gliomas, craniopharyngeomas, teratoid and metastatic tumours, the small sample size was in several cases the cause of diagnostic errors (Table 4). In large hemispheric gliomas the sample size can be increased using a larger forceps or other devices such as the biopsy needle designed by Sedan[11]. However, in functionally important deep-seated structures (basal ganglia, hypothalamus, brain stem) the removal of larger samples carries the risk of postoperative neurological deficits. In our view, the disadvantages of the small sample size can best be compensated by careful targeting of the biopsy site. To that end, the combination of rapid smear preparations with tissue embedding has been proven very useful. Smear preparations often allow the immediate recognition of tumour borders and can thus be used to guide the removal of samples for paraffin and plastic embedding. This makes it mandatory that the neuropathologist is present during the operation.

The *distinction between reactive gliosis and the infiltration zone of gliomas* constitutes another difficulty which is, however, not unique to stereotactic samples. The precise estimation of tumour borders is of great importance for the calculation of tumour volume when subsequent interstitial radiotherapy is employed. In our view, no reliable morphologic criteria can be defined to distinguish reactive astrocytes from neoplastic cells in the periphery of a differentiated astrocytoma.

Recent Advances in Histopathological Tumour Typing

In recent years considerable progress has been made in the use of immunohistochemical techniques for the location of cell and tumour markers. In the nervous system the presence of glial fibrillary acidic protein (GFAP) has been used to estimate the extent of glial differentiation and to distinguish differentiated gliomas from intracranial non-glial and metastatic tumours[3,10]. The significance of the detection of GFAP in gliomas is, however, severely reduced by the presence of this protein in both reactive and neoplastic astrocytes. The possibility exists that neoplastic glial cells possess surface antigens which can be detected immunohistochemically using monoclonal antibodies. At present specific markers have only been developed for anaplastic gliomas[2]. Identification of sarcomas and metastatic carcinomas has become possible by the use of monoclonal antibodies[7] to their cytoskeleton proteins (vimentin, cytokeratins). In the future, the advances in immunohistochemical detection of specific marker proteins will greatly reduce the limitations imposed by the small sample size of stereotactic brain tumour biopsies.

Acknowledgement

We wish to thank Drs. Mundinger, Ostertag and associates, Abteilung Stereotaxie und Neuronuklearmedizin, Neurochirurgische Klinik der Universität Freiburg, for their cooperation.

References

1. Adams, J. H., Graham, D. I., Doyle, D., Brain biopsy. The smear technique for neurosurgical biopsies. London: Chapman and Hall. 1981.
2. Carrel, S., de Tribolet, N., Mach, J.-P., Expression of neuroectodermal antigens common to melanomas, gliomas, and neuroblastomas. Acta Neuropathol. (Berl.) *57* (1982), 158—164.
3. Deck, J. H. N., Eng, L. F., Bigbee, J., Woodcock, S. M., The role of glial fibrillary acidic protein in the diagnosis of central nervous system tumors. Acta Neuropathol. (Berl.) *42* (1978), 183—190.
4. Kautzky, R., Die Schnelldiagnose intracranieller Erkrankungen mit Hilfe des supravital gefärbten Quetschpräparats. Virchows Arch. Path. Anat. *320* (1951), 495—550.
5. Kiessling, M., Anagnostopoulos, J., Lombeck, G., Kleihues, P., Diagnostic potential of stereotactic biopsy of brain tumours. A report of 400 cases. In: Tumours of the central nervous system in infancy and childhood, Vol. 1 (Voth, D., Gutjahr, P., Langmaid, C., eds.), pp. 245—256. Berlin-Heidelberg-New York: Springer. 1982.
6. Mundinger, F., CT-Stereotactic biopsy of brain tumours. In: Tumours of the central nervous system in infancy and childhood. Vol. 1 (Voth, D., Gutjahr, P., Langmaid, C., eds.), pp. 234—246. Berlin-Heidelberg-New York: Springer. 1982.
7. Osborn, M., Weber, K., Biology of disease. Tumor diagnosis by intermediate filament typing: A novel tool for surgical pathology. Laboratory Invest. *48* (1983), 372—394.

8. Ostertag, C. B., Mennel, H. D., Kiessling, M., Stereotactic biopsy of brain tumors. Surg. Neurol. *14* (1980), 275—283.
9. Pecker, J., Scarabin, J. M., Brucher, J. M., Vallée, B., Stereotactic approach to diagnosis and treatment of cerebral tumors. Paris: Laboratoires Pierre Fabre. 1979.
10. Roessmann, U., Velasco, M. E., Gambetti, P., Autilio-Gambetti, L., Neuronal and astrocytic differentiation in human neuroepithelial neoplasms. An immunohistochemical study. J. Neuropathol. exp. Neurol. *42* (1983), 113—121.
11. Sedan, R., Peragut, J.-C., Vallicioni, P., Présentation d'un appareillage original pour biopsie cérébrale et tumorale en conditions stéréotaxiques. Communication à la société de neurochirurgie de langue Française. 1975.
12. Szikla, G. (ed.), Stereotactic cerebral irradiation. Proc. INSERM Symposium on stereotactic irradiations held in Paris. Amsterdam-New York-Oxford: Elsevier/North Holland Biomedical Press. 1979.
13. Zülch, K. J., Histological typing of tumours of the central nervous system. Geneva: World Health Organization. 1979.

Section II

Cerebral Tumours

1. Stereotactic Biopsy

Acta Neurochirurgica, Suppl. 33, 185—194 (1984)

Some Correlations Between Histological and CT Aspects of Cerebral Gliomas Contributing to the Choice of Significant Trajectories for Stereotactic Biopsies

C. Daumas-Duport[1], V. Monsaingeon[1], J. P. N'Guyen[4], O. Missir[2], and G. Szikla[3]

With 4 Figures

Summary

To achieve a significant sampling in polymorphous and more or less infiltrative growths such as glial tumours is one of the major problems of stereotactic biopsies.

Authors discuss the histological and cytological criteria used by them to establish the boundaries between glioma and normal brain. Obviously peripheral areas infiltrated by outgrowing isolated tumour cells should be taken into consideration to determine the tumour volume.

Extent of such areas and relative frequency of more or less infiltrating forms are appreciated on the basis of serial biopsies obtained in a series of 100 astrocytomas, oligodendrocytomas and oligo-astrocytomas. Results show that inclusion of adjacent parenchyma infiltrated by isolated tumour cells increased considerably the tumour volume as compared to the volume of the central "tumour tissue proper".

In 24 cases of the same series preferential CT aspects corresponding to histologically different components such as "tumour tissue", infiltrated areas, tumour vascularity, peritumoural edema together with a comparison of the volume of the lesion shown by the CT and the histological tumour volume were studied.

These data are in favor of serial biopsies along trajectories corresponding to different CT aspects of the lesion.

---

[1] Department of Pathology, [2] Department of Radiology, [3] Department of Neurosurgery, C. H. Sainte-Anne, 1 rue Cabanis, F-75674 Paris Cedex, France, [4] Department of Neurosurgery, Hôpital H. Mondor, Créteil, France.

Taking into account the well known infiltrative and polymorphous nature of glial growths, this protocol might give less fragmentary and more reliable histological information necessary for therapy planning.

Keywords: Supratentorial gliomas; stereotactic biopsies; CT scan.

Introduction

How to get optimal *i.e.* as complete and reliable bioptic information as possible on polymorphous and infiltrative tumours like gliomas with a minimum of samples?

To try to answer such a question and in order to extract the pertinent information from CT scan performed prior to biopsy, we studied the correlations between histological and CT data.

As for therapeutic purposes evaluation of tumour volume is obviously of prime importance, histological criteria of tumour volume delimination will be considered first.

Histological Criteria of Tumour Volume Delimitation

1. Cytologic Criteria of Tumour Volume Delimitation

To determine the volume of gliomas, it seems indispensible to include not only tumour tissue proper (Fig. 1) but also the extent of peripheral areas infiltrated by outgrowing isolated tumour cells (Fig. 2).

At a first glance, such areas may seem to be only edematous parenchyma, but careful cytological study may reveal isolated tumour cells (Fig. 2). Isolated tumour cells can be recognized by their bulky and irregular nuclei and the apparent lack of cytoplasm, giving them a characteristic aspect of "nude nuclei cell" (Fig. 3).

Nuclear abnormalities and lack of cytoplasm allow to distinguish tumour cells from reactive astrocytes. The latter have nuclei of regular shape and a large cytoplasm with thin cytoplasmic processes (Fig. 4).

Since both the number of isolated tumour cells in the samples may be limited, and their nuclear abnormalities allowing to recognize them may be slight, detection of such cells requires optimal technical conditions, detailed elsewhere in this volume[3].

As the presence of isolated tumour cells usually coincides with edema, areas of peritumoral edema should be studied with a special attention.

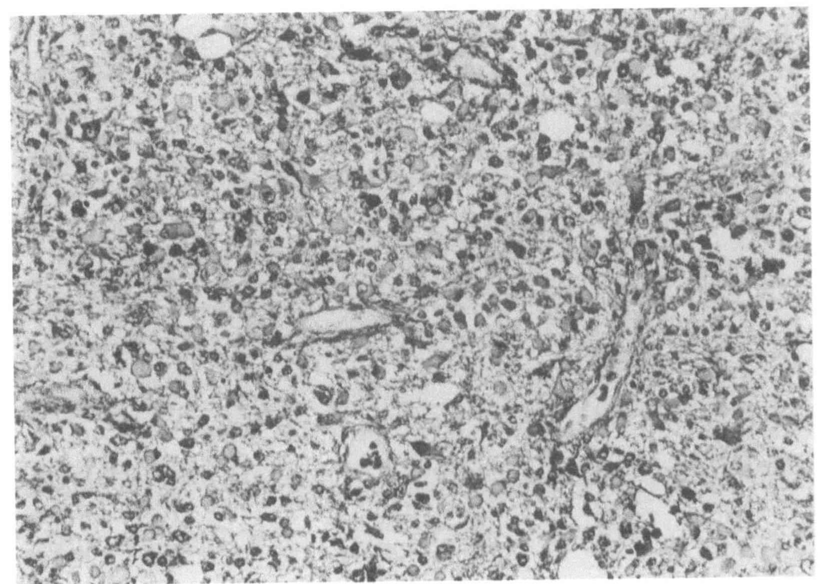

Fig. 1. Tumour tissue proper (HES × 1,000)

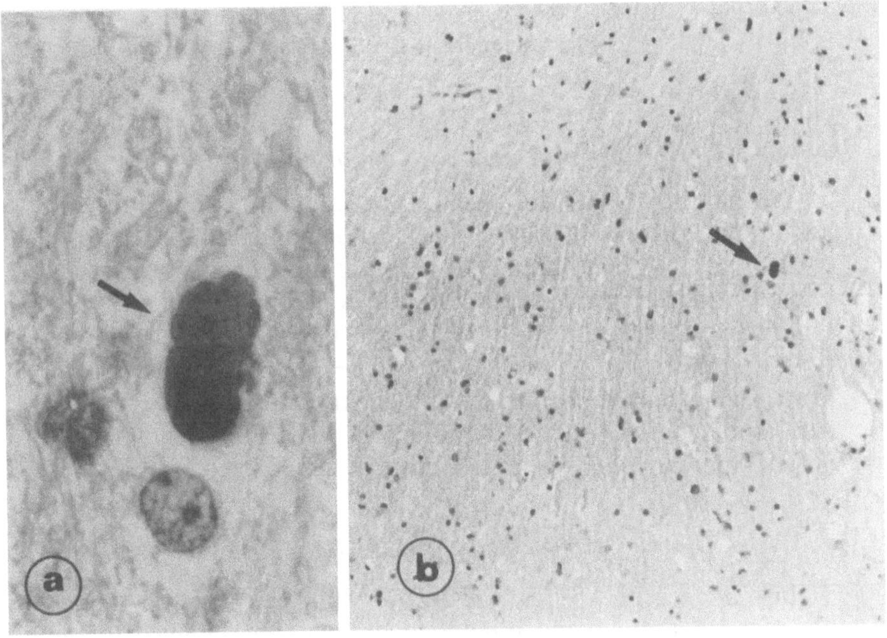

Fig. 2. Edematous parenchyma infiltrated by "isolated tumour cells". (a) HES × 4,000; (b) HES × 325

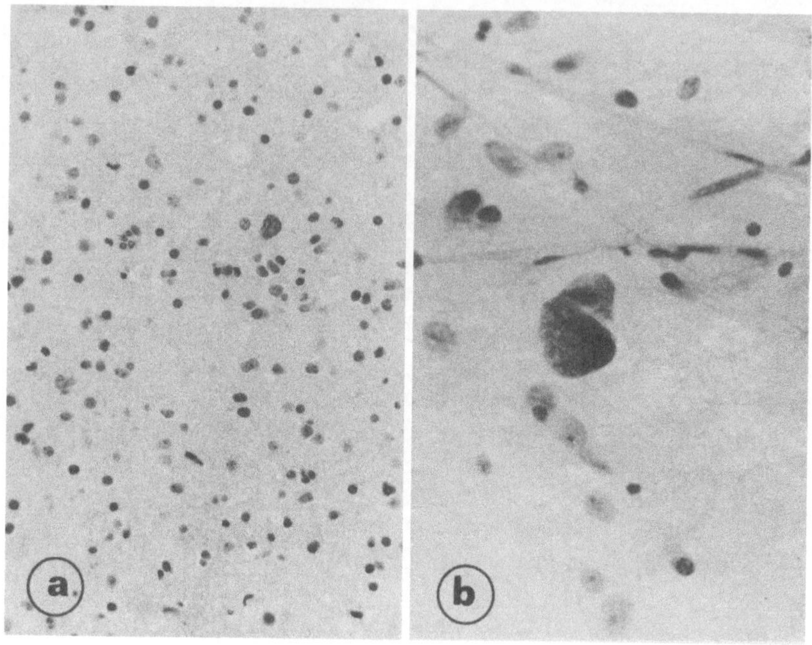

Fig. 3. Isolated tumour cells ("nude cell nuclei"). a) paraffin (HES × 1,000), b) smears technique (HES × 4,000)

2. *Spatial Configuration of Gliomas*

Distinction of two histological aspects: "tumour tissue proper", and "isolated tumour cells" lead us to distinguish three types of gliomas according to their 3D configuration (Table 1): type I: gliomas which appear as tumour tissue proper, with no or only very limited peripheral infiltration beyond the main core of the tumour; type II: infiltrating gliomas showing, beyond the tumour tissue proper, an extensive peripheral area infiltrated by isolated tumour cells, and type III: isolated tumour cells infiltrating recognizable nervous parenchyma, without tumour tissue proper.

3. *Tumour Volume*

In a recent series of 100 biopsied astrocytomas, oligodendrocytomas and oligoastrocytomas, 60 belonged to the infiltrating group (3D type II), 25 to type I, 15 to type III. In the sixty gliomas type II, inclusion of adjacent parenchyma infiltrated

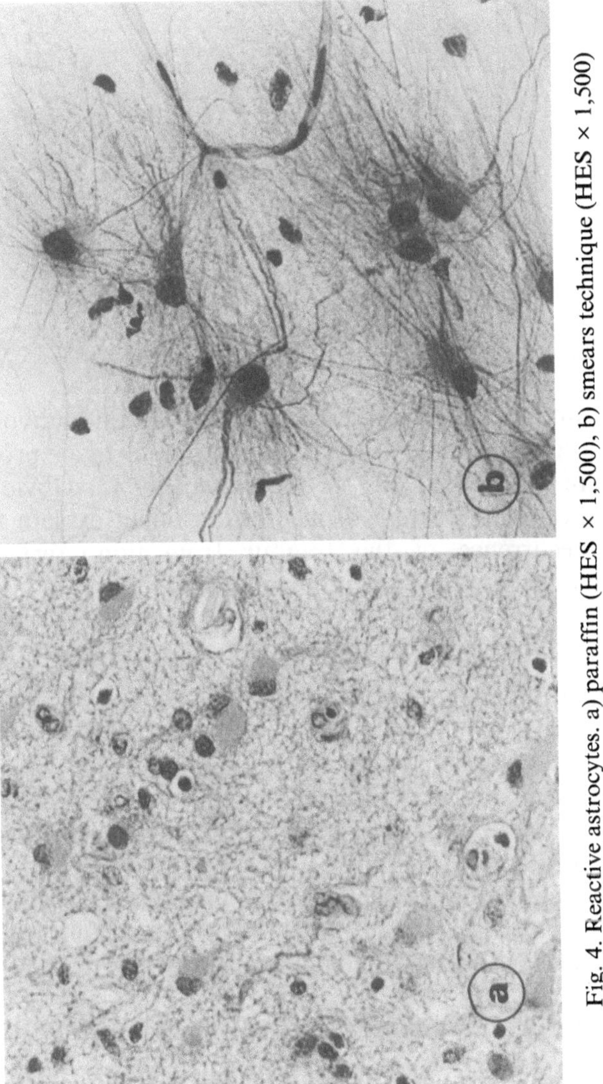

Fig. 4. Reactive astrocytes. a) paraffin (HES × 1,500), b) smears technique (HES × 1,500)

Table 1. *Spatial Configuration of Gliomas*

Spatial configuration	Tumour tissue	Isolated tumour cells
Type I	+	0
Type II	+	+
Type III	0	+

by isolated tumour cells increased considerably the tumour volume as compared to the volume of the central "tumour tissue proper" (× 2 or more in ~80%, × 3 or more in ~40%). Obviously, underestimation of the extent of infiltration might explain for a great part recurrence of the tumour from non-resected or insufficiently irradiated peripheral areas.

Correlative Study of Histological and CT Data

For a better understanding of correlations between histological and CT aspects of gliomas, it might be useful to recall the following main histological characteristics (see Figs. 1 and 2).

The "tumour tissue" component has new formed microscopic blood vessels, tumour cells are in contact and the parenchyma is no longer recognizable.

Areas corresponding to "isolated tumour cells" are devoid of new formed blood vessels, and presence of isolated tumour cells usually coincides with parenchymal edema.

1. "Qualitative" Comparison Between Histological and CT Data

In a preliminary study[1] contrast enhancement has been compared with the following histological parameters: microscopic tumour vascularity, 3 D configuration and malignancy.

This study concerned 50 gliomas (astrocytomas, oligo-astrocytomas and oligodendrocytomas) explored by serial stereotactic biopsies.

Only presence or absence of contrast enhancement was considered. Malignancy and 3 D configuration was evaluated according to our double histologic codification of gliomas[2]. Tumour vascularity (TV) was subjectively graded 0 to + + + + (TV = 0: lack of neovascularization). Results are shown in Tables 2 to 4.

Table 2 shows that there is no contrast enhancement in tumours graded TV = 0 and TV = +, while contrast enhancement is

Table 2. *Contrast enhancement—tumour microscopic vascularity (T. V.)*

Tumour vascularity	Contrast enhancement	No contrast enhancement	Hyperdensity on plain scan	Total
TV = 0	0	8		8
TV = +	1 (limited + +)	4		5
TV = + +	6	7	1	14
TV = + + +	15	0	4	19
TV = + + + +	4	0		4
Total	26	24		50

constant in tumours graded TV = + + + and TV = + + + + (except in calcified tumours with hyperdensity on plain scan).

Correlation between tumour vascularity and contrast enhancement seems fairly constant.

Table 3 shows that contrast enhancement is constant in gliomas 3 D type I, (except in 1 case with hyperdensity on plain scan), it is absent in gliomas 3 D type III, and variable in gliomas 3 D type II. In this last group contrast enhancement appeared linked to tumour vascularity.

There appears a relationship between CT contrast enhancement and histological 3 D configuration of gliomas.

In Table 4, contrast enhancement is compared with malignancy. Contrast enhancement is constant in malignant gliomas, but is also present in all other grades. *Apparently there is no direct correlation between malignancy and contrast enhancement.*

Table 3. *Contrast Enhancement—3 D Configuration (N = 50)*

3 D Configuration	n	Contrast enhancement	No contrast enhancement	% Contrast enhancement
Type I	16	15	0 + 1 hyperdensity on plain scan	~ 100%
Type II	26	11	15	42%
Type III	8	0	8	0%

Table 4. *Contrast Enhancement—Malignancy (N = 50)*

Malignancy	N	Contrast enhancement	No contrast enhancement	% Contrast enhancement
A (~ grade 1)	14	10*	4	70%
B (~ grade 2)	20	6	14	30%
C (~ grade 3)	10	4	6	40%
Malignant (~ grade 4)	6	6	0	100%

* Including 8 Pilocytic Astrocytomas.

2. Topographic Comparison Between CT and Bioptic Data

Few days after bioptic examination, biopsy tracks may be visualised on post contrast CT scan as a rectilinear contrast enhancement.

In 26 post contrast CT studies where previous biopsy tracks were clearly recognizable the topographic relationship of histological and CT aspects could be established with precision.

In six type I gliomas, contrast enhancement coincided with "tumour tissue proper", low attenuation areas with edema.

In sixteen type II cases, areas with contrast enhancement present in 12 cases corresponded to tumour tissue while low attenuation areas corresponded to edematous parenchyma infiltrated by isolated tumour cells and partially to plain edema. Samples taken in normal density areas did not contain tumour cells.

In four 3D type III cases, the low attenuation area corresponded to edematous parenchyma, with no tumour cells in normal density areas. This latter finding *i.e.* absence of infiltrating tumour cells in normal density areas is however based on a limited number of samples (9) and needs therefore confirmation in further cases.

The above data show that enhanced areas correspond to tumour tissue proper and that peripheral low attenuation areas often called "peritumoral edema", though actually related to edema, may correspond either to plain edema or to edematous infiltrated parenchyma.

This observation confirms that the tumour volume cannot be determined from CT data alone. Our data suggest however that in gliomas "3 D type I" the enhanced area is likely to correspond to the tumour volume. The same might be true for 3 D type III lesions where the low attenuation areas seem to coincide with the presence of scattered tumour cells, at least in the four cases where a more detailed correlation could be established.

Choice of Biopsy Trajectories

Stereotactic biopsies aim to provide optimal histological information for therapy planning; for most gliomas, beyond data on the histological type and grade of malignancy, information on 3 D configuration and tumour volume may be of practical interest.

In order to get optimal histological information, trajectories should provide samples from different attenuation areas in post-contrast CT. Along these tracks serial biopsy samples should be taken from the periphery to the tumour central core, including peripheral low attenuation areas. Intra-operative histology of each sample by smear preparation[3] allows to check the necessity of further biopsies.

In our experience, the use of intraoperative smears and better knowledge of CT-histological correlations contribute to obtain optimal bioptic information with a minimum of trajectories.

Reliability of serial stereotactic biopsies has been studied in a recent series of 268 patients (January 1979 to October 1982). Detailed results are given elsewhere in this volume[3].

As a conclusion we feel that biopsy procedures performed according to the above mentioned data furnish useful and reliable information contributing to therapy planning.

References

1. Daumas-Duport, C., Meder, J. F., Monsaingeon, V., Missir, O., Aubin, M. L., Szikla, G., Cerebral gliomas: malignancy, limits and spatial configuration. Comparative data from serial stereotactic biopsies and computed tomography (a preliminary study based on 50 cases). J. Neuroradiology *10* (1983), 51—80.
2. Daumas-Duport, C., Monsaingeon, V., Szenthe, L., Szikla, G., Serial stereotactic biopsies: a double histological code of gliomas according to malignancy and 3 D-configuration, as an aid to therapeutic decision and assessment of results. Proc. 8th Meeting World Soc. Stereotactic and Functional Neurosurgery, Part III, Zurich 1981, Appl. Neurophysiol. *45* (1982), 431—437.
3. Monsaingeon, V., Daumas-Duport, C., Mann, M., Miyahara, S., Szikla, G., Stereotactic sampling biopsies in a series of 268 consecutive cases—validity and technical aspects. 6th Meeting European Soc. Stereotactic and Functional Neurosurgery Rome 1983 (in this volume). In: Advances in Stereotactic and Functional Neurosurgery 6 (Gybels, J., *et al.,* eds), pp. 193—198. Acta Neurochir. (Wien) Suppl. *33*. Wien-New York: Springer. 1984.

Acta Neurochirurgica, Suppl. 33, 195—200 (1984)

Stereotactic Sampling Biopsies in a Series of 268 Consecutive Cases—Validity and Technical Aspects

V. Monsaingeon[1], C. Daumas-Duport[1], M. Mann[1], S. Miyahara[2], and G. Szikla[2]

With 2 Figures

Summary

Reliability of bioptic informations is obviously related to technical aspects. In our experience:

The Sedan-Vallicioni "guillotine" trocar yields bigger and more satisfactory samples than biopsy forceps.

Routinely performed extemporaneous smears on each sample give useful cytologic data and may help to reorient biopsies.

Glutaraldehyde fixation of the remaining material, allowing light and electron microscope study, gives cytological details of paramount importance (differential diagnosis of glioma with gliosis).

Reliability of histological data, in a series of 268 consecutive cases, is assessed by comparison with histology after subsequent surgical removal and with follow-up data (non tumoral lesions).

Keywords: Stereotactic sampling biopsies; histological technique.

Serial stereotactic biopsies, performed to establish histological type—and malignancy—of tumours, can contribute to 3D localization of tumour limits[1].

Reliability of bioptic informations depends essentially on adequate localization of samples[2], but is obviously related to histological technique.

---

[1] Department of Pathology, [2] Department of Neurosurgery, C. H. Sainte Anne, 1 rue Cabanis, F-75014 Paris Cedex, France.

Technique

At our unit, biopsies are sampled with the Sedan-Vallicioni "guillotine" trocar. Their size is 15 mm long and 1 to 1.5 mm diametre.

Systematic extemporaneous smears of each sample are made, cutting off a small piece at both ends.

After absolute alcohol fixation (30 sec min) smears are stained with Hematein-Phloxin (one minute each) and examined.

Samples are fixed in glutaraldehyde (6.5% of a basic solution of 23%, diluted in Sörensen buffer) and kept at 4 °C for at least 3 hours.

After a 3 hours minimum rinsing in Sörensen buffer, small samples are taken for electron microscopy. The remaining tissue is deshydrated and embedded in paraffin in the usual way.

Results

Between january 1979 and october 1982, stereotactic sampling biopsies have been achieved in 268 consecutive patients, according to our bioptic protocol[3] and to this technique. Systematic extemporaneous smears are used only since 1981.

Diagnosis are given in Table 1.

Table 1. *Results*. N: 268 stereotactic bioptic examination (1979–1982)

Tumors		207–77%
Gliomas	160	
Ependymomas	6	
Pineal tumours	10	
Meningiomas	8	
Metastasis	5	
Other tumours	6	
Unclassified tumours	12	
Cysts, dysplasia, hamartomas		9– 4%
Non tumoral lesions		44–16%
Gliosis—glioma?		5– 2%
False negative*		3– 1%

* Previously to routine smears.

Reliability of results may be studied by comparison with:

a) histology after subsequent surgical removal (Table 2),

b) follow-up data: amongst 43 non tumoral lesions, follow-up of 35 patients is known (24 longer than 1 year). One patient died two

Table 2. *Reliability. Surgical Removal (n = 24)*

Concordant diagnosis (including grading of gliomas)		22
Gliomas	12	
Other tumours	7	
Non tumoral lesions	3*	
Previously non classified tumour**		1**
Discordant diagnosis (gliosis-glioma done previously to routine smears)		1

* Epilepsy surgery.

** Non significant sampling: very hard tissue.

months after biopsy, and no necropsy was performed. The other 34 patients are improved or stabilized without clinical and CT data suggesting tumour growth.

Discussion

According to our experience:

The Sedan-Vallicioni "guillotine" trocar yields large size samples, not distorded by compression, in opposition to forceps samples. Such specimens provide more reliable histological informations, and avoid artefacts which hinder reading and might induce misinterpretation.

Glutaraldehyde fixation is preferable to formaldehyde (Fig. 1). At first, it gives more cytological details (cytoplasm and nuclei) of paramount importance, especially for precise delimitation of gliomas and differential diagnosis of glioma with gliosis. Secondly, such a fixation allows to use the same sample as well for optic as for electron microscopy.

Routinely performed extemporaneous smears give useful cytologic data, complementary to those obtained with paraffin-embedding (Fig. 2). Hematein-Phloxin stain of the smears demonstrates entire cells with more cytological details than Methylen-Blue.

Immediate control allows to check the necessity of further samples, contributing to get optimal informations with a minimum of samples[2]. It may help to reorient biopsies (small CT lesions might be missed).

Actually, our three "false negatives" have been diagnosed previously to routine smears.

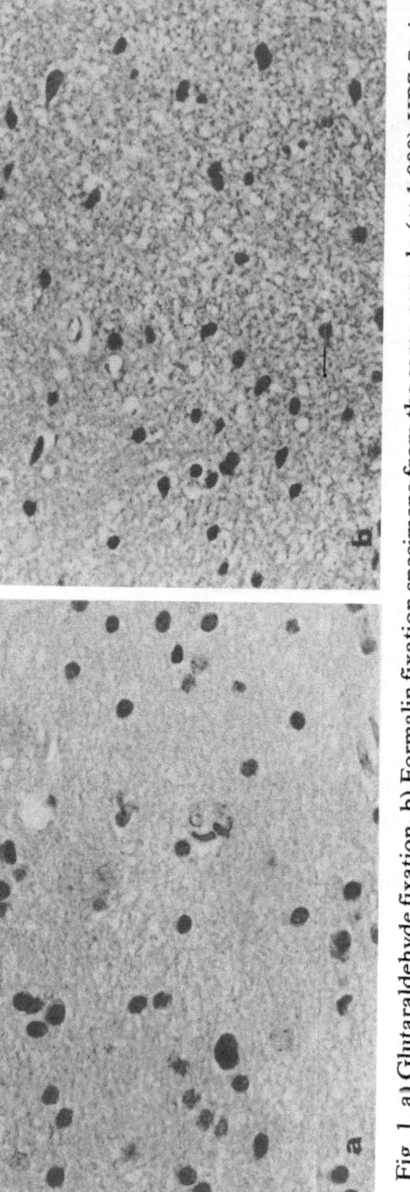

Fig. 1. a) Glutaraldehyde fixation, b) Formalin fixation specimens from the same sample (× 1,000) HPS Stain

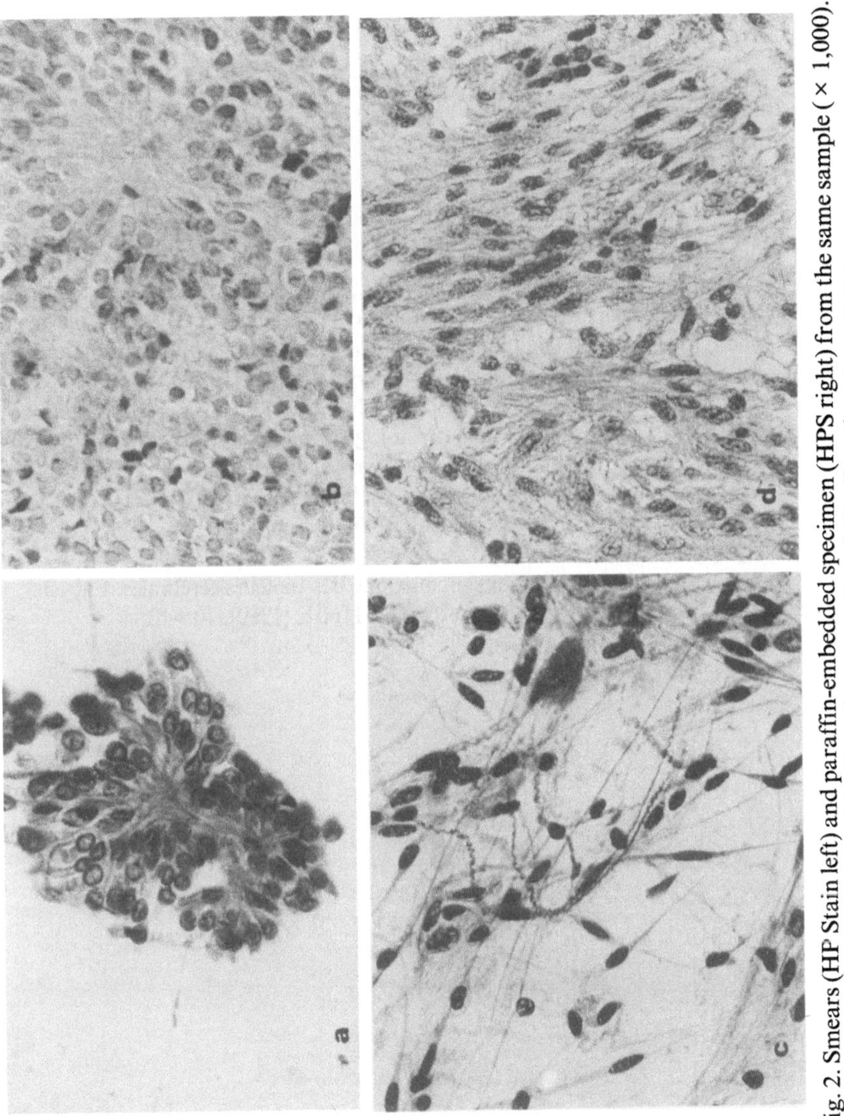

Fig. 2. Smears (HP Stain left) and paraffin-embedded specimen (HPS right) from the same sample (× 1,000). a) and b) Ependymoma, c) and d) pilocytic astrocytoma

Conclusion

CT oriented serial stereotactic sampling biopsies performed with:

— Sedan trocar,

— Glutaraldehyde fixation,

— Routine extemporaneous smears yield as reliable histological informations as craniotomy specimens, and furthermore give significant data on tumour volume and 3 D delimitation.

References

1. Daumas-Duport, C., Monsaingeon, V., Szenthe, L., Szikla, G., Serial stereotactic biopsies: a double histological code of gliomas according to malignancy and 3 D configuration, as an aid to therapeutic decision and assessment of results. Appl. Neuro. Physiol. *45* (1982), 431—437.
2. Daumas-Duport, C., Monsaingeon, V., N'Guyen, J. P., Missir, O., Szikla, G., Some correlations between histological and CT aspects of cerebral gliomas, contributing to the choice of significant biopsy tracks. In: Advances in Stereotactic and Functional Neurosurgery 6 (Gybels, J., *et al.*, eds.), pp. 183—192. Acta Neurochir. (Wien), Suppl. 33. Wien-New York: Springer. 1984.
3. Szikla, G., Blond, S., Bilan stéréotaxique des tumeurs cérébrales. Encycl. Med. Chir. Paris, Radiodiagnostic II, 31160 E (1980), 10—12.

Acta Neurochirurgica, Suppl. 33, 201—205 (1984)

The Reliability of Stereotactic Biopsy

M. Scerrati[1] and G. F. Rossi

Summary

The reliability of the informations provided by stereotactic biopsy of expanding cerebral lesions was analyzed. Out of 68 patients, studied with stereotactic biopsy, 14 were subsequently submitted to surgery and 5 to autopsy. In 18 cases there was a perfect correspondence between the diagnosis based on biopsy and that based on surgery or autopsy. In one case the tumor was missed at biopsy. The reliability of stereotactic biopsy seems related to the modality of its planning and execution and to the experience of the neuropathologist.

Keywords: Cerebral tumors; stereotactic biopsy.

Introduction

The appropriate treatment of intracranial space occupying lesions should be based on the knowledge of their nature. Clinical and radiological findings cannot be sufficient[3,8]. Stereotactic biopsy seems to be apt to reach such a knowledge[2-8]. However, taking into account the well known polymorphism of certain cerebral tumors, the objection can be raised that stereotactic biopsy might not provide complete and, therefore, reliable informations[1]. We thought it useful to check the consistency of such a risk on our personal material.

Material and Method

Sixty-eigth stereotactic biopsies performed from October 1979 to May 1983 in patients harbouring brain expanding lesions are considered. 41 patients were male, 27 female, the age ranging between 5 and 73 years. The Talairach or Leksell stereotactic apparatus were used. The biopsy was carried out after a series of neuroradiological investigations (CT scan, cerebral angiography, and in certain

[1] Istituto di Neurochirurgia, Università Cattolica del Sacro Cuore, Largo A. Gemelli, 8, I-00168 Roma, Italy.

cases ventriculography) aiming at: 1. the accurate spatial definition of the lesion; 2. the precise spatial relation between the lesion and the stereotactic instrument[4-8].

The biopsies were performed along 1 or more (up to 3) tracks. Specimens were taken stepwise at a distance of 5 to 10 mm. The central and the peripheral parts of the lesion as well as the surrounding brain tissue were explored. The forceps we used was designed in our laboratory by Dr. Gentilomo[5]: it works by combining aspiration and section. The cylinders of the tissue obtained have a length of about 10–12 mm and a diameter of 1.5–2 mm. The specimens were fixed in 10% formalin, embedded in paraffin and cut at 4 μ; they were then stained with standard or, if necessary, special methods.

Results

The histological diagnosis of the lesions explored by stereotactic biopsy is shown in Table 1. The majority of them were tumors derived from neuroepithelial tissue (54 cases), among which astrocytomas were the most frequent. Non glial tumors were found in 8 cases. In 5 cases the lesions were non-neoplastic. In one case, the biopsy was negative.

The location of the biopsied lesions was the cerebral hemispheres in 48 cases, the third ventricle and diencephalon in 17 cases, and in 3 cases the region of the midbrain, pons and IV ventricle.

A comparison between the histological diagnosis based on the stereotactic specimens and on the corresponding surgical or autoptical material could be made in 19 patients (Table 2). A full agreement was achieved in all operated patients (14 patients) and in 4 out of the 5 who underwent autopsy. In the remaining case, the one with negative biopsy, it turned out at autopsy that the bioptic forceps had missed a small pontine glioma.

In 21 patients the informations obtained through the stereotactic biopsy gave the opportunity of utilizing the stereotactic procedure itself as a means of treatment: drainage of a neoplastic cyst (9 cases) and interstitial tumoral implant of radioisotopes (12 cases).

Complications

Transient worsening of the patient's neurological status after stereotactic biopsy occurred in 2 patients: the postoperative CT scan revealed a small intralesional hemorrhage.

One patient died 5 days after biopsy: he was suffering from a diffuse astrocytoma involving most of the left hemisphere. The autopsy did not show any evidence of bleeding, but a diffuse and very impressive brain edema.

Table 1. *Diagnosis of 68 Stereotactically Biopsied Lesions (October 1979–May 1983)*

Diagnosis		Number of cases
Tumors of Neuroepithelial Tissue		
Pilocytic Astrocytoma (I)		2
Astrocytoma (II)		18
Oligodendroglioma (II)		8
Mixed Oligoastrocytoma (II)		5
Ganglioglioma (I, II)		1
Anaplastic Astrocytoma (III)		7
Glioblastoma (IV)		12
Anaplastic Plexuspapilloma (III, IV)		1
	Total	54
Tumors of other tissues		
Meningioma (I)		1
Craniopharyngioma (I)		2
Germinoma (II–III)		3
Metastasis		1
Primary malignant lymphoma (III, IV)		1
	Total	8
Non-neoplastic Lesions		
Encephalitis		1
Pseudotumoral Infarct		1
Hystiocytosis X		1
Gliosis		2
	Total	5
Negative		1

Discussion

The results of our study seem to indicate that the risk of obtaining biopsy material from a cerebral expanding lesion is not so high. The similarity of the findings obtained on the material removed through the stereotactic biopsy and on that removed with open surgery or autopsy is quite satisfactory. Though only 19 out of 68 cases in our series could be checked surgically or autoptically, it

Table 2. *Verified Biopsies (October 1979–May 1983)*

Biopsy	Operation	Number of cases
Pilocytic Astrocytoma (I)	Pilocytic Astrocytoma (I)	2
Astrocytoma (II)	Astrocytoma (II)	2
Oligodendroglioma (II)	Oligodendroglioma (II)	4
Oligoastrocytoma (II)	Oligoastrocytoma (II)	3
Ganglioglioma (I, II)	Ganglioglioma (I, II)	1
Meningioma (I)	Meningioma (I)	1
Craniopharyngioma (I)	Craniopharyngioma (I)	1
	Total	14

Biopsy	Autopsy	Number of cases
Astrocytoma (II)	Astrocytoma (II)	1
Oligodendroglioma (II)	Oligodendroglioma (II)	1
Glioblastoma (IV)	Glioblastoma (IV)	2
Negative	Astrocytoma (II)	1
	Total	5

has to be noticed that 17 of them were gliomas, *i.e.* the brain tumors presenting most of the difficulties to the neuropathologist. In our opinion the risks of a misdiagnosis by stereotactic biopsy are low. They are related to the modality of execution of the procedure as well as to the ability of analysis of the bioptic material. The risk can be consistently reduced by carefully planning the biopsy on the basis of the various neuroradiological characteristics. A standard procedure for stereotactic biopsy does not exist. The technique has to be adapted to the single patient. In certain patients a single track with few specimens can be sufficient; this might be the case of extracerebral tumors, which are usually homogeneous. In other cases, multiple sampling of specimens often along more than one track is mandatory. In any case the bioptic material has to be submitted to an expert and very interested neuropathologist.

When the above conditions are satisfied, it is our opinion that stereotactic biopsy represents a real progress in the diagnosis of intracranial lesions and a means which should be available to anyone dealing with the difficult problems of neurooncology.

Acknowledgements

The authors are grateful to Prof. Dr. Giorgio Macchi (Neurological Institute of Catholic University, Rome) for his kind assistance in the neuropathological examinations.

References

1. Gullotta, F., Morphological and biological bases for the classification of brain tumors. In: Advances and Technical Standards in Neurosurgery, Vol. 8 (Krayenbuehl, H., *et al.*, eds.), pp. 122—165. Wien: Springer. 1981.
2. Mundinger, F., The treatment of brain tumors with interstitially applied radioisotopes. In: Radionuclide Applications in Neurology and Neurosurgery (Wang, Y., Paoletti, F., eds.), pp. 199—265. Springfield, Ill.: Ch. C Thomas. 1970.
3. Ostertag, C. B., Mennel, H. D., Kiessling, M., Stereotactic biopsy of brain tumors. Surg. Neurol. *14* (1980), 275—283.
4. Pecker, J., Scarabin, J. M., Brucher, J. M., Vallée, B., Démarche stéréotaxique en neurochirurgie tumorale, pp. 1—301. Paris: Pierre Fabre. 1979.
5. Scerrati, M., Gentilomo, A., Pizzolato, G. P., The role of the stereotactic biopsy in the diagnosis and treatment of brain tumors. Acta Neurol. *2* (1980), 429.
6. Scerrati, M., Pizzolato, G. P., The role of stereotactic biopsy in the 3-dimensional localization of cerebral tumors. Acta Neurochir. (Wien) *57* (1981), 305—306.
7. Scerrati, M., Arcovito, G., D'Abramo, G., Montemaggi, P., Pastore, G., Piermattei, A., Romanini, A., Rossi, G. F., Stereotactic interstitial irradiation of brain tumors: preliminary report. Rays *7* (1982), 93—99.
8. Szikla, G., Stereotactic cerebral irradiation, pp. 1—340. Amsterdam-New York-Oxford: Elsevier, North Holland. 1979.
9. Zülch, K. J., Types histologiques des tumeurs du système nerveux central. Classification histologique internationale des tumeurs. Genève: OMS. 1979.

Acta Neurochirurgica, Suppl. 33, 207—210 (1984)

Intra-Encephalic Stereotactic Biopsies (309 Patients/318 Biopsies)

R. Sedan[1], J. C. Peragut[1], Ph. Farnarier[1], J. Hassoun[2], and M. Sethian[1]

Summary

The authors report their experience of the intra-encephalic stereotactic biopsies.

Their principal aim is the neuropathologic determination of the nature of the lesion.

In a large number of cases (25%), the diagnosis made before biopsy was fundamentally altered by this examination.

Keywords: Sterotaxy; stereotactic biopsies.

At our department, intra-encephalic stereotactic biopsies have been performed since 1976 in order to:

— determine the anatomo-pathological type of the intracranial lesion when its type was not clearly defined by other investigations or when confirmation was necessary before deciding on a purely medical treatment;

— and/or evacuate liquid collections (blood, cystic liquid, pus);

— and/or establish the location of the lesion in order to preserve functional areas or vessels at surgical removal.

These biopsies were performed under the following conditions:

— in order to reduce the risk of complications, the number of biopsy-tracks and of samples were as limited as possible;

— general anesthesia and transcutaneous fixation of the stereotactic frame (without shaving the head) contributed to reduce the surgical stress.

Such stereotactic biopsies carried out according to Talairach's

---

[1] Service de Neurochirurgie Fonctionnelle, [2] Laboratoire de Neuropathologie, Hôpital de la Timone, Marseille, France.

technique with a systematic cerebral angiography do not last more than 1 hour 30 minutes.

Stereotactic angiography allows one to choose a safe avascular area for cerebral puncture.

It allows also one to draw a natural size map of the cerebral cortex which facilitates planning of subsequent open surgery. Samples are systematically investigated extemporaneously essentially to verify that they do correspond to the lesion. They are secondarily investigated in detail (light and electron microscopy). The determination of tumoral volume to plan radioactive isotope implantation was not attempted.

Our original biopsy instrument is constructed on the principle of an aspiration cannula. Cylindrical samples taken by this device measure 1 cm × 2 mm, allowing for detailed anatomo-pathological investigation.

Material

Three hundred and eighteen biopsies were performed in 318 patients. 62% were male patients and 47% were under 50 (20% under 30) years old.

Complications

Complications were rarely observed. This might be explained as follows:

The number of biopsy trajectories was limited, only one trajectory was used in 279 patients (87% cases).

The shortest route was chosen (lateral orthogonal route perpendicular to the median plane of the skull in 289 patients (79.5 cases).

The number of samples was limited, less than 4 in 268 patients (84% cases).

In 14 patients (4.5% cases) haemorrhage occured through the cannula, without any consequence in 13 cases. This was accompanied by a transient paresis in one case.

Two patients died and one presented a regressive hemiplegia, related to biopsy. Fifteen transient complications were observed (hemiparesis: 10, meningitis: 2, miscellaneous: 3).

The patients were selected based on the location of the lesion. In 122 patients (39%), the lesion was situated in a highly functional area and in 119 patients (38%) in a deep cerebral zone.

In 19.5% of cases, biopsy was performed to confirm the diagnosis of glioblastoma and to justify chemotherapy without surgical excision.

In Marseilles, since 1976, the criteria for selecting patients lead us to perform biopsy in only one out of three intracerebral tumours.

The patients who did not undergo stereotactic biopsy had lesions in surgically accessible regions or there was no doubt as to their neuropathological diagnosis.

Results

In most cases, the prebioptic diagnosis was given by the confrontation of clinical, radiological, CT, isotope and angiographic investigations.

1. Biopsy failed in 27 cases: either because interpretation of specimens was impossible (necrosis), or because nervous tissue was normal (the tumour area was missed).

Neuropathological interpretation of specimens was erroneous in 2 cases. Thus it can be claimed that this method was inefficient in 29 cases (9%).

2. Biopsy merely confirmed the previously suspected histological diagnosis in 86 cases (27%) (malignant glioma: 62 cases, 19.5%).

In most cases of this group biopsy was carried out to obtain a neuropathological proof before deciding that only chemotherapy should be applied.

3. Biopsy documented the previously undetermined malignancy grade of gliomas in 123 cases (39%): malignant glioma in 75 cases and benign glioma in 48 cases.

4. Biopsy modified the diagnosis in an important manner, changing the type of treatment in 79 cases (25%). In 18.5% of cases the mistake was serious.

Prebioptic Diagnosis Modified

Prebioptic diagnosis	Nbr	Biopsy diagnosis
Benign tumor	7	Malignant tumor
Malignant tumor	6	Benign tumor
No tumor	13	tumor
Tumor	29	no tumor
Tumor	3	nothing
	58 (18.5%)	

Conclusion

Until new completely atraumatic and reliable methods of cerebral tumour diagnosis become available, carefully performed stereotactic biopsy appears to be an efficient and low risk diagnostic method, which provides important information for therapeutic decisions in problematic cases.

References

1. Broggi, G., Franzini, A., Value of serial stereotactic biopsies and impedance monitoring in the treatment of deep brain tumors. J. Neurol. Neurosurg. Psychiat. *44* (1981), 397—401.
2. Chirossel, J. P., Méthodologie stéréotaxique dans l'approche des tumeurs cérébrales sustentorielles. Thèse, Grenoble. 1977.
3. Daumas-Duport, C., Vedrenne, C., Szikla, G., Contribution of stereotactic biopsies to the 3 D localization of brain tumors, gliomas in particular. In: Stereotactic Cerebral Irradiation (Szikla, G., ed.), pp. 33—41. North Holland-Amsterdam: Elsevier. 1979.
4. Ellis, W. G., Youmans, J. R., Dreyfus, P. M., Diagnostic biopsy for neurological disease. In: Neurological Surgery, Vol. 1 (Youmans, J. R., ed.), pp. 382—422. Philadelphia: W. B. Saunders Company. 1982.
5. Hahn, J. F., Levy, W. J., Weinstein, M. J., Needle biopsy of intracranial lesions guided by computerized tomography. Neurosurgery *5* (1979), 11—15.
6. Ostertag, C. B., Mennel, M. D., Kiessling, M., Stereotactic biopsy of brain tumors. Surg. Neurol. *14* (1980), 275—283.
7. Pecker, J., Scarabin, J. M., Brucher, J. M., Vallee, B., Démarche stéréotaxique en neurochirurgie tumorale. Paris: Laboratoires Pierre Fabre. 1979.
8. Pecker, J., Scarabin, J. M., Brucher, J. M., Vallee, B., Apport des techniques stéréotaxiques au diagnostic et au traitement des tumeurs de la région pinéale. Rev. Neurol. *134* (1978), 287—295.
9. Rushworth, R. G., Stereotactic guided biopsy in the computerized tomographic scanner. Surg. Neurol. *14* (1980), 451—454.
10. Sedan, R., Peragut, J. C., Farnarier, Ph., Hassoun, J., Torres, T., Place de la biopsie en condition stéréotaxique dans le tactique thérapeutique des gliomes malins. Neurochirurgie *27* (1981), 285—286.
11. Sedan, R., Peragut, J. C., Farnarier, Ph., Hassoun, J., Torres-Garcia, T., La biopsie stéréotaxique. Sa place dans le diagnostic des néoformations intracrâniennes. J. Méd. Marseille *2* (1982), 87—88.
12. Waltregny, A., Petrov, V., Brotchi, J., Serial stereotaxic biopsies. Acta Neurochir. (Wien), Suppl. *21* (1974), 221—226.

Acta Neurochirurgica, Suppl. 33, 211—212 (1984)

Diagnostic Accuracy and Multimodal Approach in Stereotactic Biopsies of Deep Brain Tumours

G. Broggi[1], A. Franzini[1], C. Giorgi[1], and A. Allegranza[2]

Introduction

The diagnostic value of stereotactic biopsies of deep brain tumours depends on the accuracy of the target. It is necessary to investigate the different components of pathologic tissue in order to obtain an idea of the spatial extension of the tumour and its boundaries[3]. In 200 stereotactic brain tumour biopsies performed since 1978, the sampling of tissue was guided by a multimodal technique including neuroradiological and neurophysiological investigations.

Methods

After reconstruction of the CT images of a tumour on the stereotactic plain X-ray, the following procedures were performed along the estimated trajectories:

1. Continuous monitoring of tissue impedance was carried out from the cortex to the deeper boundaries of the neoplasm. If it was possible, the impedance recording was performed until healthy tissue beyond the tumor limits was encountered[1].

2. Depth-EEG recording was carried out along the same transtumoral trajectory on the purpose to localize the sites where clearly pathological activity or electric silence were present. In this procedure it was useful to reach tissue with normal activity beyond the tumour in order to obtain more data about the deeper boundaries of the growth[2,3]. At this point of the operation the impedance and EEG data were correlated with the CT scans in order to establish preoperatively the gross structure and extension of the neoplasm and to select the most promising biopsy tracts. The necrotic areas were easily disclosed when low impedance and electrical silence were recorded. The same goes for cystic areas where the impedance was similar to C.S.F. values. The neoplastic proliferating tissue was localized when a clear correspondence existed between these data derived from

[1] Department of Neurosurgery and [2] Division of Neuropathology, Istituto Neurologico "C. Besta", Milano, Italy.

depth measurements and the neuroradiological data including CT scan and angiography. The correct choice of the target was confirmed by intraoperative smear examinations which in our series showed a high diagnostic accuracy.

Results

The correlation of intraoperative smear examinations with paraffin embedded specimens yielded a diagnostic accuracy of about 85% in our series of 200 patients. The histological diagnosis could be verified after the stereotactic procedure in 36 patients who underwent open surgery or had postmortem autoptic examinations. An error in the histological grading of glial tumours was found in two patients with low grade astrocytomas, in one patient with an anaplastic glioma and in one patient with a glioblastoma[4]. The diagnosis of a glioma was correct in 24 cases. In eight patients extra-axial tumours were found and in four patients metastatic tumours. In all of them these diagnoses were in agreement with the biopsy.

References

1. Broggi, G., Franzini, A., Passerini, A., Impedance monitoring during stereotactic biopsy of deep brain tumours. In: Stereotactic Cerebral Irradiation. INSERM symp. no. 12 (Szikla, G., ed.). Amsterdam: Elsevier North Holland. Biomedical press. 1979.
2. Broggi, G., Franzini, A., Giorgi, C., Servello, D., Spreafico, R., Avanzini, G., Focal C.T. hypodense lesions and epilepsy. Depth EEG study and stereotactic biopsy. Acta Neurochir. (1983) in press.
3. Szikla, G., Blond, S., Bilan stéréotaxique des tumeurs cérébrales. Encyclopédie Médico-Chirurgicale, 31660 E, 1981.
4. W.H.O. Histological classification of tumours of the nervous system. Geneva 1979.

Acta Neurochirurgica, Suppl. 33, 213—217 (1984)

Stereotactic Biopsy of Brainstem Tumors

M. Galanda[1,*], **P. Nádvorník**[1], **M. Šramka**[1], and **M. Basandova**[1]

With 4 Figures

Summary

Based upon their experience with 158 stereotactic biopsies from brain tumors, authors consider that their technique of stereotactic biopsy can be applied to brainstem tumors as well. Though the risk of brainstem biopsy seems to be higher, no significant complication has been observed in 12 cases. The transtentorial approach was usually chosen. The tissue sample was obtained by a specially designed needle, allowing to adjust the size of the sample, which is cut off by the outer part of the needle. Previous stimulation of biopsied area is considered useful. In the past pneumoencephalography was used for localization of the lesion, to-day computed tomography makes biopsy more precise. The tissue samples are examined in smear preparations (cytology) and by conventional histological methods.

Keywords: Stereotactic surgery; brainstem tumor biopsy; cytological examination.

Introduction

The brainstem tumors pose serious problems for neurosurgeons. They are usually inoperable, but for radiation therapy the nature of the tumor must be defined. Precise stereotactic biopsy-technique with smear preparation proved to be a suitable approach for deep-seated cerebral lesions (Ostertag *et al.* 1980[2], Nádvorník *et al.* 1976[1]): the same seems to be the case for the brainstem tumors.

[1] Research Institute of Medical Bionic, Bratislava, Czechoslovakia.
* Present address: Kunz, 97400 Banska Bystrica, ČSSR.

Material and Methods

Stereotactic biopsies were taken in 12 patients aged 4 to 55 years.

Previously pneumoencephalography, now mostly CT, angiography, neurological examination and isotope brain scan were used for tumor localization. Biopsy was transtentorially taken with a specially designed cannula using the Mundinger-Riechert stereotactic instrument (Fig. 1). The inner part of the cannula

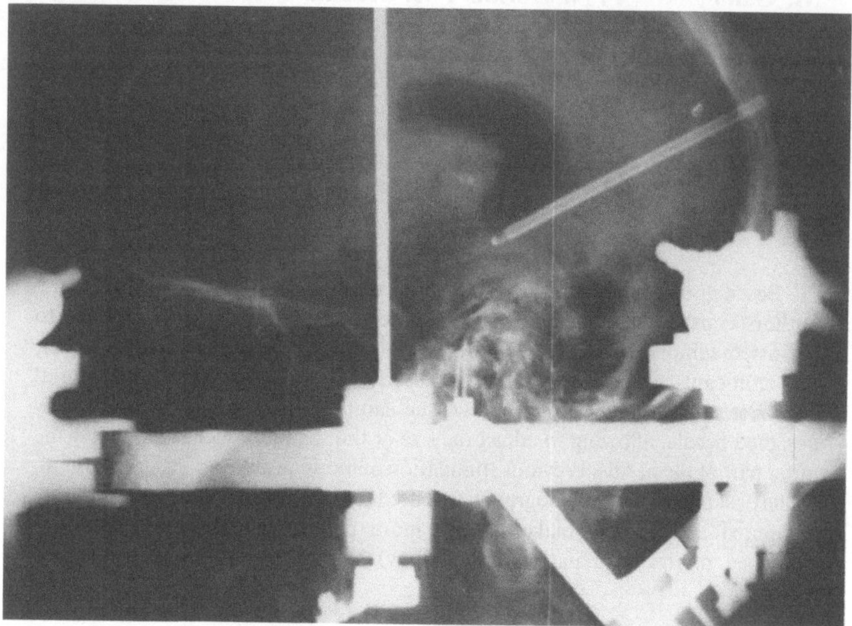

Fig. 1. Transtentorial approach to the brainstem

can be fixed to the stereotactic frame by a special device (Fig. 2). After aspiration of the adjacent brain into the opening, the outer part of the cannula will cut off the sample from the brain instead of tearing it off (Fig. 3). Previous stimulation of the biopsied area is considered useful. After biopsy, the outer part of the cannula remains in place and keeps the region under control. Depending of the size of the lesion several biopsies were stepwise done. The samples were immediately examined cytologically using Loefflers methylene blue stain (Fig. 4) and later histologically.

Results

The method was used for brainstems biopsies in 12 patients. Gliomas were found in 5 patients, clival meningiomas in 2, pituitary

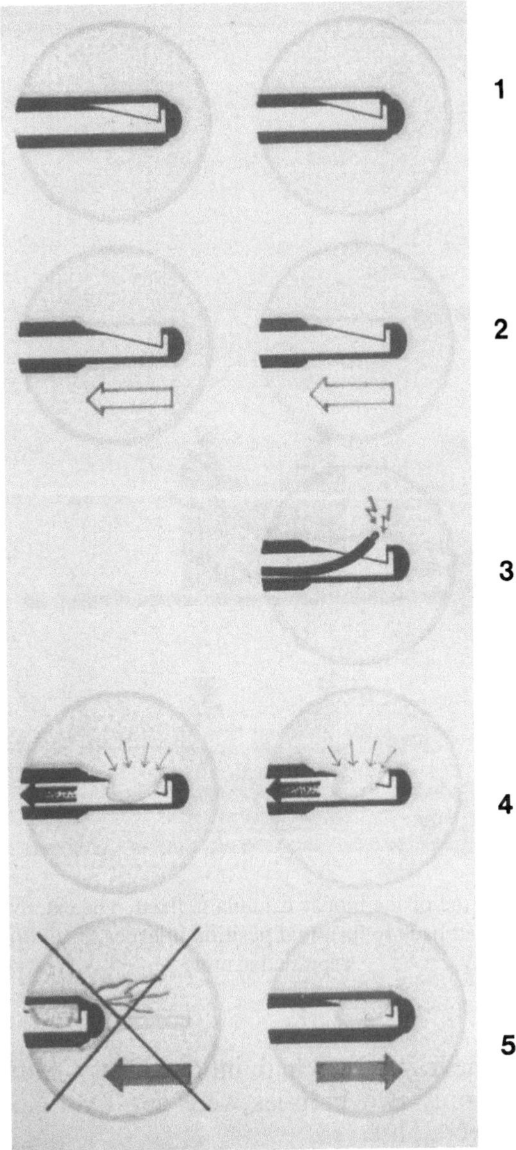

Fig. 2. Biopsy technique. *1* Initial position of biopsy instrument; *2* Withdrawal of the outer part of the cannula; *3* Electrical stimulation; *4* Aspiration of tissue into the open inner tube; *5* Sample is cut off by external tube pushed back to its initial position. Inner tube is withdrawn with the sample. The external tube remains at the biopsy site. Left bottom: tearing of the sample from the brain by pulling out the inner tube should be avoided

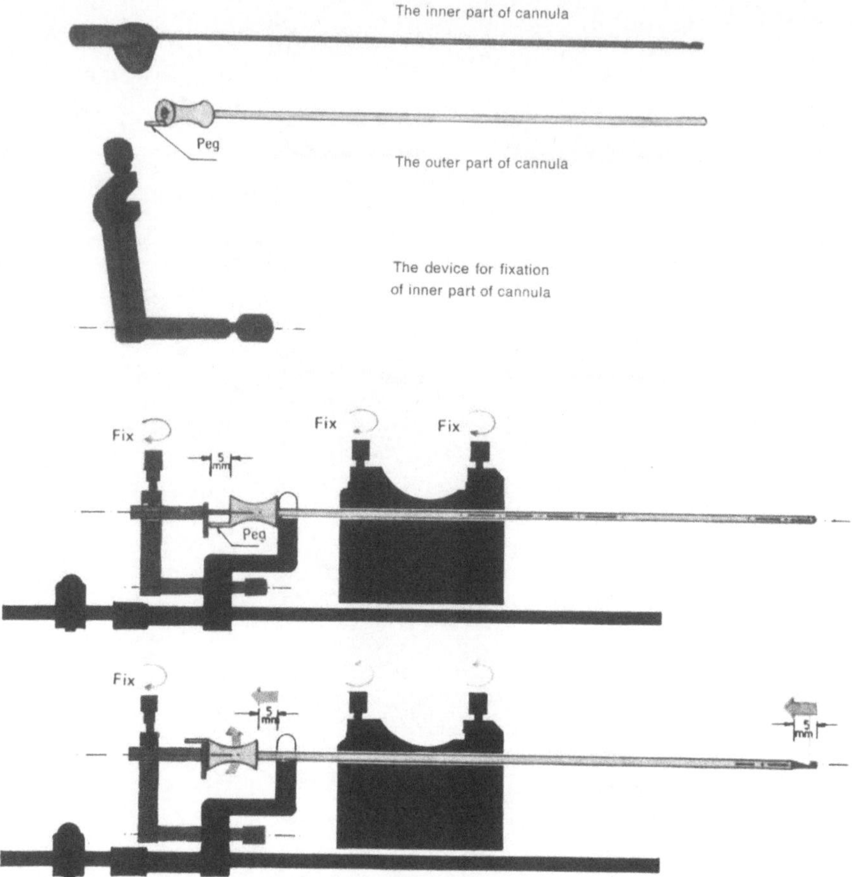

Fig. 3. The inner tube of the biopsy cannula is fixed. The external tube can be withdrawn or pushed back to its initial position in order to cut off smoothly the aspirated sample

adenoma in one case, two had inflammatory changes in the brainstem and only two biopsies were negative. No significant complications were observed.

Discussion

Because of the theoretical risk of possible complications stereotactic biopsy of brainstem lesions is only rarely performed (about 10% in our material). The transtentorial approach however allows direct introduction of the bioptic needle into the lesion with

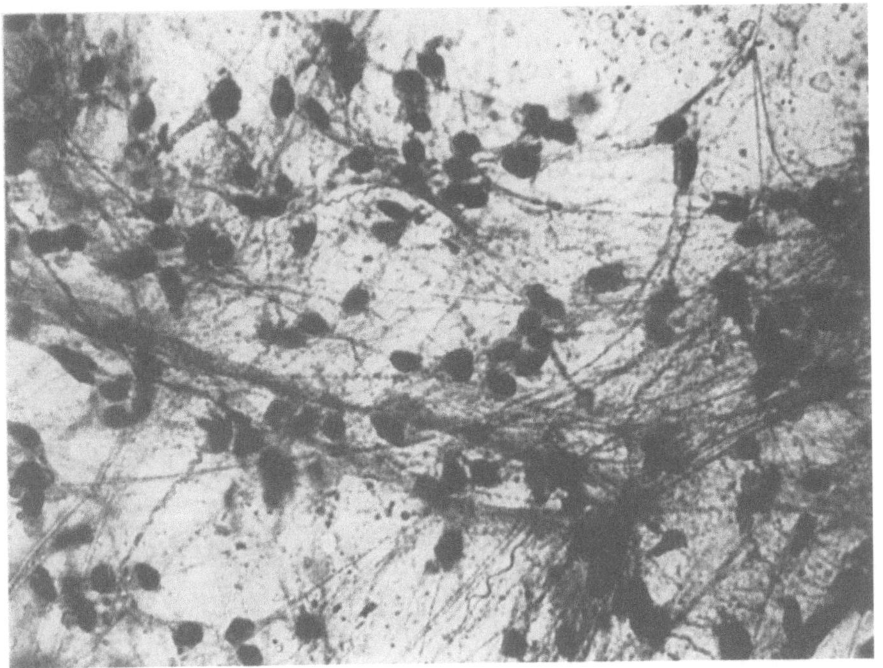

Fig. 4. See text

minimal damage to other brainstem structures. Our specially designed needle makes biopsy safer. According to our experience brainstem biopsy should be considered an adequate method for determination of the nature of lesions in this area of brain.

References

1. Nádvorník, P., Šramka, M., Galanda, M., Stereobiopsia, Rozhl. Chir. 55 (1976), 331—336.
2. Ostertag, C. B., Mennel, H. D., Kiessling, M., Stereotactic biopsy of brain tumors. Surg. Neurol. *14* (1980), 275—283.

Acta Neurochirurgica, Suppl. 33, 219—224 (1984)

Stereotactic Biopsy of Intracranial Processes

F. Mundinger[1] and **W. Birg**[1]

With 8 Figures

For CT-stereotaxis many methods are in use. Here we present our CT-stereotaxis method. The stereotactic device developed by Riechert and Mundinger in the computer compatible version of Mundinger and Birg is fixed at the CT-table by means of a special adjustable holder (Figs. 1 and 2). If the center point of our stereotactic device coincides with the image haircross of the scanner and the headring is plane parallel to the CT-scanning plane (Fig. 3), all the coordinates measured at the CT-screen also hold true for the stereotactic device: no calculation for any stereotactic coordinate, no further reference frame are necessary!

The accuracy of the method was tested with our stereotactic phantom: the measurements showed a maximum deviation of 0.6 mm from the predetermined position. For functional and non-functional interventions, our method is very easy to use. In the case of stereotactic biopsy, implantation of radionuclides, of catheter or DBS-systems we take CT-slices of 1.5–5 mm. Then, with the CT-program, the structure in question (tumor, cyst) (Fig. 4) is traced and the target points are measured and marked. At the sagittal and coronal reconstructions the trepanation point is determined (Figs. 5, 6). For control purposes all coordinates measured on the CT are transferred to the X-rays (Figs. 7 and 8). Then the computer gives us the setting parameters for our stereotactic device and the operation begins.

The same procedure applies for the case of functional stereotactic interventions. Here the area of the diencephalon is

[1] Abteilung Stereotaxie und Neuronuklearmedizin, Neurochirurgische Universitätsklinik, Hugstetter Strasse 55, D-7800 Freiburg im Breisgau, Federal Republic of Germany.

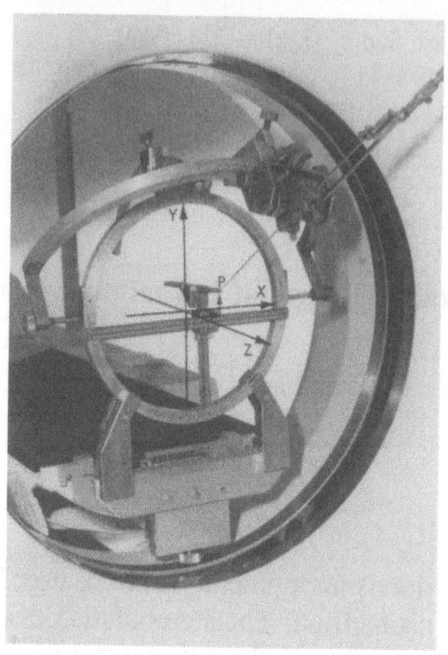

Fig. 1. Presentation of the CT scanner gantry with the stereotaxic device developed by Riechert and Mundinger in the computer compatible modification by Mundinger and Birg. The cartesian target point coordinates of the stereotaxic device are identical with the coordinates of the CT scanner when the 0-point of the stereotaxic device is in the origin of the CT scanner

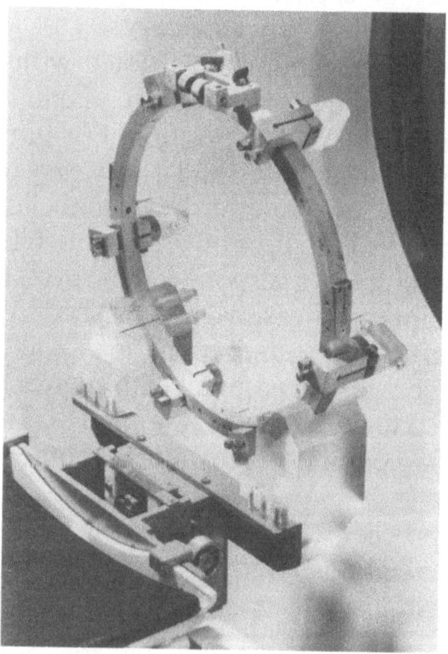

Fig. 2. Stereotactic base ring is fixed by means of the fixer apparatus on the CT table, which is vertically and horizontally adjustable with vernier micrometer screws. This makes it possible to superimpose the zero points of the base ring and gantry quickly

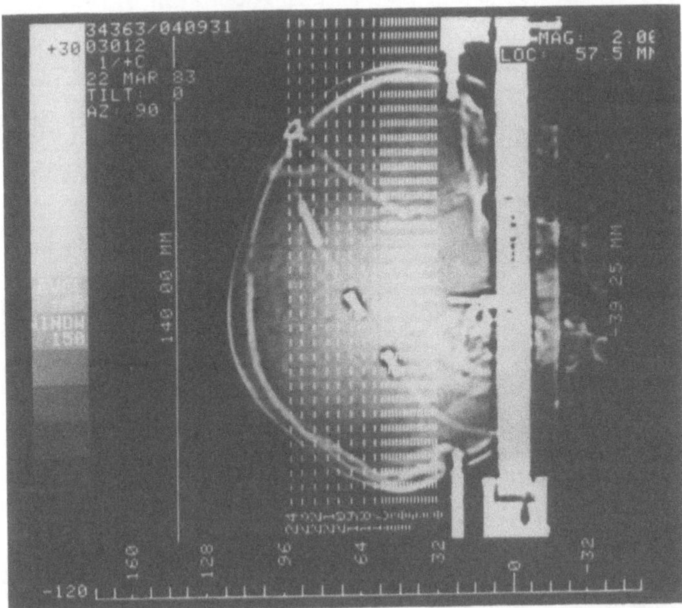

Fig. 3. The CT scan is taken parallel to the stereotactic base ring with distances between the layers of 1.5–5.0 mm. The lowest CT layer is in the 0 plane of the stereotactic base ring (z = 0) (see Fig. 4)

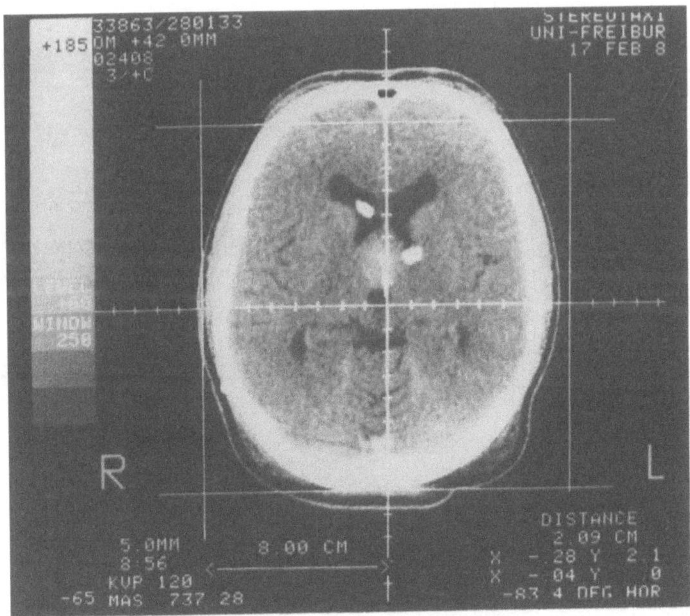

Fig. 4. The target point for the biopsy is determined and the x- and y-coordinates are calculated using the CT-computer (see lower right corner). The z-coordinate corresponds with the slice location (in this case 42 mm above the 0-plane of the base ring)

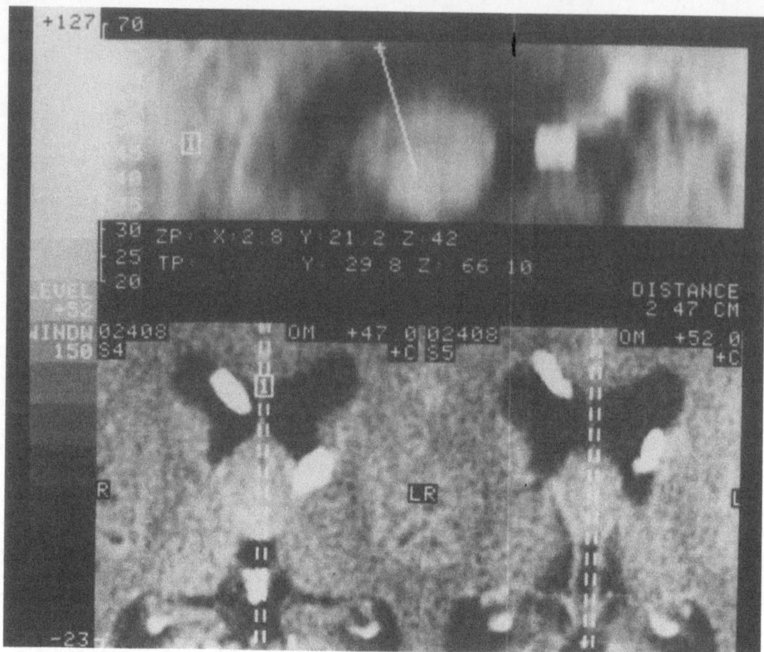

Fig. 5. Sagittal reconstruction. The target in the hyperdense space occupying process (*ZP*) is marked. The x-, y- and z-coordinates are immediately given by the CT-computer. The y- and z-coordinates of the second point (*TP*) for the approach of the cannula are determined in the same way and displayed on the screen

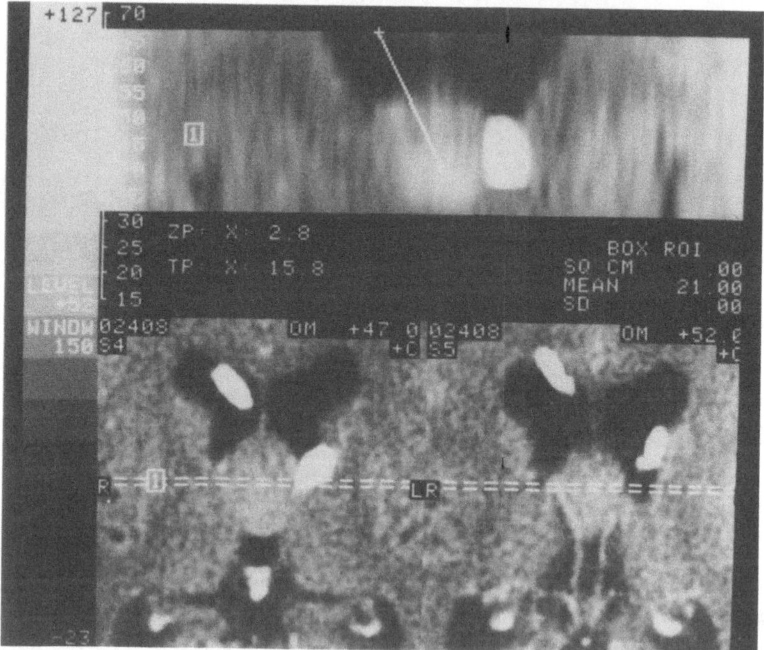

Fig. 6. Coronal reconstruction. The x-coordinates of target (*ZP*) and direction point (*TP*) are determined (see Fig. 5)

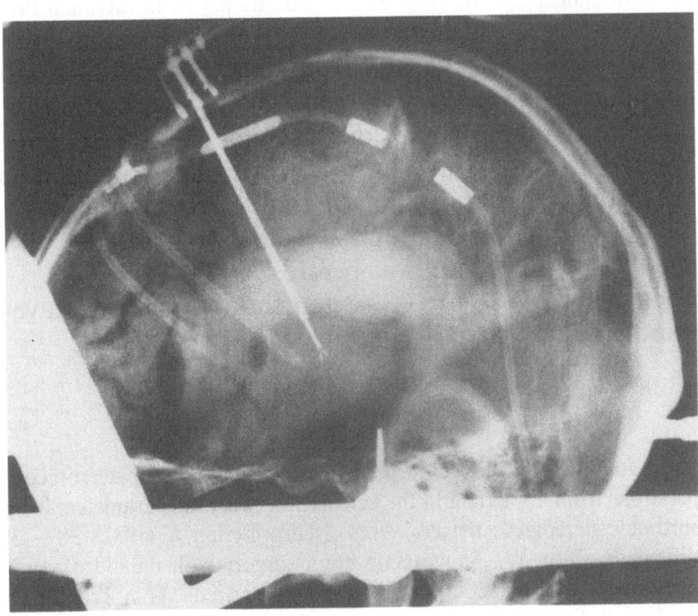

Fig. 7. The stereotactically guided biopsy probe is exactly in the precalculated position for draining the colloidal cyst of the foramen Monroe

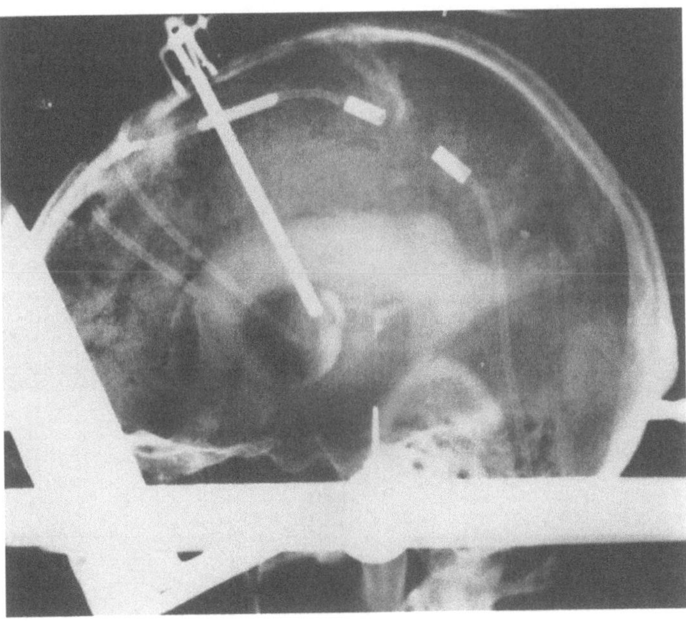

Fig. 8. In this case the colloid of the cyst in stereotactically drained

scanned with 1.5 mm layers. Using the CT-computer we measure the coordinates of Monro's foramen or of the anterior or posterior commissure and the height of the thalamus. With these structures and the relative coordinates of the target structure in question, we get the absolute target coordinate at the CT-screen. However, these are also the coordinates on our stereotactic device.

The further procedure is as before.

Since January 1981, 475 CT-stereotactic biopsy-cases have been done using this method at our department of Freiburg.

References

Birg, W., Mundinger, F., Direct target point determination for stereotactic brain operations from CT data and the calculation of setting parameters for polar-coordinate stereotactic devices. Appl. Neurophysiol. *45* (1982), 387—395.

Mundinger, F., Birg, W., Stereotactic brain surgery with the aid of computed tomography (CT-stereotaxy). In: Computerized Tomography, Brain Metabolism, Spinal Injuries. Advances in Neurosurgery, Vol. 10 (Driesen, W., Brock, M., Klinger, M., eds.), pp. 17—24. Berlin-Heidelberg-New York: Springer. 1982.

Acta Neurochirurgica, Suppl. 33, 225—232 (1984)

A Global 3-D Image of the Blood Vessels, Tumor and Simulated Electrode

P. Suetens[1], **J. Gybels**[1], **P. Jansen**[2], **A. Oosterlinck**[2], **A. Haegemans**[3], and **P. Dierckx**[3]

With 4 Figures

Summary

A method is developed yielding an integrated stereoscopic image of the cerebral blood vessels, CT view of tumor and simulated electrode, allowing the surgeon to choose any electrode direction that looks convenient to him. The method is especially of interest when the tumor is not visible on the original angiogram.

Keywords: 3-D imaging; cerebral tumors; digital radiography.

Introduction

Computerized tomography and cerebral angiography are two techniques to derive a spatial definition of cerebral tumors. On the one hand, a stereoscopic pair of angiograms enables the surgeon to have a depth impression of the cerebral vessels either by direct viewing or by means of a stereoscope. This stereoscopic image can give some information on the position of the lesion, because of the pathological course of certain blood vessels. Computerized tomography on the other hand yields a series of—two-dimensional—parallel transverse sections of the tumor. However, it is quite impossible to combine the stereoscopic image of the blood

[1] Department of Neurology and Neurosurgery, A. Z. Sint Rafaël, Kapucijnenvoer 33, B-3000 Leuven, Belgium.

[2] Center for Human Genetics, A. Z. Sint Rafaël, Kapucijnenvoer 33, B-3000 Leuven, Belgium.

[3] Department of Computer Sciences, Celestijnenlaan 200 A, B-3030 Heverlee, Belgium.

vessels and the CT view of the lesion into one integrated three-dimensional image.

We have developed a method yielding such an integrated stereoscopic image of the cerebral blood vessels, tumor and simulated electrode.

Method

A full description of the method can be found in Suetens *et al.*[1]. In short, the method consists of generating three stereoscopic image pairs, one of the blood vessels, one of the tumor and one of the electrode. These stereoscopic images are then integrated into one stereoscopic image.

The stereoscopic image pair of the blood vessels is available from stereoscopic angiography. The stereoscopic image pair of the tumor has to be computed from the CT image data. These two stereoscopic image pairs are then combined so that the tumor can be viewed in relationship with the surrounding blood vessels. A stereoscopic image of the electrode is then projected on the 3-D image of the tumor and the blood vessels. By varying the position of this simulated electrode, an appropriate path can be discovered.

Since the three image pairs must be superposed, simulated viewing conditions must be identical to the angiographic viewing conditions. This implies that the relationship between the patient's head position during angiography, CT and stereotactic intervention must exactly be known. We assume that the angiograms are made at the moment of the stereotactic operation, the patient being fixed in the stereotactic frame. Both the position of the electrode and of the blood vessels are then defined in the same stereotactic space. Consequently, only a spatial transformation from CT image data into the stereotactic space is needed.

The principle of our method is simple: a point in the three-dimensional space is defined unambiguously when its position is known in relation to three reference points with known spatial variables.

In a first step, the lesion boundaries are outlined on the CT image data. Each of the boundaries on the successive CT images can then be represented as a set of neighboring points. During the CT examination, each of these points will be determined with respect to three reference points which are clearly visible on the CT images and which are also distinguishable on radiographs.

Afterwards, at the moment of the stereotactic operation, the stereotactic coordinates of these three reference points can then be calculated by means of stereometry from a stereoscopic pair of radiographs. Since the tumor boundary points are related to these three reference points, their stereotactic coordinates can also be computed.

However, there are some practical difficulties. First, the reference points must be distinguishable both on CT image data and on radiographs, but such points do not naturally exist. Second, the patient's head has to remain fixed during the CT examination.

The first problem can be solved by putting three little metal (*e.g.* platinum) balls of about 0.5 to 1.0 mm diameter in the cranial bone.

To solve the second problem, a plastic mask is made, which clings perfectly to the patient's head, and which can be attached to the headrest of the CT scanner. In this way the patient is unable to move his head.

Extracting the tumor boundary points from CT image data and calculating their stereotactic coordinates are essential intermediate steps to achieve a three-dimensional display of the tumor structure. By three-dimensional display we mean a stereoscopic image pair of the tumor that can be superposed on the stereoscopic angiogram.

A surface description of the tumor can be obtained by means of a B-spline function, fitted to the set of tumor boundary points. The tumor can then be displayed as a netlike surface, which can simply be drawn on the original subtraction angiogram, or as a smooth-shaded transparent object, which can be superposed on the stereoscopic angiogram by means of a digital image processor. In order to accomplish this last display possibility, it is imperative that the X-ray data are converted to digital form, since computers can process only digital images. At present we digitize our film angiograms by means of a camera. In future, however, we hope to use a digital radiography device, which makes the use of film superfluous.

Results

We have applied our technique to a 28 year old man with an intracranial tumor visible on CT images. A normal angiogram showed displacement of the intracranial blood vessels, but the tumor itself was not visible. A tumor biopsy was indicated to obtain accurate information concerning the nature of the tumor in order to apply the most adequate treatment.

Fig. 1 shows a digitized stereoscopic pair of subtraction angiograms in the arterial phase. Note that the tumor is not visible on these images. Fig. 2 shows the CT slices through the tumor.

Figs. 3 and 4 show the integrated 3-D image of blood vessels, CT view of tumor and simulated electrode trajectories. In Fig. 3 the tumor is represented as a meshwork of curves and is simply drawn onto the original stereoscopic angiogram. In Fig. 4 the tumor is represented as a glass-like object. Therefore superposition could only be performed on digitized angiograms.

Conclusion

A method has been discussed that yields an integrated stereoscopic image of the cerebral blood vessels, CT view of tumor and simulated electrode trajectory. The practical implementation is relatively easy and economically feasible. A drawback of the method is that the observer cannot look around the object. Blood vessels, tumor and electrode can only be viewed from one direction.

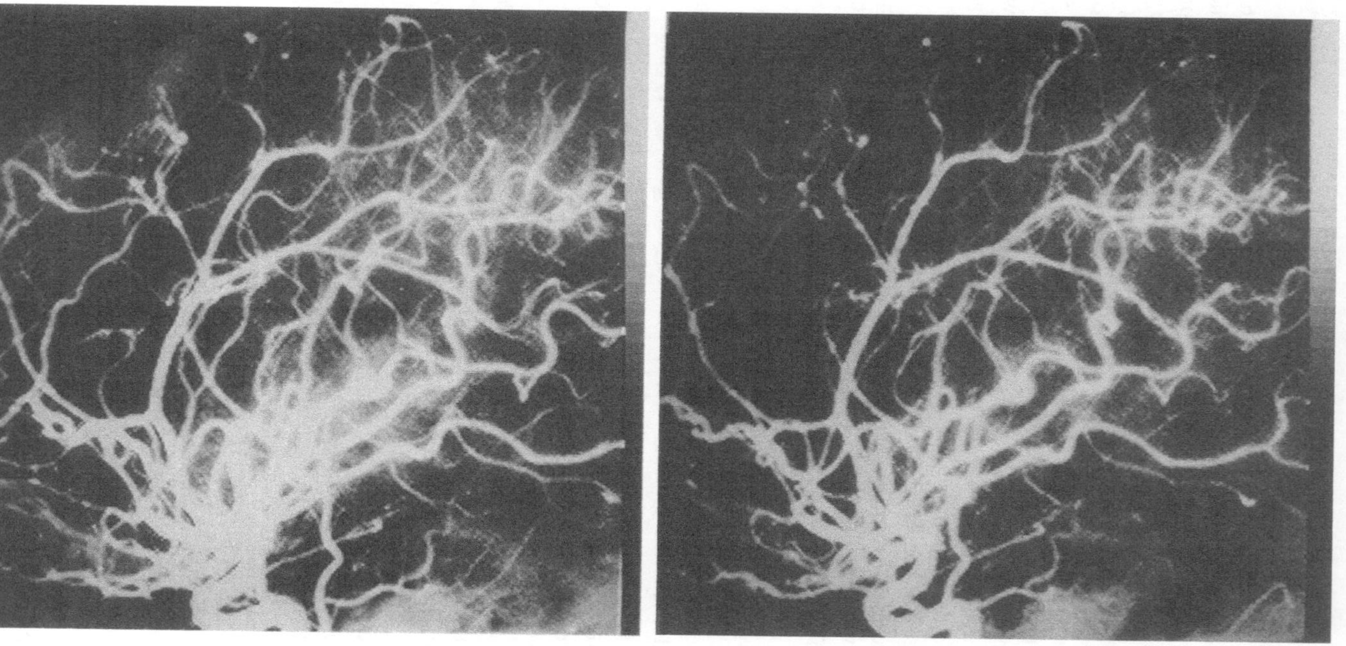

Fig. 1. Digitized stereoscopic pair of subtraction angiograms

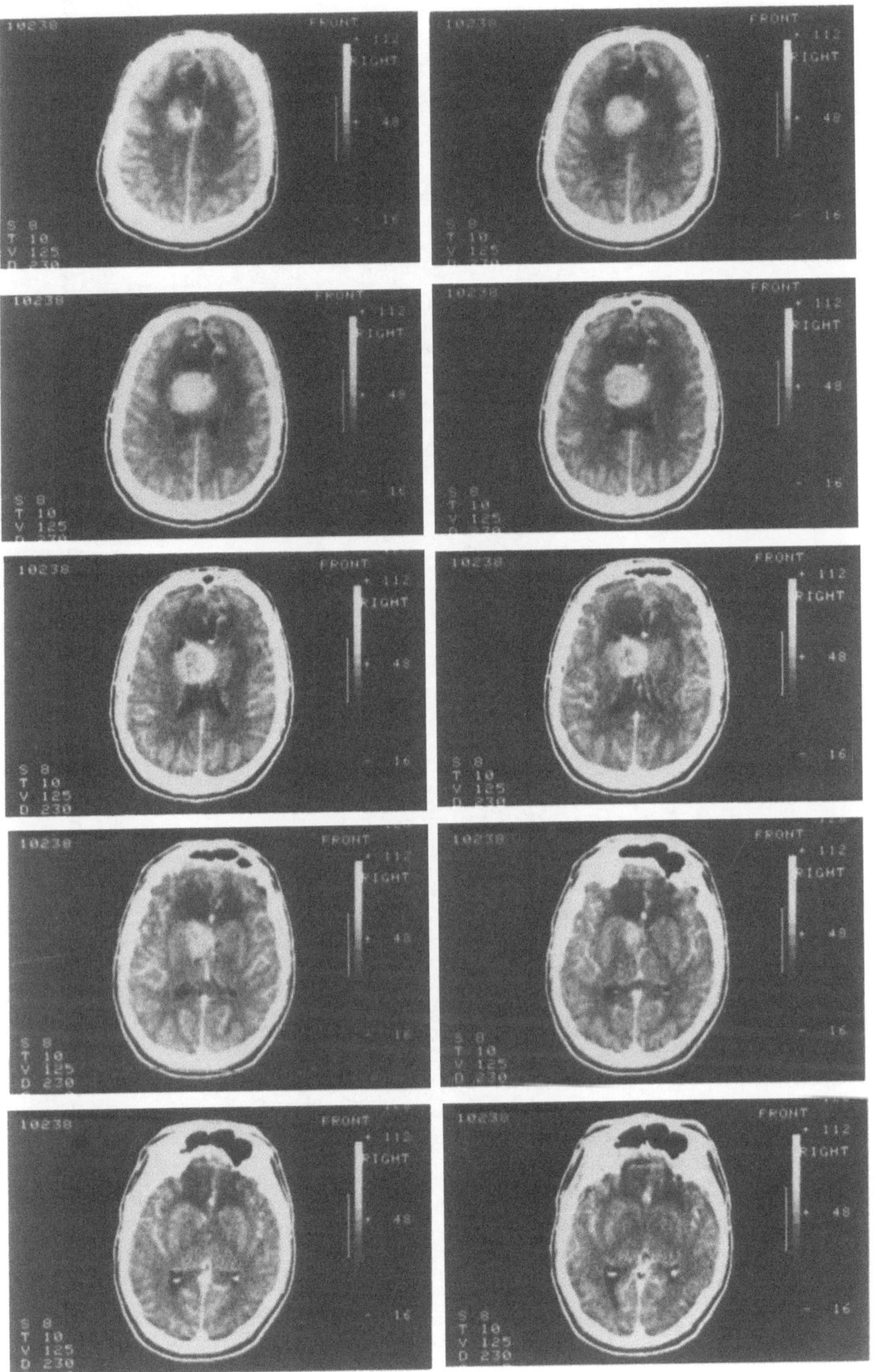

Fig. 2. CT slices through the tumor

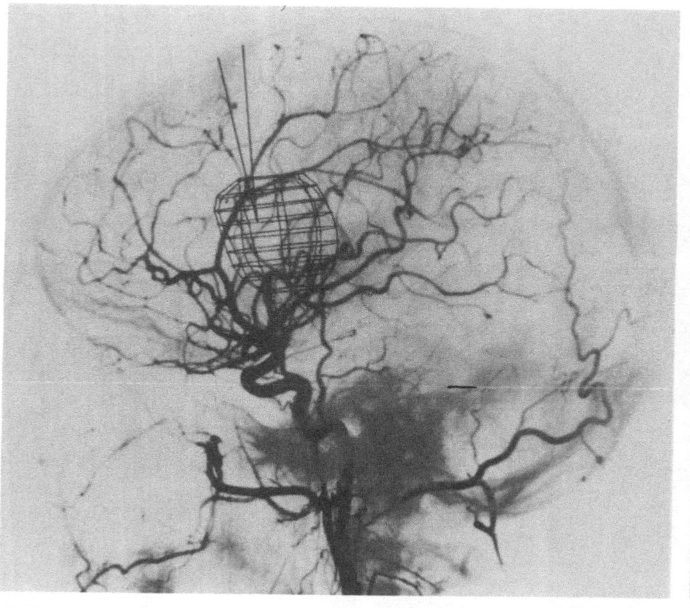

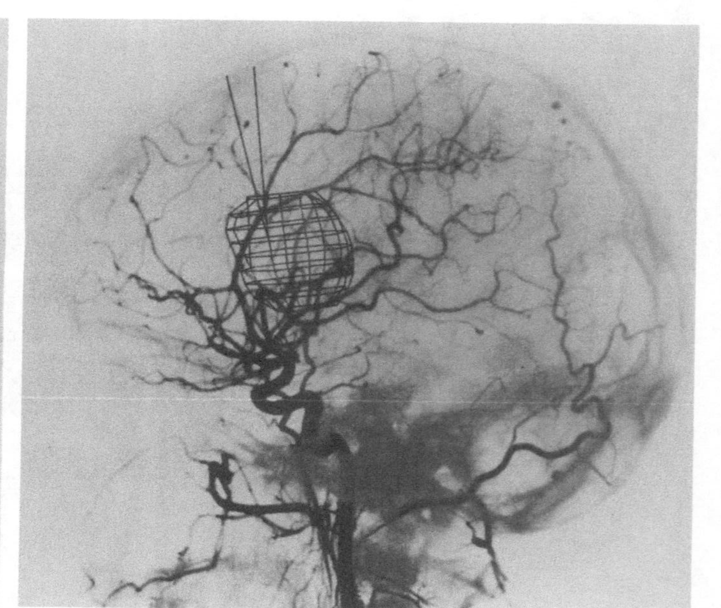

Fig. 3. Integrated 3-D image of blood vessels, CT view of tumor and two simulated electrode trajectories. The tumour is represented as a meshwork of curves

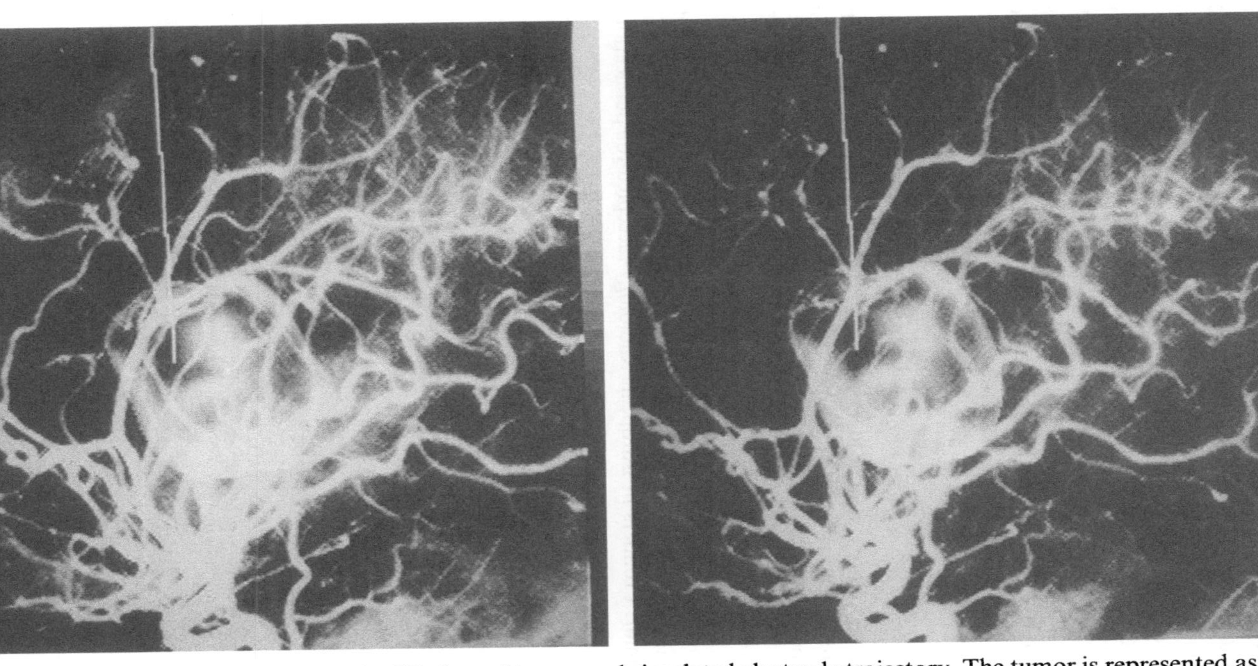

Fig. 4. Integrated 3-D image of blood vessels, CT view of tumor and simulated electrode trajectory. The tumor is represented as a glass-like object

This disadvantage can partially be removed when more than two angiograms are made from various side-by-side angles of view. Any two of these images constitute a stereoscopic pair. Multiple stereoscopic images of the tumor and simulated electrode can also be generated and superposed on the corresponding stereoscopic pairs of angiograms. The integrated image can then be displayed on an autostereoscopic screen. This technique allows the observer to move his head laterally and, in a restricted zone, to look around the object as in natural vision.

Acknowledgements

The authors would like to thank Mrs. Feytons-Heeren for typing the manuscript. This research is supported by the F.G.W.O. (Belgium) under grant number 3.0021.81.

Reference

1. Suetens, P., Baert, A., Gybels, J., Haegemans, A., Jansen, P., Oosterlinck, A., Wilms, G., An integrated 3-D image of cerebral blood vessels and CT view of tumor. Frontiers in European Radiology (accepted for publication).

Acta Neurochirurgica, Suppl. 33, 233—235 (1984)

Computer Assisted Stereotactic Biopsies Utilizing CT and Digitized Arteriographic Data

P. J. Kelly[1], **B. A. Kall,** and **S. G. Goerss**

Summary

This report describes a computer based method for stereotactic biopsy of intracranial lesions detected by CT scanning. Points within a tumor or an entire interpolated tumor volume are created from digitized CT slices and suspended within a 3-dimensional computer matrix. Vessel segments from digitized stereoscopic cerebral angiograms obtained under stereotactic conditions may also be included in the computer matrix. The computer calculates the mechanical adjustments on an arc-quadrant stereotactic frame which place the center of a tumor volume or digitized point within the tumor into the focal point of the frame and define an avascular trajectory by which the tumor may be biopsied. Stereotactic biopsies have been performed on eighty-six (86) patients without mortality or neurologic morbidity.

Keywords: Stereotactic techniques; cerebral neoplasm; arteriography; computers; CT scanning.

Introduction

CT based stereotactic biopsies of deep-seated intracranial neoplasms can obtain a histologic diagnosis with minimal risk to the patient. In addition, information derived from stereotactic serial biopsies indicates the true histologic boundaries of a neoplasm and can be used to modify computer volumetric data derived from stereotactic CT scanning. Utilization of an operating room computer allows the precise determination of tumor volume and can display its three dimensional configuration[3]. In addition, the three dimensional position of cerebral blood vessels may be calculated from stereotactic stereoangiography. The computer may similate biopsy trajectories to ensure that no important vascular structures will be injured by biopsy probe or forceps.

[1] Department of Neurosurgery, State University of New York at Buffalo, 2121 Main Street, Buffalo, NY 14214, U.S.A.

Method

Stereotactic CT data is obtained utilizing a GE 8800 CT scanner and a method described elsewhere in this volume and previously[2,3]. The CT data tape is input to the operating room computer system (Data General Eclipse S-140). Serial CT slices are displayed on the display terminal. The stereotactic reference marks, a point within a tumor or multiple points on serial tumor outlines are digitized utilizing cursor and trackball, for incorporation of a point or interpolated tumor volume into a three dimensional computer matrix, respectively.

A stereotactic 6° stereoscopic arteriogram is performed utilizing an arteriographic reference system (ARS). The ARS creates four (4) reference marks on each radiograph which define zero planes in X, Y and Z. The position of the reference marks and points of inflection on important blood vessels are digitized from stereo pairs utilizing a digitizing board. Interpolated vessel segments are suspended within the 3-dimensional computer matrix.

Stereotactic frame settings are calculated by computer from a point selected within the tumor volume. Trajectory angles on the arc-quadrant stereotactic frame are determined from an avascular digitized point from antero-posterior and lateral views of the orthogonal arteriogram. If necessary, the computer can simulate the biopsy trajectory to ensure that no vessels lie within its path. In addition the position of the biopsy trajectory and biopsy sites are displayed on contiguous CT slices.

Biopsies are performed utilizing a 1.6 mm insulated canula through which a 1 mm cup biopsy forceps is inserted. Consecutive serial biopsies are obtained at 5 mm intervals up to, through and beyond the CT defined limits of the tumor volume. The position of each biopsy is documented by AP and lateral teleradiographs.

Results

Eighty-six (86) patients with deep seated intracranial neoplasms have undergone stereotactic biopsy procedures. Tumors were located in the basal ganglia in 9 patients, thalamus in 20 patients and within the posterior fossa in 5 patients. The remainder had tumors located deep within the subcortical white matter. Histologically, there were 23 glioblastomas, 25 astrocytomas, 13 metastatic tumors, 6 meningiomas, 4 infarctions, 3 abcesses and 10 miscellaneous lesions. No histological diagnosis was possible from the specimens obtained in 2 patients. There were no instances of neurological morbidity or mortality following these procedures in this series.

Discussion

The method described is a low risk procedure which effectively obtains a histologic diagnosis in patients with deep seated intracranial neoplasms. In addition histologic information on the limits of an intracranial neoplasm may be used to modify CT data.

Although computer reconstruction of CT data allows the representation of a tumor volume in stereotactic space utilizing a three-dimensional computer matrix, the histologic limits of the tumor may not necessarily correspond to the boundaries of the tumor derived from CT scanning[1]. Utilizing an operating room computer system, the CT defined tumor volume within the matrix may be stretched or contracted along the plane of each biopsy trajectory. Thus the tumor volume described within the computer matrix can be more representative of the actual tumor volume in the patient.

References

1. Daumas-Duport, C., Monsaingeon, V., Szenthe, L., Szikla, G., Serial stereotactic biopsies: a double histological code of gliomas according to malignancy and 3D configuration as an aid to therapeutic decision and assessment of results. Appl. Neurophysiol. *45* (1982), 431—437.
2. Goerss, S., Kelly, P. J., Kall, B., Alker, G. J., jr., A computed tomographic adaptation system. Neurosurgery *10* (1982), 375—379.
3. Kelly, P. J., Alker, G. J., jr., Goerss, S., Computer-assisted stereotactic laser microsurgery for the treatment of intracranial neoplasms. Neurosurgery *10* (1982), 324—331.

Acta Neurochirurgica, Suppl. 33, 237 (1984)

Stereo-EEG Contribution to the Three-Dimensional Definition of the Hemispheric Astrocytomas

C. Munari[1,2], **A. Musolino**[2], **S. Kochen**[3], **G. Szikla**[2], **J. Bancaud**[1,2], and **J. Talairach**[2]

In the past years, 30 cases of hemispheric astrocytomas underwent a stereo-EEG exploration in our unit.

CT scan data concerning the topography and the supposed limits of the lesion were synthetized with the stereotactic neuroradiological data (angiography and ventriculography). 4 to 7 intracerebral multilead electrodes were introduced with the double aim: to contribute to define the limits of the tumor and to precise (with electrical stimulation) the "anatomo-functional" organization of neighboring brain structures.

In our experience, stereo-EEG data can contribute to the interpretation of CT findings in terms of the underlying pathological processes such as brain edema, brain necrosis, tumoral infiltration and tumoral tissue.

According to our experience, the use of only one deep electrode does not permit valid correlations with the spatial reconstruction of the CT scan data. It proved useful to record three or more electrodes, oriented in different plans.

Moreover, the electrical stimulations permit to identify intracerebral connections (*e.g.* motor or visual pathways, etc.) which may or may not be displaced by the space occupying process.

Possible signification of the different stereo-EEG patterns should be discussed in the light of neuroradiological, CT and histopathological data.

---

[1] Unité 97 de recherches sur l'épilepsie, INSERM, 2ter rue d'Alésia, F-75014 Paris, France.

[2] Service de Neurochirurgie B, Hôpital Sainte Anne, 1 rue Cabanis, F-75014 Paris, France.

[3] Antartida Hospital, Buenos Aires 1424, Argentine.

Acta Neurochirurgica, Suppl. 33, 239—241 (1984)

Depth-EEG in Stereotactic Biopsy

L. Ravagnati[1], V. A. Sironi[1], E. Cappricci[1], G. Ettorre[1], M. Farabola[2], and F. Marossero[1]

Summary

This paper presents the results of the use of depth electrode mapping of EEG signals in and around the lesions to be biopsied in 40 patients. The correlation between histological findings and depth-EEG patterns are discussed. Special emphasis is placed on cases with hypodense CT lesions which were usually large and confined to one or more cerebral lobes, did not enhance with contrast media, were angiographically silent, and manifested clinically with occasional epileptic fits.

Keywords: Depth-EEG; stereotactic biopsy; CT scan hypodense lesions; brain tumors.

Stereotactic biopsy can offer conclusive informations regarding the histological nature of different cerebral lesions, thus giving the opportunity to plan the most appropriate therapy[3]. Bioptic specimens, however, can introduce elements of doubt or even errors, when they are taken from parts of the lesion which are not diagnostically significant. In order to reduce the degree of error, many techniques and devices have been proposed and used[1,2].

This paper presents the results of the use of depth electrode mapping of EEG signals in and around the lesions to be biopsied. The histological findings and depth-EEG patterns in 40 patients are correlated.

Material and Methods

Depth-EEG recordings were performed in 40 patients (aged from 15 to 73 years, mean: 32 years) with cerebral lesions demonstrated by CT scan.

[1] Institute of Neurosurgery, and [2] Service of Neuroradiology, School of Medicine, University of Milan, Via F. Sforza, 35, I-20122 Milano, Italy.

The material can be subdivided in two groups, according to the CT features and the clinical symptomatology. The first group is composed of 21 cases of small or medium size CT lesions which were seated in deep brain structures and had usually manifested either by signs of increased intracranial pressure or neurological deficits. The second group includes 19 cases of non-enhancing hypodense CT lesions which were mostly large and confined to one or more cerebral lobes. The lesions were angiographically silent and manifested clinically in most cases by occasional partial epileptic seizures.

The Talairach's apparatus has been used for the stereotactic positioning of the recording electrodes and biopsy instruments.

The volume of the tissue specimens varied from 1 to 4 cubic millimeters. The bioptic specimens were either frozen, cut and stained for immediate examination or embedded in paraffin for later study.

Results

Small deeply seated lesions: When the recording electrode was gradually advanced from the cortex of the convexity toward the radiological site of the lesion, different modifications of the depth-EEG activity (frequency, amplitude) were observed, varying from normality to depressed, slow wave abnormality, irritative activity, and electrical silence.

Serial bioptic specimens were taken at the sites corresponding to the different depth-EEG patterns. The results of the correlation between depth-EEG and histology can be summarized as follows: at the side where depth-EEG activity changed from normality to depressed, slow-wave activity, an abnormal tissue was usually found, *i.e.* perilesional edema, glial reaction. At the site of electrical silence abnormal tissue was always found, which usually showed the highest degree of pathology. Electrical silence was found to be not pathognomonic since it was recorded in lesions of different nature (tumors, necroses, benign cysts).

The histological specimens showed astrocytoma in 6 cases (2 grade I and 4 grade II), astro-oligodendroglioma grade II in 1 case, oligodendroglioma grade II and grade III in 2 cases, 1 glioblastoma, 1 plexuspapilloma, 1 craniopharyngioma, 1 metastasis, 1 nontumoral cystic lesion, 1 necrosis, 3 cases with edema only and 3 abscesses.

Large hypodense CT lesions: Various depth-EEG patterns, ranging from normal or almost normal activity to depressed, slow-wave abnormality and electrical silence, were recorded in different areas of hypodense CT lesions, even in those that had homogenous CT characteristics in all their parts (measured in Hounsfield units).

The histology of the specimens taken from these areas, homogenously hypodense but electrically different, has shown different features, with a correlation between depth-EEG abnormalities and pathology.

There were 8 astrocytomas (4 grade I and 4 grade II), 1 astro-oligodendroglioma, 1 spongioblastoma, 4 cases with glioma or gliosis, 4 cases with edema only and 1 case with normal brain tissue.

Discussion

The target for biopsy of small lesions is often reconstructed from CT scan data on stereotactic films, since it is not directly or indirectly by angiography and pneumencephalography visualized. The accuracy of the target can be improved by depth-EEG recording, which allows the recording of abnormal signals from pathologic tissue.

In cases of large hypodense lesions in one or more cerebral lobes, the data of depth-EEG are even more valuable, since these data make biopsies possible in diagnostically significant sites. In fact, depth-EEG is able to demonstrate, inside the homogenous CT lesion, areas with different electrical characteristics and corresponding tissue of different histological nature.

References

1. Bancaud, J., Talairach, J., Geier, S., Scarabin, J. M., EEG et SEEG dans les tumeurs cérébrales et l'épilepsie. Paris: Edifor. 1973.
2. Benabid, A. L., Persat, J. C., Chirossel, J. P., Rougemont, J., Barge, M., Délimitation des tumeurs cérébrales par stéréo-impedo-encéphalographie (SIEG). Neurochirurgie *24* (1978), 3—14.
3. Conway, L. W., Stereotactic biopsy of deep intracranial tumors. In: Current Techniques in Operative Neurosurgery (Schmiedek, H., Sweet, W. H., eds.), pp. 187—198. Berlin-Heidelberg-New York: Springer. 1976.

Acta Neurochirurgica, Suppl. 33, 243—245 (1984)

A Simple Method for the Growth of Cell Cultures from Small Biopsies of Brain Tumours Taken During CT-directed Stereotactic Procedures

D. G. T. Thomas[1], **J. L. Darling, B. A. Watkins,** and **Maria C. Hine**

With 1 Figure

Summary

An adaption of a simple method for the growth of small (< 50 mg wet weight) biopsies of human brain tumours taken during stereotactic neurosurgical procedures is described.

Keywords: Stereotactic surgery; brain tumour; biopsy; cell culture; explant.

Introduction

Computerised tomographic (CT) directed stereotactic biopsy of brain tumours is now widely used in neurosurgery. It would be of great value to be able routinely to examine the biopsied tumour in cell culture as well as histologically. However, pieces of tissue removed by these techniques are usually small and conventional collagenase digestion of biopsies this small is often unsuccessful. In this communication, we describe an adaption of a simple method (Warren and de la Cruz 1972) for the culture of small brain tumour fragments.

Materials and Methods

Biopsies were collected using BRW (Brown, Roberts and Wells) stereotactic system (Radionics Limited, Burlington, MA, U.S.A.). The procedures involved in the collection of tumour biopsies have been reported in detail elsewhere (Anderson *et al.* 1983).

---

[1] Gough-Cooper Department of Neurological Surgery, Institute of Neurology, Queen Square, London, WC1N 3BG, U.K.

After removal, biopsies were placed in Hams F-10 plus 200 units/ml penicillin, 100 µg/ml streptomycin, 50 µg/ml Kanamycin and 2.5 µg/ml fungizone (Flow Laboratories, Irvine, Scotland) and immediately transferred to the cell culture laboratory. Biopsies were washed in biopsy collection medium and then transferred to growth medium (Hams F-10 with 20 mM HEPES supplemented with 10% foetal calf serum, 50 units/ml penicillin and 50 µg/ml streptomycin). For collagenase digestion, 0.5 ml of collagenase solution (2,000 units/ml, Worthington CLS or Sigma Grade I A) was added to 4.5 mls of Hams F-10 containing the tissue fragments in a cell culture flask. After 24 hours incubation at 37 °C, the tissue was gently disaggregated by pipetting, centrifuged to remove the enzyme preparation, counted with Coulter Counter, resuspended 5–10 mls of growth medium, and

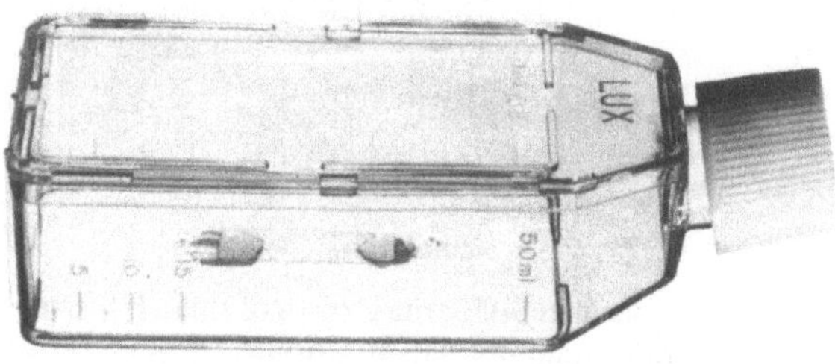

Fig. 1. Coverslip overlay method: Tissue culture flask with coverglass held in place by silicone grease. Approx. 0.5 × life size

replated in a fresh culture flask. For mechanical disaggregation, fragments of tissue were suspended in growth medium and pipetted rapidly for 10–15 seconds. The cell suspension was then transferred to a cell culture flask.

For the new coverslip overlay method, biopsies were washed in biopsy collection medium. Using a sterile 1 ml pipette, two small spots of silicone grease (Edwards High Vacuum grease) were placed about 1 cm apart on the base of a 25 cm² plastic cell culture flask. Using sterile dental forceps (College Pattern) a piece of tumour biopsy or the whole of the stereotactic biopsy was placed between the spots of silicone grease in a drop of biopsy collection medium. A sterile glass coverslip (9 × 22 mm) was placed over the biopsy and gently pressed down using sterile forceps until the edges of the coverslip were held down by the silicone grease (Fig. 1). Finally, 5 mls of growth medium was carefully added down the side of the flask. Coverslip overlays were examined at weekly intervals. When there were signs of significant cell proliferation from the biopsy, the coverslip and remains of the biopsy were removed and the cultures were refed with fresh medium. When a large area of cells had developed, the cultures were trypsinised and replated in the normal way.

Results and Discussion

In our hands, the use of mechanical methods and collagenase have proved unsatisfactory for the preparation of cultures from small (< 50 mg wet weight) biopsies. Culture of seven consecutive glioma biopsies by these methods failed. The principal reason for the failure was probably the small yield of cells produced in this way (range $2.5–5 \times 10^5$ cells/biopsy). Table 1 shows the overall success

Table 1. *Preparation of Coverslip Overlay Cultures from Stereotactic Biopsies*

Culture success	Mean weight of biopsies (mg)	Range (mg)	Success rate (% in brackets)	
No growth (n = 3)	9.5	2.5–22.9	3/34 (8.8)	
Growth in primary culture (n = 14*)	11.2	3.0–34	14/34 (41.2)	overall 91.2%
Growth in secondary culture (n = 17)	22.5	4.5–52.3	17/34 (50)	

* Includes 6 cultures which have substantial growth and will continue to secondary culture.

rate of the coverslip overlay technique when applied to the following 34 consecutive biopsies taken during stereotactic neurosurgery. There was no evidence of toxicity of the silicone grease, indeed cells were often observed directly touching the grease.

In conclusion, the technique is useful for the culture of small brain tumour biopsies derived from stereotactic surgery and may also be useful in other occasions when only a small sample is available for tissue culture study.

The authors are grateful to the Cancer Research Campaign, Medical Research Council, Brain Research Trust and Mr. Basil Samuel for their support for this project.

References

Anderson, R. E., Thomas, D. G. T., du Boulay, G. H., Radiological aspects of CT-guided stereotactic neurosurgical procedures. Neuroradiol. *24* (1983), 163—166.

Warren, R. J., de la Cruz, C., Fibroblasts from biopsies.—An easier way. Exp. Cell Res. *71* (1972), 238.

Acta Neurochirurgica, Suppl. 33, 247—251 (1984)

Tissue Mechanical Resistance Measurements and Records in Stereotactic Biopsy Procedures

F. Colombo[1], **F. Angrilli**[2], **R. Basso**[2], **L. Casentini**[1], and **A. Benedetti**[1]

With 3 Figures

Introduction

In previous reports the authors have described a fully motorized, computer driven, stereotactic apparatus[1,5]. In a following step a constant velocity dynamometer was built[6], and connected with the aim of recording the thrust exerted by the motor while pushing the stereotactic tool on its way to the target. The output of the instrument was plotted into a bidimensional diagram (X probe track in millimeters; Y force in Newton).

Measuring Apparatus and Method

The measuring apparatus is composed of the following main components: 1. constant-velocity probe-pusher; 2. tool's displacement meter; 3. low-friction dynamometer; 4. X, Y recorder (Fig. 1).

The fundamental performances aimed at were: linearity and repeatibility; possibility of using the instrument in any direction; minimization of size and weight; absolute safety during the use; probe axis coincident with that of other stereotactic probes.

The apparatus in its final form is represented in Fig. 2.

The probe, constituted by a little stainless steel rod, moves with rectilinear constant speed on a length of 120 mm as maximum stroke.

The velocity can be set in the range 0.5–150 mm/s. The records presented here were obtained with 10 mm/s velocity. The probe displacement is recorded on X-

[1] Division of Neurosurgery, City Hospital, Via Rodolfi, I-36100 Vicenza, Italy.

[2] Institute of Applied Mechanics, Padua University, Via Venezia n. 1, I-35100 Padova, Italy.

axis by means of a proper transducer. The uncertainty in the probe extremity location is ± 0.1 mm.

In the dynamometer, the internal frictions of the moving equipment do not interfere with the measure, so that the lowest detectable force is 10^{-5} N. The full-

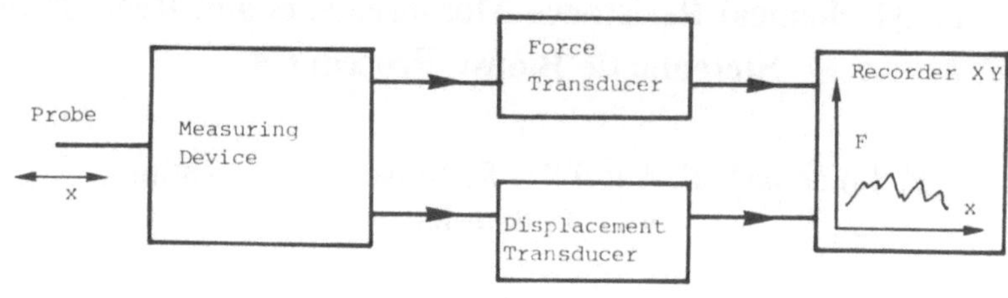

Fig. 1

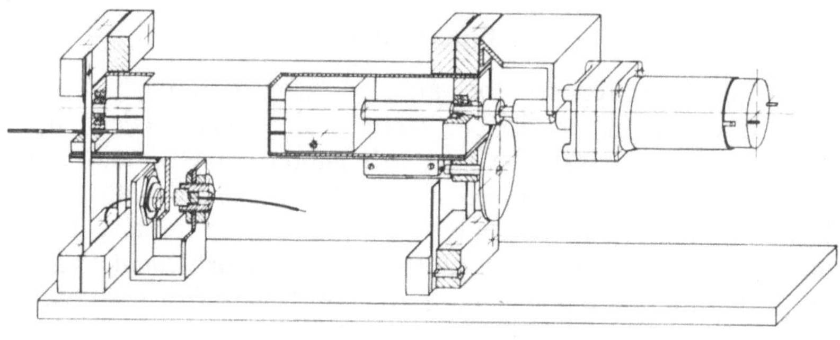

Fig. 2

scale force is 10 N and the sensitivity can be set in a wide range. The maximum linearity error was 1.4% of full-scale for any selected range.

Since June 1982 we have recorded the Tissue Mechanical Resistance (TMR) during more than 20 biopsy procedures. TMR data were compared with bioptic samples obtained in pathologic areas.

Results

Some characteristics TMR records are shown in Fig. 3.

Discussion

TMR registration affords a new information on line with the progression of the stereotactic probe. This information is comparable but not superimposable to those given by CT examination[3], SEEG recording[2], or tissue impedance recording[4].

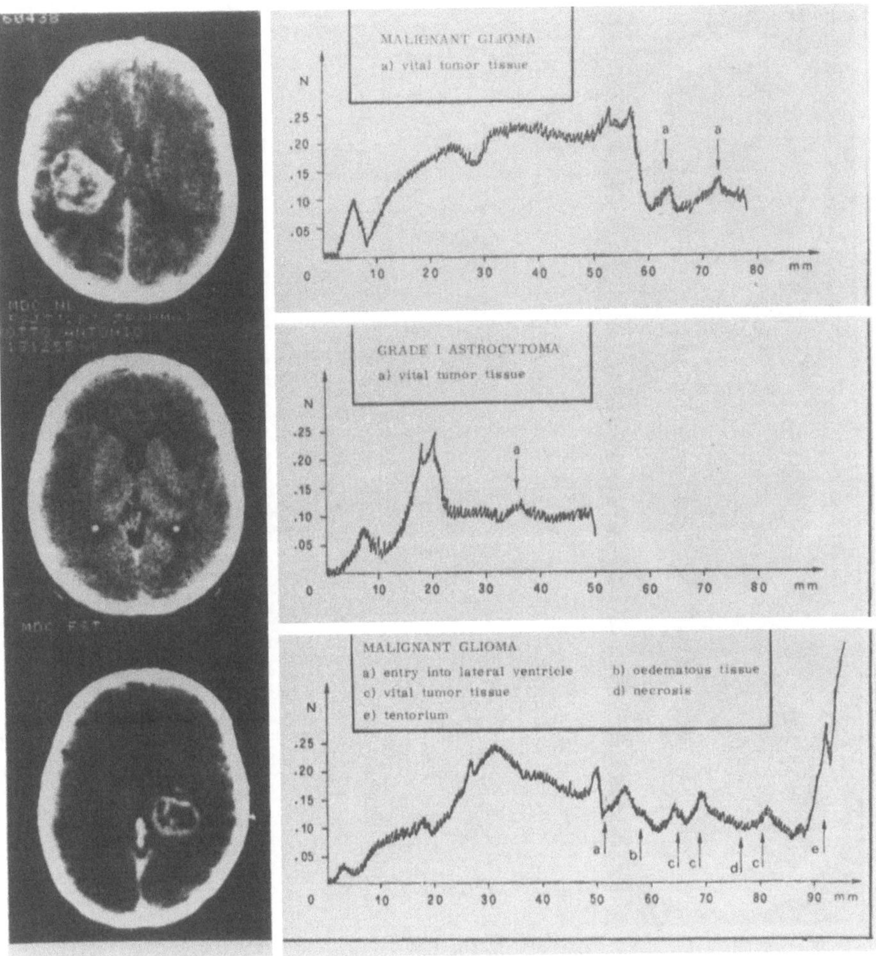

Fig. 3a

In our opinion it is particularly useful to determine the border zone of the pathological area.

TMR is significantly modified by the presence of edema (progressively decreasing TMR), necrosis, hemorrhage (low TMR), fluid filled cyst (TMR nil). With respect to the last three pathological conditions, vital tumor tissue displays an enhanced TMR.

Characteristic patterns of TMR records can be described for some kinds of intracranial tumors. Low grade astrocytomas are

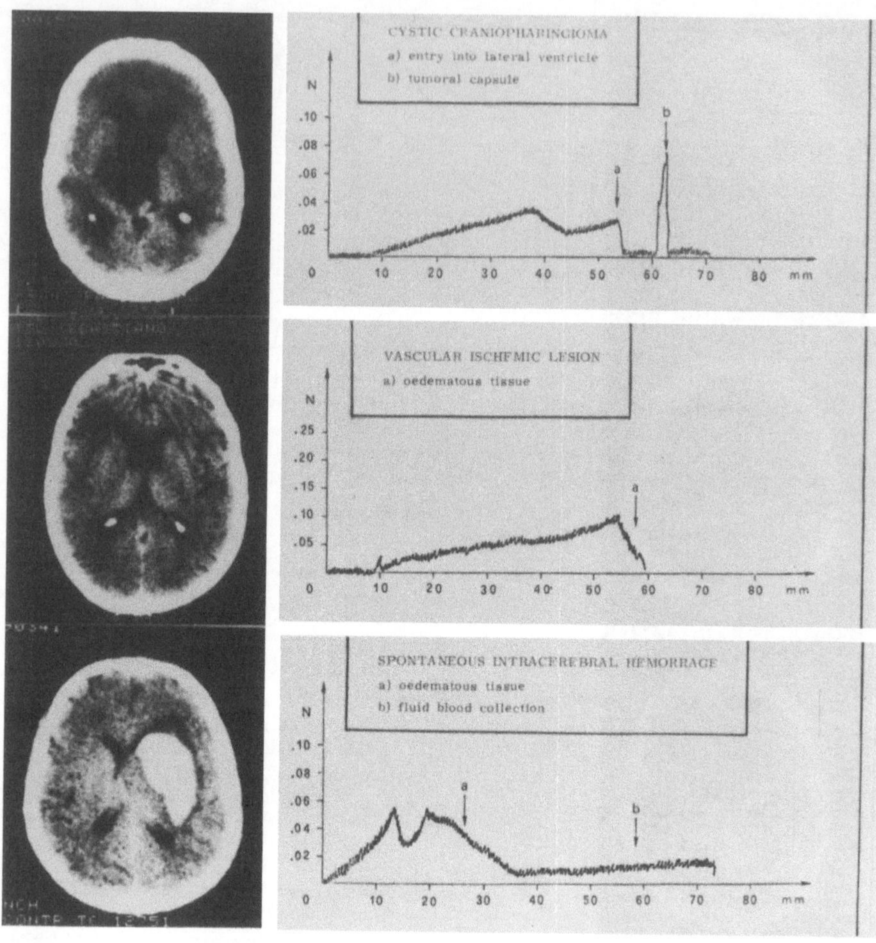

Fig. 3b

detectable by a uniformely low TMR, circumscribed by a clear-cut margin. Malignant gliomas are surrounded by a zone of decreasing TMR (edema); in the tumor bulk TMR displays alternating areas of enhanced and lowered TMR. Cystic lesion always show an abrupt rise and fall of TMR corresponding to the piercing of the capsule. We found TMR particularly useful for selecting a proper biopsy target and for avoiding less significative areas (hemorrhage, necrosis). In our experience the total number of samples, necessary for an exhaustive histological diagnosis was always reduced.

References

1. Angrilli, F., Colombo, F., Zanardo, A., Nuovo apparato per il posizionamento e la guida di attrezzi chirurgici a cielo coperto. Ingegneria n. 9 (1982), 2—7.
2. Bancaud, J., Talairach, J., Szikla, G., Stereo-EEG exploration in interstitial irradiation of gliomas. In: Stereotactic Cerebral Irradiation (Szikla, G., ed.), pp. 57—62. Amsterdam: Elsevier. 1979.
3. Birg, W., Mundinger, F., Direct target point determination for stereotactic operations from CT data. Appl. Neurophysiol. *45* (1982), 387—395.
4. Broggi, G., Franzini, A., Passerini, A., Correlation between impedance values and deep brain tumors during stereotactic biopsies. In: Stereotactic Cerebral Irradiation (Szikla, G., ed.), pp. 51—56. Amsterdam: Elsevier. 1979.
5. Colombo, F., Angrilli, F., Zanardo, A., *et al.*, A universal method to employ CT spatial information in stereotactic surgery. Appl. Neurophysiol. *45* (1982), 352—364.
6. Colombo, F., Angrilli, F., Basso, R., Benedetti, A., A new dynamometric technique to measure and locate endocranial structures. Ricerche e Studi n. 52 dell'Istituto di Meccanica Applicata alle Macchine. Padova. 1982.

Acta Neurochirurgica, Suppl. 33, 253—255 (1984)

Preliminary Experiences with Intraoperative Ultrasonography in Cerebral Tumor Biopsy

V. A. Fasano[1], **W. Liboni**[2], **G. Broggi**[1], **M. De Mattei**[3], and **A. Sguazzi**[1]

With 3 Figures

Recent technological advances in ultrasound instrumentation (gray scale "B" mode units) have resulted in equipment that image, in "real time", slices of the human brain which are similar in quality to computerized tomography. The use of this technique in the operating room, after a small portion of the skull has been removed, shows the advantages of ultrasonography over the CT scan:

— little equipment is required,

— the possibility of imaging the lesion without radiation exposure,

— the resolution of cystic and solid lesions[2].

A real-time sector scanning device with a transducer operating at 3.5–7.5–10 MHz and a sector angle from 18° to 90° (High Stoy Technol. Corpor., Neuro Sector Ultras. syst., A. L. TL, Ashington) was used for biopsy in 10 cases of deep cerebral tumors, *i.e.* 4 parieto-occipital glioblastomas, 2 thalamic astrocytomas (Fig. 2), 2 pineal astrocytomas, 2 pinealocytomas (Fig. 3). The ultrasonic transducer with a special guide for biopsy, provides precise data to guide biopsy needles (Fig. 1) and to confirm their exact location within the lesion[1]. The spatial resolution of this ultrasound apparatus permits a bioptic approach with respect to the real volume of the tumor. It is independent of the three cartesian axes

[1] Neurosurgical Institute, [2] Neuroradiological Service and [3] I. Neurological Clinic of the University of Turin, Via Cherasco, 15, I-10126 Torino, Italy.

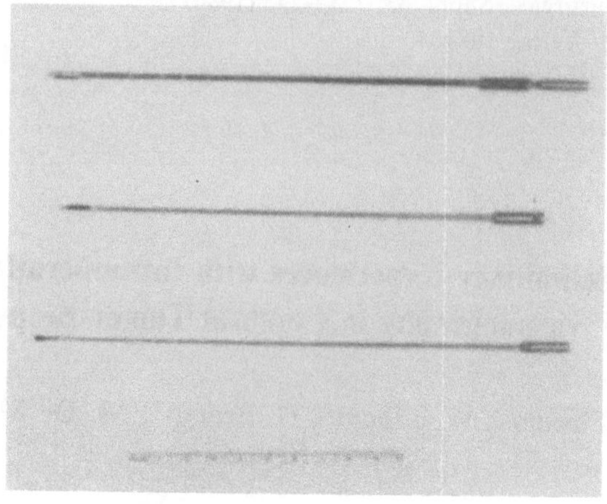

Fig. 1. Original biopsy needles

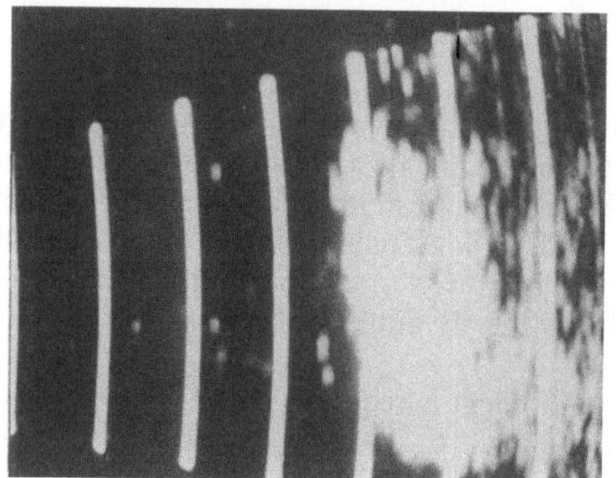

Fig. 2. Ultrasonographic aspect of thalamic astrocytoma

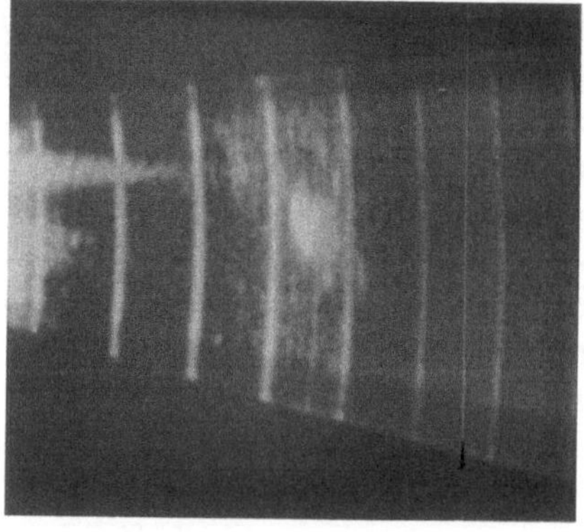

Fig. 3. Ultrasonographic biopsy of pinealocytoma

which are typical of stereotactic techniques. The great advantage over other bioptic techniques is the extreme flexibility of the method which permits exploration of all tumor regions. The preliminary results are satisfactory.

References

1. Fasano, V. A., Broggi, G., Barolat-Romana, G., The stereotactic approach to the biopsy and freezing of deep and invasive cerebral gliomas. Excerpta Medica—Intern. Congr. Series, No. 413 (1977), 72.
2. Fasano, V. A., Liboni, W., Ponzio, R., De Mattei, M., Preliminary experiences with "real time" intraoperative ultrasonography associated to laser sources and ultrasonic aspirator in neurosurgery. Surg. Neurol. (1983) (in press).

Acta Neurochirurgica, Suppl. 33, 257—259 (1984)

CT Assisted Stereotactic Biopsy of Deep Cerebral Lesions and the Results

C. Ohye[1], H. Nakajima, T. Matsushima, T. Komatsu, M. Hirato, and Y. Kawashima

Introduction

Various methods for CT assisted stereotactic biopsy of deep seated cerebral lesions have been reported on. We here describe our simple method of stereotactic biopsy and the results of long term follow-up of our patients.

Methods and Material

Twenty patients were included in this study. Fourteen were males and six females. The patients age was between 6 and 55 years. Fourteen patients had epileptic seizures at least once in their early history. Four showed symptoms of increased intracranial pressure. One patient had a motor paresis and one had involuntary movements. In diagnostic CT scans all patients had either high density (7 cases), low density (9 cases), isodensity (2 cases), or mixed low and high density (2 cases) supratentorial lesions. In two isodensity lesions, angiography or metrizamide ventriculography revealed an abnormal mass. Lesions were found in the right frontal region (5 cases), left frontal (2 cases), left temporal (2 cases), right parietal (1 case), left parietal (1 case), 3rd ventricle (3 cases), paraventricular (1 case), basal ganglia (4 cases) and corpus callosum (1 case).

When an intracranial lesion was visible, for example by calcificiation on plain X-ray, CT slices were made through the center of the lesion. We prefered a frontal approach. Based on the angle of CT slicing and Reid's base line, the approximate burr hole site for biopsy was determined and marked on the patient's scalp. When the lesion was not visible, the extent of the lesion was determined on the plain X-ray using a two-plane CT method[1], *i.e.* several CT slices were made along a plane passing the center of the lesion and through prefrontal region. The predetermined burr hole site was marked on the patient's scalp as mentioned above. A burr hole

[1] Address for Correspondence: Department of Neurosurgery, Gunma University School of Medicine, 3-39 Showa-machi, Maebashi, Gunma, Japan.

Table 1. *Summary of Cases*

Case No.	Age	Sex	Follow up interval after biopsy (months)		Histology
1	27	M	O ———————	65 M	Degen. Tiss.
2	53	M	O* Chem ——————— †	33 M	Ast. G 2
3	34	M	O ———————	60 M	Ang. Malf.
4	34	F	O* IR ———————	54 M	Ast. G 2
5	54	M	O* IR — †	7 M	Ast. G 4
6	6	F	O* IR ——————— †	22 M	Ependymoma
7	35	M	O ——— *OR + IR ———————	43 M	Ast. G 3
8	55	F	O ——— * IR * OR ———	50 M	Ast. G 3
9	10	M	O* IR ———————	37 M	Ast. G 2
10	16	M	O* OR + IR ———————	33 M	Ast. G 2
11	24	F	O* OR + IR ———————	33 M	Ast. G 2
12	26	M	O ———————	28 M	Gliosis
13	16	M	O ———————	33 M	Gliosis
14	8	M	O* IR ———————	30 M	Germinoma
15	13	M	O* IR ———————	18 M	Ast. G 2
16	14	F	O* IR ———————	18 M	Ast. G 2
17	21	F	O ———————	17 M	Gliosis
18	39	M	O ———————	10 M	Calc.
19	10	M	O* IR ———————	3 M	Germinoma
20	42	M	O* OR + IR ———————	7 M	Ast. G 2

O = biopsy, * = treatment, IR = irradiation, OR = operative removal, Ast. G 2 = astrocytoma grade 2, G 3 = grade 3, G 4 = grade 4, M = months, † = dead, Chem = chemotherapy.

was made at the already marked point and a recording or biopsy needle was introduced along a plane corresponding with the CT scan by adjusting the angle of the needle. This procedure served as a reliable guide to introduce the needle toward the target point. Using a high resolution CT scanner (GE CT/T for example) subcortical structures such as cortical gray, white matter, basal ganglia, thalamus and ventricles are well distinguished. Furthermore, prior to biopsy, electrical activity of subcortical structures was recorded by a semimicroelectrode to distinguish each structure according to the characteristic electrical pattern and to overcome intrinsic inaccuracy of CT images[2]. It was noteworthy that abnormal density areas, namely the target area, exhibited no electrical activity. Finally, the specimen was taken from this silent zone by suction or with a special forceps.

Results

The results are tabulated in Tab. 1. Among twenty cases, fourteen cases were diagnosed as neoplasms and six cases as being non-neoplastic. There were eleven cases of astrocytoma Grade II–IV, three cases of gliosis without neoplastic change, two germinomas, and one case of degenerative tissue, one angiomatous malformation, one ependymoma and one calcification ("brain stone"). Out of fourteen tumors, one astrocytoma of the corpus callosum (Grade IV) and one ependymoma of the 3rd ventricle died within several months in spite of radiation therapy. Treatment consisted in chemotherapy (1 case), radiation therapy (6 cases), partial removal of the tumor followed by radiation therapy (3 cases) and no treatment at all (2 cases). The patient treated by chemotherapy only deteriorated and died 33 months later. In two patients not treated initially partial removal of the tumor and radiation therapy were carried out 2 years later because of tumor growth (astrocytoma grade III).

Eleven patients with tumors are still alive. Six patients without a neoplasm are doing well. Stereotactic biopsy is an useful method to decide on the basis of histological findings which therapeutic procedure is appropriate for small deep seated lesions in the brain.

References

1. Ohye, C., Nagaseki, Y., Shibazaki, T., Hirai, T., Imai, S., Physiologically guided stereotactic biopsy for symptomatic epileptic patients with CT scan abnormality. In: Stereotactic Cerebral Irradiation (Szikla, G., ed.), pp. 69—74. North Holland, Amsterdam: Elsevier. 1979.
2. Ohye, C., Nakajima, H., Kawashima, Y., Miyazaki, M., Stereotactic CT scan and its correlation with the neural activity of the deep structure. Appl. Neurophysiol. *43* (1980), 183—188.

Acta Neurochirurgica, Suppl. 33, 261—263 (1984)

Observations with the Utilization of the Brown-Roberts-Wells Stereotactic System in the Management of Intracranial Mass Lesions

M. L. J. Apuzzo[1], **V. Zelman**[1], **J. Jepson**[2], and **P. Chandrasoma**[3]

A prototype Brown-Roberts-Wells (BRW) stereotactic instrument (production model now available, Radionics, Inc., Burlington, MA, U.S.A.) has been employed as both a diagnostic and surgical adjunct in intracranial mass lesions. This data represents the first one hundred consecutive cases (167 point placements) requiring computerized guidance of stereotaxy at our institution employing this technique. The system, which is comprised of four major functional units (a base ring, a localizer, a phantom base, and arc system) was employed with a GE 8800 scanner (General Electric Company, Medical Systems Division, Milwaukee, WI, U.S.A.) for data collection and a Hewlett Packard (HP41 CV) (Hewlett Packard, Palo Alto, CA, U.S.A.) programable calculator for data processing. In all procedures the so called BRWT program which allows for entry point selection by the surgeon was used. These components accomplished point access within one hour with an accuracy of more that one millimeter. All cases were completed under local anesthesia in the operating theater with only data collection accomplished in the scanner area. Scanner utilization times were generally 15 minutes or less.

The pathological processes included 66 neoplasms, 9 vascular events and 25 infections or infestations affecting deep regions of the cerebral hemispheres, midline structures, ventricular cavities, cerebellum or brain stem (Table 1). Biopsy (> 400 point specimens), culture, evacuation, aspiration, endoscopic excision

[1] Departments of Neurosurgery, [2] Radiation Medicine, and [3] Pathology University of Southern California School of Medicine, Los Angeles, California and Kenneth R. Norris, Jr. Cancer Hospital and Research Institute.

Table 1. *Localization of Target Masses (100 Cases)*

A. *Cerebral (77)*	
Dominant hemisphere	43
Nondominant hemisphere	34
Centrum, basal gangia	51
Para III ventricular	9
Temporal lobe	9
III ventricular	5
Pineal region	4
B. *Cerebellar (9)* (transtentorial)	
C. *Diencephalic—mesencephalic (14)*	

Table 2. *Procedural Complications (100 Cases)*—2%*

A. Deaths	0
B. Hematoma (1)	temporal tip
C. Infection (1)	

* 167 point placements.
400 point tissue specimens.

and implantation of isotopes were successfully completed with an overall complication rate of 2% (Table 2) and a tissue recovery adequate to establish criteria for subsequent patient management in 96% of cases.

Biopsy was accomplished mainly by utilization of flexible forceps (Olympus Corp. of America, New Hyde Park, New York, NY, U.S.A.) through a 13 gauge cannula introduced to the target area (82 cases).

Posterior fossa masses were approached transtentorially with the tentorium being perforated following ultra short-acting barbiturate administration (9 cases).

Intraventricular, cisternal and intraparenchymatous endoscopy was performed with a 6.8 mm sheathed instrument (Karl Storz, Endoscopy-America Inc. Southboro, MA, U.S.A.) which allows for visualization, irrigation, aspiration, tissue removal and fiberoptic laser introduction (12 cases).

Isotope implantation was designed to assure irradiation of extensive tumor target areas. Multiple transcutaneous catheter arrays (four to nine units) were employed with multiple point sources (40–94) of iridium-192 (14 cases).

The safety and reliability of the method and its applications appear to be related to the inherent design accuracy of the BRW system, patient selection, intrumentation at the target point, selection of the target point, proper preoperative planning, and adjunctive professional support (*i.e.* anesthesiology, pathology, cytology, microbiology, radiation physics, radiation therapy, laser physics, and radiology).

The system appears to be adaptable for utilization with NMR and PET imaging, and has been employed in conjunction with real time ultrasonography. Its value for use in combination with laser endoscopy, photodynamic agents via laser fiberoptics and microwave antenna placement for hyperthermia therapy are being evaluated. More complex programs relating instrumentation to imaging data are being developed.

Acta Neurochirurgica, Suppl. 33, 265—267 (1984)

CAT Scan-directed Stereotactic Brain Biopsy: With Template Produced by Computer Graphics

B. L. Wise[1] **and C. Gleason**

Summary

Stereotactic biopsy of inaccessible deep cerebral lesions based on and directed by the CT scan is a safe and effective method of biopsying cerebral lesions. It also has a potential for treatment of certain deep cerebral lesions and for instillation of antibiotics, tapping cysts, etc. The coordinates for the stereotactic procedure may be obtained by measuring the location of the lesion on CAT scan of the head and inputting these measurements into special BASIC computer program. The computer printer makes a template which is superimposed on the lateral radiograph of the head with stereotactic frame in place, and the coordinates read off from the scales. The potential for possible stereotactic RF lesioning of deep brain tumors, after other methods have failed, deserves further investigation.

We have found stereotactic biopsy of deep cerebral lesions, using a modified Leksell stereotactic frame[1] with specially designed biopsy needles, to be an effective and safe method to obtain adequate tissue to diagnose deep cerebral lesions. We started doing these procedures before CT scanning was available; then, the procedure required pneumo-encephalography or ventriculography for localization of the lesion prior to biopsy.

Since CT scanning became available, both we and others have adopted it to stereotactic biopsy, thereby obviating the need for pneumography. Most other techniques require CT scanning with the stereotactic frame on the patient, and some require the entire procedure to be done with the patient in the scanner. While these techniques are accurate, they require considerable CT scan time or even a dedicated CT scanner and software program, which may not be possible in a busy general hospital.

[1] Department of Neurosciences, Mount Zion Hospital and Medical Center, 1600 Divisadero St., San Francisco, California, U.S.A.

In our technique, the previously recorded CT scan is extrapolated on to the AP and lateral radiographs taken with the stereotactic frame on the patient's head and the stereotactic X and Y coordinates of the lesion are read off from the scales on the film. (Appropriate corrections are made for X-ray magnification and X-ray beam center.) The Z coordinate is scaled from the CT scan which is recorded with an overlying grid so the distances may be measured directly[2].

Our latest modification involves a computer program which takes the measurements of the location of the lesion on the CT scan, does all the necessary calculations including correction for X-ray magnification, and prints a template which is superimposed on the lateral X-ray of the skull taken with the frame in place. The lesion is drawn on the film and the stereotactic coordinates are then read off directly from the scales. We have used the DEC PDP 11/34 computer, but any computer using BASIC can be used.

A burr hole is placed in an appropriate position and the biopsy needle (a specially designed long No. 14 needle with stylet) is passed through the electrode carrier of the stereotactic frame to the appropriate position. Aspiration via syringe is maintained during the passage through the lesion and on withdrawal. Frozen section examination of the removed tissue is done immediately. Further specimens may be taken as needed for further frozen or permanent section. Our procedures have all been done under general anesthesia although local anesthesia is feasible.

To date, sixteen (16) stereotactic biopsies of brain lesions have been done.

The diagnosis are as follows:

Table 1

Glioma	7
Malignant lymphoma of the brain ("microglioma")	2
"Inflammatory" lesion	2
"Degenerative" lesion—no tumor	1
Brain abscess	1
Metastatic carcinoma	2
Germinoma of brain	1

Two of the gliomas were multicentric. The patients with "inflammatory" and "degenerative" lesions were followed for several years, so it does not appear that tumors were missed. There were no serious permanent complications and no deaths. In two patients, there was a transient increase in neurological deficit which cleared.

Our recent policy has been to begin steroid administration at the time of the biopsy, but not before, and to stop it within several days if there is no worsening of the patient's condition, unless it is continued as part of the management of the lesion.

The same technique was used to treat lesions in two instances; in one, to tap a brain abscess and instill antibiotics[3] and the other, to make RF lesions in a glioma which had recurred after radiation.

References

1. Feinstein, B., Alberts, W. W., Wright, E. W., jr., Levin, G., A stereotaxic technique in man allowing multiple spatial and temporal approaches to intracranial targets. J. Neurosurg. *17* (1960), 708—720.
2. Gleason, C. A., Wise, B. L., Feinstein, B., Stereotactic localization (with computerized tomographic scanning), biopsy, and radiofrequency treatment of deep brain lesions. Neurosurgery *2* (1978), 217—222.
3. Wise, B. L., Gleason, C. A., CT directed stereotactic surgery in the management of brain abscess. Ann. Neurol. *6* (1979), 457.

patients, there was a transient increase in neurological deficit which cleared.

Our recent policy has been to begin steroid administration at the time of the biopsy, but not before, and to stop it within several days if there is no worsening of the patient's condition, unless it is continued as part of the management of the lesion.

The stereotactic technique was also used therapeutically in two instances: in one, to tap a brain abscess and instill antibiotics, and the other to make RF lesions in a [illegible] which had recurred after [illegible].

References

1. [illegible], B., Abrams?, W., [illegible], W., and Leksell?, L.: A stereotactic technique in [illegible] ... and temporal approaches to intracranial [illegible]. Neurosurg. 37 (1980) 205–[illegible].
2. [illegible], A., [illegible], R., [illegible], S., [illegible]: [illegible] ... and [illegible] of deep brain [illegible]. [illegible] (19[illegible]) [illegible].
3. [illegible], B. [illegible], A., [illegible]: [illegible] ... of brain [illegible] ... 6–17.

Section II

Cerebral Tumors

2. Stereotactic Focal Irradiation

Acta Neurochirurgica, Suppl. 33, 271—280 (1984)

I. Effects on Tumour and Brain

Experimental Data on Early and Late Morphologic Effects of Permanently Implanted Gamma and Beta Sources (Iridium-192, Iodine-125 and Yttrium-90) in the Brain

Ch. B. Ostertag[1], **D. Groothuis**[2], and **P. Kleihues**[3]

With 3 Figures

Summary

To study the radiation response of normal brain tissue to interstitial irradiation Iodine-125 seeds and Iridium-192 wire pieces were permanently implanted into the subcortical white matter in beagle dogs. Sequential observations on physiologic and morphologic changes were carried out up to one year after implantation. To study the radiation effects of Iodine-125 implants on neoplastic tissue, Avian-sarcoma-virus induced gliomas and sarcomas in beagle brains were permanently implanted with Iodine-125 seeds under CT stereotactic conditions. The intratumoral placement produced sharply defined necroses with central mineralization.

Keywords: Interstitial irradiation; Iodine-125; Iridium-192; experimental brain tumor; Avian-sarcoma-virus; quantitative autoradiography.

---

[1] Abteilung Stereotaxie and Neuronuklearmedizin, Neurochirurgische Klinik, Universität Freiburg, Hugstetter Strasse 55, D-7800 Freiburg im Breisgau, Federal Republic of Germany.

[2] Department of Neurology, Evanston Hospital, Northwestern University, Evanston, Illinois, U.S.A.

[3] Abteilung Neuropathologie, Pathologisches Institut, Universität Freiburg, Hugstetter Strasse 55, D-7800 Freiburg im Breisgau, Federal Republic of Germany.

Introduction

Local interstitial radiation therapy of intrinsic and inaccessible brain tumors is confronted with two major problems:

1. The tolerance of normal brain tissue, which is usually involved in local tumor irradiation, *i.e.* perifocal white matter edema and demyelinating effects, is crucial.

2. Data on radiation effects of implanted radioactive sources on neoplastic tissue, *i.e.* data on the radiosensitivity and on the biology of tumors, are still widely unavailable.

In clinical practice the dose with which to achieve a given volume of tumor necrosis is roughly estimated. This report deals with the experimental findings of Iodine-125 and Iridium-192 permanent implants in healthy and neoplastic brain tissue. Our own experimental findings are correlated with experimental data on Yttrium-90 irradiation from the literature. The study is directed to collect data on the tolerance non-tumoral brain tissue and to attempt to establish a dose-response relationship.

Morphologic Changes in the Dog Brain Following Interstitial Iodine-125 Irradiation

Iodine-125 seeds (manufactured by 3 M Company, St. Paul, M. N.) with an activity of 3.55 mCi were permanently implanted under stereotactic conditions into the subcortical white matter of the gyrus coronalis of the left hemisphere in 6 beagle dogs.

One animal with a non-radioactive seed implanted under similar operative conditions served as a control. The animals were allowed to survive 25, 46, 71, 94, 248, 368 days, respectively, after the implantation. The control animal survived 46 days. A detailed description of the experimental procedure is given elsewhere[16,17].

The accumulated doses were calculated in cGy from a point source reflecting the radioactive decay with respect to time. The dose rate constant used was 1.35 ($\pm$ 3.5%) rad $\cdot$ $cm^2/mCi \cdot h$[12–14]. The calculated doses at a 5 mm distance ranged from 7,900 cGy in 25 days to 32,000 cGy in 368 days*.

In all of the experimental animals, the radioactive seeds were surrounded by a zone of calcified necross (Fig. 1). In the initial stages (up to 70 days survival), the necrotic area was usually dumb-

---

* Thanks go to K. Schlegel of the Deutsche Krebsforschungsinstitut, Heidelberg, for providing the dosimetry calculations.

bell shaped with larger extensions at both ends of the seed. In later stages, necroses were increasingly oval-shaped and almost entirely calcified. Reaction in the adjacent brain tissue differed distinctly in the grey and the white matter. In the cortex, there was a very limited astrocytic reaction in the immediate vicinity of the seed. Neurons, even at a distance of less than ·2 mm from the necrotic zone, were morphologically normal. In contrast to the grey matter, the white matter reaction extended more deeply into the adjacent structures.

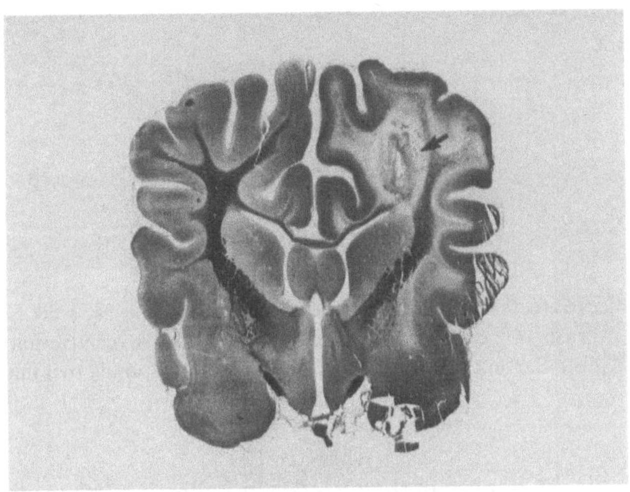

Fig. 1. Coronal section through the brain of a dog surviving 18 days after implantation of an Iodine-125 seed (10.3 mCi). The accumulated dose at 5 mm distance perpendicular to the seed's axis was 20,000 cGy. Note the calcified necrosis (↑) around the removed seed, the perifocal demyelination and the diffuse vasogenic edema of the homolateral white matter (Klüver-Barrera stain, 1.5 ×)

There was an extensive astrocytic reaction with numerous, often densely packed GFAP positive cells[9].

The perifocal white matter was usually microcystic and the Heidenhain-Woelcke stain revealed a small zone of demyelination with an extension of up to 3 mm from the central radionecrosis (Fig. 2). Blood vessels with radiation damage could not be detected in the animals surviving more than 70 days. Immunohistochemical stainings using antiserum against dog serum proteins showed an extensive vasogenic edema, both perifocally and in the homolateral white matter.

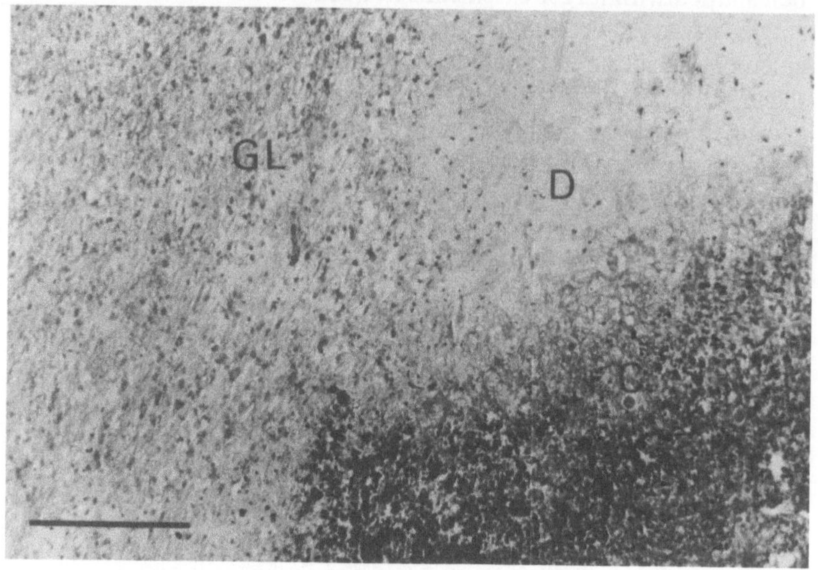

Fig. 2. Enlarged section of a tissue necrosis around an Iodine-125 seed: Next to the calcified necrosis (*C*), a zone of demyelination (*D*) and a reactive gliosis (*GL*). (Klüver-Barrera stain. The horizontal bar corresponds to 1 mm)

Physiological Changes in the Dog Brain Following Interstitial I-125 Irradiation

Single Iodine-125 seeds with activities ranging between 6 and 8 mCi were permanently implanted into the subcortical white matter of 18 beagle dogs. The seeds were left in place for duration of 16 to 175 days. Permeability changes attributed to the radionecrosis were studied using quantitative autoradiography with C^{14}-alpha-aminoisobutyric acid (AIB). A unidirectional blood-to-tissue transfer constant (K) of AIB was measured, which under these conditions is an estimate of the capillary permeability-surface area product[3]. The transfer constant of AIB in normal brain is approx. 0.002 ml/g/min.

In all dogs, regardless of time of exposure, there was around the implant a clearly demarcated sphere of blood-brain-barrier breakdown. The highest values for the transfer constant were found in the rim of vital brain around the necrosis, and ranged from 0.02 to 0.05 ml/g/min, *i.e.* an increase of 10 to 25 times that of normal brain. The values showed a rapid return to normal brain values over distances of millimeters from the necrosis. The values were higher in the white matter than in grey matter along the edge of the necrosis. There was no increase in the contralateral hemisphere.

Morphologic Changes in the Dog Brain Following Interstitial Iridium-192 Irradiation

Single pieces of Iridium-192 wire (2.6 mm length, 1.05 mCi) were permanently implanted into the subcortical white matter of the left hemispheres of 6 dogs. As in the preceding Iodine-125 experiment, the animals were allowed to survive 25, 46, 70, 120, 250 and 365 days, respectively. After sacrifice of the dogs, morphological studies were carried out as described in the I-125 experiment.

Already in the initial stages (up to 46 days) the radioactive wires were surrounded by a delineated calcifying necrosis. After 70 days the central necrosis was liquified with a perifocal small rim of clacification (up to .3 mm). The necrosis was almost spherical and had a diameter of 5.5 mm. The transistional zone (up to 2 mm) was characterized by an extensive gliosis and numerous blood vessels with enlarged diameter and thickening of the vessel wall. The perifocal white matter was microcystic. Heidenhain-Woelcke stains revealed a perifocal demyelination, which was not sharply demarcated. There was an extensive vasogenic edema in the homolateral white matter.

Radiation Effects of Iodine-125 in Virally-Induced Dog Brain Tumors

Brain tumors were induced by intracerebral inoculation of 7 three day old thoroughbread beagle puppies with .05 ml Avian-sarcoma virus (ASV) suspension. The ASV suspension was donated by D. A. Bigner, Durham, North Carolina. Injections were given percutanously into the left hemisphere using an automatic injection device. At the time of the first tumor postive CT control, a single Iodine-125 seed (8.5–10.5 mCi activity) was placed into the lesion. The animals were observed until severe neurological deficits occured and death was assumed to be imminent. The dogs were sacrificed after survival times ranging from 15 to 97 days. Morphologic studies were carried out as described in the previous experiments. The inoculation produced solitary or multiple sarcomas in three dogs and intraventricular anaplastic gliomas in four dogs.

The intratumoral placement of Iodine-125 seeds in anaplastic gliomas produced sharply defined calcifying necroses with unaffected vital tumor tissue outside the necrosis (Fig. 3). The

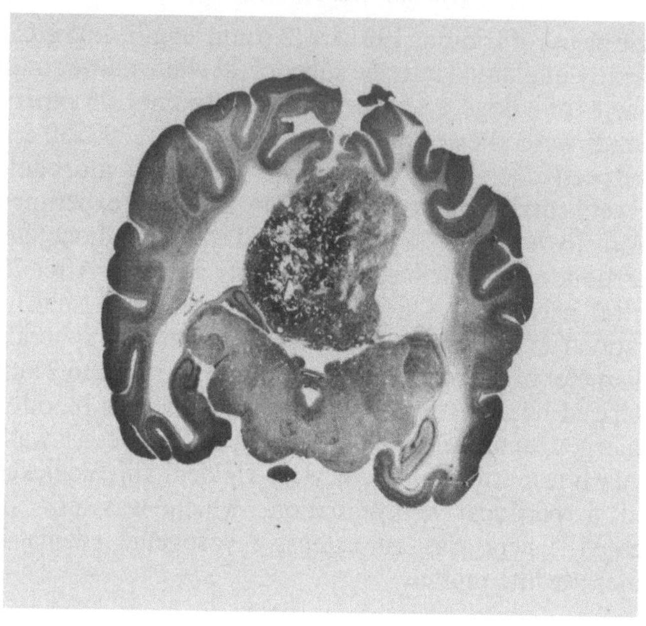

Fig. 3. Coronal section through the brain of a dog with an Avian-sarcoma-virus induced anaplastic glioma which was implanted with an Iodine-125 seed (10.5 mCi, 18 days). Note the sharply delineated calcified necrosis with vital tumor outside the necrosis (Klüver-Barrera, 1.5 ×)

necrotizing and calcifying effect was already apparent after 18 days with a transitional zone of up to 4 mm. The calcified necrosis was complete after 97 days when the transitional zone was no longer detectable. The calcification pattern of the necrosis was distinctly different from tumor calcifications in non-irradiated tumor parts. The maximum resulting volume of necrosis was 2.14 ml after 97 days and 10.5 mCi implanted activity. In all cases, a considerable shrinkage of radionecrotic tumor parts was evident in consecutive CT controls.

Discussion

The rationale of interstitial irradiation is to deliver a high local dose with a rapid fall off outside the target volume, thereby avoiding damage to the surrounding healthy brain.

Experimental studies on interstitial radiation effects in brain tissue are fragmentary and deal mostly with the effects of Radium-226[8,18,23], Radon-222[10,11,19], Gold-198[1,21] and the beta emitting Yttrium-90[5-7].

The low energy gamma radiation of I-125 and the absence of beta radiation cause tissue reactions which are different from either beta emitting sources like Yttrium-90 or the gamma and beta emitting sources like Radon-222, Gold-198 and Iridium-192.

Due to the low photon energy of I-125, much of the energy is absorbed by the tissue next to the implant. Accordingly, we found around the implanted seed a necrosis which was always calcified and was observed as early as 25 days after the implantation and reached its maximum after approx. 70 days. The size of the necrosis did not increase further after 70 days (18,000 cGy). The dose which accumulated later apparently did not contribute to the necrotizing effect. The conspicuous calcification around the seed diminishes the absorbed radiation considerably. In the animal surviving one year, the resultant tissue defect was almost spherical, *i.e.* the non-isotropic dose distribution of the I-125 seeds was no longer recognizable. A regular feature was the presence of a widespread vasogenic edema, which was restricted to the homolateral hemisphere. The "breakdown" of the blood-brain-barrier that occurs around an Iodine-125 implant is restricted. Delayed radiation damage outside the perifocal demyelinated zone, which is frequently observed after conventional external irradiation, was not detected[4].

The morphologic changes in I-125 implants differed in many aspects from those resulting from either pure beta radiation or high energy gamma radiation. In a previous paper, we reported on the effects of short time (up to 35 days) Iridium-192 permanent implants in the cat brain[15]. Long term implants (up to 120 days) yielded both calcifying and liquifying necroses. The transition zone between the area of destruction and the healthy brain was not as sharply demarcated as that around I-125 implants. The high energy gamma radiation of Ir-192 (half-life 74.5 d, 300–610 keV), which has also been extensively used for interstitial irradiation of gliomas, is absorbed by brain tissue to a much lesser degree than the low energy gamma radiation of I-125.

On the other hand, Y-90, being a pure beta emitter like Pd-109, causes small, sharply defined, sometimes fluid-filled cystic brain lesions due to the finite range of beta particles[6,7]. A fluid-filled cystic lesion was never observed after I-125 permanent implantation, reither experimental nor human. Instead, there was always a calcifying necrosis. Another prominent feature of Y-90 irradiation is an acute widespread vasogenic brain edema and delayed demyelination. Due to the rapid absorption of beta rays by brain tissue, low or high activity Y-90 sources effect necroses which do not differ much in size but in permeability changes in the perifocal zone[6].

Experimental Gold-198 implants, having physical characteristics which make them strongly resemble Radon-222 implants, cause tissue changes of both types, focal necrosis, and more distant tissue reactions[1].

To gain an idea of the necrotizing effect of interstitially implanted Iodine-125 and of the radiation dosage necessary to destroy a given tumor volume, morphologic changes were correlated with the accumulated radiation dose. Avian sarcoma virus (ASV)-induced dog brain tumors were chosen to serve as a primary model for human brain tumors[2,22]. These tumors are autochtonous, *i.e.* their blood supply and growth are characteristic of a primary brain tumor. Apart from sarcomas, the most often found tumor type is an anaplastic glioma, which is similar to the most often found human brain tumor[22].

The most striking feature observed after intra-tumoral placement of I-125 seeds was the resulting volume of tumor necrosis, which was almost spherical and 3–5 times greater than comparable necroses in healthy brain tissue. The calculated accumulated dose at the surface of the necrotic volume ranged between 10–12,000 cGy. This estimation of the absorbed dose applies only for a medium in which the attenation coefficient is known. The perifocal calcification, however, is assumed to absorb as much as 30% of the radiation energy.

Conclusions

1. Implants of Iodine-125 in the dog brain effect sharply delineated calcifying necroses with a small perifocal zone of demyelination and an ipsilateral vasogenic edema. The edema is most prominent after 120 days, whereas the necrosis does not

increase in size any further after 70 days. The total size of the necrosis depends on the implanted activity.

2. Implants of Iridium-192 wire pieces in the healthy dog brain produce liquifying and calcifying defined necroses. The transitional zone with vessel damage, gliosis, and demyelination is considerably wider when compared with Iodine-125 induced necroses.

3. Yttrium-90 rods within days provoke the most acute perifocal edema of the vasogenic type with a progressive focal demyelinating process. The size of the resulting, often liquifying necrosis is more or less irrespective of the implanted activity. The speed and the degree of spreading of the vasogenic edema, however, depend on the activity implanted.

4. Iodine-125 implants in virally-induced anaplastic gliomas and sarcomas in dogs effect sharply delineated clacifying necroses. The response of tumor tissue and tumor vessels to low dose rate gamma radiation is distinctly different in terms of the necrotic volume but not of the necrobiotic characteristics when compared with Iodine-125 radio-necroses in healthy brain tissue.

References

1. Ajuriaguerra, J. D. E., Bende, P., Constans, J., David, M., Tubiana, M., Étude expérimentale des lésions provoquées par l'implantation intracérébrale de fragments d'or radioactif: Incidences thérapeutiques. Rev. Neurol. (Paris) *91* (1954), 260—285.
2. Bigner, D. D., Odem, G. L., Mahaley, M. S., Day, E. D., Brain tumor induced in dogs by the Schmidt-Ruppin strain of rour sarcoma virus. J. Neuropath. exp. Neurol. *28* (1969), 648.
3. Blasberg, R. G., Groothuis, D., Molnar, P., Application of quantitative autoradiographic measurements in experimental brain tumor models. Seminars in Neurology *1* (1981), 203—221.
4. Caveness, W. F., Experimental observations: Delayed necrosis in normal monkey brain. Radiation Damage to the Nervous-System (Gilbert, H. A., Kagan, A. R., eds.). New York: Raven Press. 1980.
5. Clayton, B. E., Langmead, W. A., Worden, J. M., Implantation of radioactive Yttrium in the pituitary fossa of the guinea pig. Br. J. Radiol. *34* (1961), 120—128.
6. Csanda, E., Radiation brain edema. Advances in Neurology, Vol. 28: Brain Edema (Cervós-Navarro, J., Ferszt, R., eds.). New York: Raven Press. 1980.
7. Csanda, E., Komoly, S., Takáts, A., Szücs, A., Neuropathological characteristics of Beta irradiation induced brain edeme. Acta Neuropathol. Suppl. VII, pp. 67—69. Berlin-Heidelberg-New York: Springer. 1981.
8. Davis, L., Goldstein, S. L., The therapeutic use of the radioactive isotopes in intracranial tumors. Ann. Surg. *136* (1952), 381—391.

9. Eng, L. F., DeArmond, S. J., Glial fibrillary acidic (GFA) protein immunocytochemistry in development and neuropathology. Eleventh international congress of anatomy: Glial and neuronal cell biology, pp. 65—79. New York: Alan R. Liss. 1981.
10. Edwards, D. J., Bagg, H. J., Lesions of the corpus striatum by radium emanation and the accompanying structural and functional changes. Amer. J. Physiol. *65* (1923), 162—183.
11. Globus, J. H., Wang, S. C., Radon implantation in the medulla oblongata of the dog; effects on the degree and extent of cellular reactions. J. Neuropathol. exp. Neurol. *11* (1952), 429—442.
12. Hartmann, G. H., Schlegel, W., Scharfenberg, H., The three dimensional dose distribution of ^{125}J Seeds in tissue. Phys. Med. Biol. *28* (1983), 693—699.
13. Hilaris, B. S., Handbook of interstitial brachytherapy. Acton, Mass.: Publishing Sciences Group. 1975.
14. Kirshnaswamy, V., Dose distribution around an ^{125}I seed source in tissue. Radiol. *126* (1978), 489—491.
15. Ostertag, C. B., Hossmann, K. A., v. d. Kerckhoff, W., Radiation effects of Iridium-192 implants in the cat brain. Nucl.-Med. *21* (1982), 99—104.
16. Ostertag, Ch. B., Weigel, K., Technical note: Three-dimensional CT scanning of the dog brain. J. Computer Ass. Tomography *6* (5) (1982), 1036—1037.
17. Ostertag, Ch. B., Weigel, K., Warnke, P., Lombeck, G., Kleihues, P., Sequential morphological changes in the dog brain following interstitial Iodine-125 irradiation. Neurosurgery *13* (1983), 523—528.
18. Pendergrass, E. P., Hayman, J. M., Houser, K. M., Rambo, V. C., The effect of radium on the normal tissue of the brain and spinal cord of dogs, and its therapeutic application. Amer. J. Roentgenol. *9* (1922), 553—569.
19. Stein, S. N., Peterson, E. W., The use of radon seeds to produce deep cerebral lesions. Proc. Soc. Exp. Biol. Med. *74* (1950), 583—585.
20. Szikla, G., Stereotactic cerebral irradiation. Proceedings of the INSERM Symposium on Stereotactic Irradiations held in Paris (France), 13. July 1979. Amsterdam: Elsevier/North Holland Biomedical Press. 1979.
21. Talairach, J., Ruggiero, G., Aboulker, J., David, M., A new method of treatment of inoperable brain tumours by stereotaxic implantation of radioactive Gold—A preliminary report. Br. J. Radiol. *28* (1955), 62—74.
22. Vick, N. A., Bigner, D. D., Kvedar, J. P., The fine structure of canine gliomas and intracranial sarcomas induced by the Schmidt-Ruppin strain of the rous sarcoma virus. J. Neuropathol. exp. Neurol. *30* (1971), 354—367.
23. Williamson, C. S., Brown, R. O., Butler, J. W., A study of the effects of radium on normal brain tissue. A preliminary report. Surg. Gynaec. Obstet. *31* (1920), 239—242.

Acta Neurochirurgica, Suppl. 33, 281—289 (1984)

Morphology of Intracranial Tumours and Adjacent Brain Structures Following Interstitial Iodine-125 Radiotherapy

M. Kiessling[1], **P. Kleihues**[1,*], **E. Gessaga**[3], **F. Mundinger**[2], **Ch. B. Ostertag**[2], and **K. Weigel**[2]

With 2 Figures

Summary

Analysis of 8 autopsied cases with permanent ^{125}I implantation demonstrates that interstitial irradiation of CNS neoplasms causes extensive focal tumour necroses. In some cases, complete tumour regression resulted, with no viable neoplastic cells detectable at autopsy. In large gliomas of the cerebral hemispheres and basal ganglia, central radiation-induced necroses were present, but peripheral tumour masses progressed and ultimately determined the clinical outcome. In patients with tumours located in basal midline structures, interstitial ^{125}I produced areas of delayed radionecrosis extending into the adjacent normal brain tissue. All of these patients were treated with external radiation in addition to interstitial implantation, indicating cumulative radiation toxicity.

Introduction

Focal application of radioactive sources for the cure of malignant tumours has been used for several decades in a variety of tissues and neoplasms[1]. In the nervous system this approach was pioneered by Talairach[10], Mundinger[5] and Szikla[9] who developed stereotactic techniques for interstitial radiotherapy of brain tumours. With the advancement of computerized tomography the diagnostic potential of stereotactic brain tumour biopsies[3] is being

---

[1] Abteilung Neuropathologie, Pathologisches Institut, [2] Abteilung Stereotaxie und Neuronuklearmedizin, Neurochirurgische Klinik, Universität Freiburg, Federal Republic of Germany, and [3] Pathologisches Institut, Kantonsspital Aarau, Switzerland.

* Address for Correspondence: Dr. P. Kleihues, Institut für Pathologie, Universitätsspital, CH-8091 Zürich, Switzerland.

recognized by an increasing number of neurosurgical oncologists and this technique is now frequently used to introduce radioactive seeds into various intracranial tumours for temporary or permanent interstitial radiation. During recent years, low energy-γ emitting ^{125}I has been preferentially used and clinical follow-up studies indicate that this treatment constitutes an effective adjuvant therapy of CNS tumours[6]. There is, however, little information on the morphological effects of ^{125}I irradiation on tumour tissue and adjacent brain structures. The present study is the first report on postmortem findings in patients with permanent implantation of ^{125}I seeds.

Case Reports

Case 1

History. A 16 year old male patient presented with right hemiparesis and aphasia. The CT-scan showed a fairly well demarcated space-occupying lesion in the left Sylvian fissure.

Stereotactic biopsy revealed a highly cellular, undifferentiated tumour, histopathologically classified as malignant Non-Hodgkin-lymphoma. A single ^{125}I seed (15.4 mCi) was implanted.

Postoperative course. A CT-scan performed $2\,^1/_2$ months later showed extensive tumour regression. A few days later the patient died with clinical signs of cardiac failure.

Autopsy. Only a brain autopsy was permitted. The radioactive seed was located in the left insular region and surrounded by a small radionecrosis. The subcortical white matter revealed foci of demyelinization with reactive gliosis. Occasionally, small vessels in the vicinity of the seed showed fibrinoid necroses. Remnants of the tumour were not detectable.

Case 2

CT-Scan of the 53-year old male patient showed an extensive hypodense space-occupying lesion in the left frontal lobe extending into the rostral basal ganglia.

Stereotactic biopsy revealed an anaplastic astrocytoma (WHO Grade III). Three ^{125}I seeds (total activity 68 mCi) were implanted into different areas of the tumour (Fig. 1, lower), followed by postoperative external radiation (7,500 rads).

Postoperative Course. Approximately 6 months later, the condition of the patient deteriorated and the CT showed signs of tumour progression. A further therapeutic attempt was made using temporary irradiation with ^{125}I (15.3 mCi) but the patient died the following day with symptoms of increased intracranial pressure.

Autopsy. The implanted ^{125}I seeds were surrounded by extensive tumour necroses (Fig. 1, upper) with radiation-induced fibrinoid degeneration of vessel

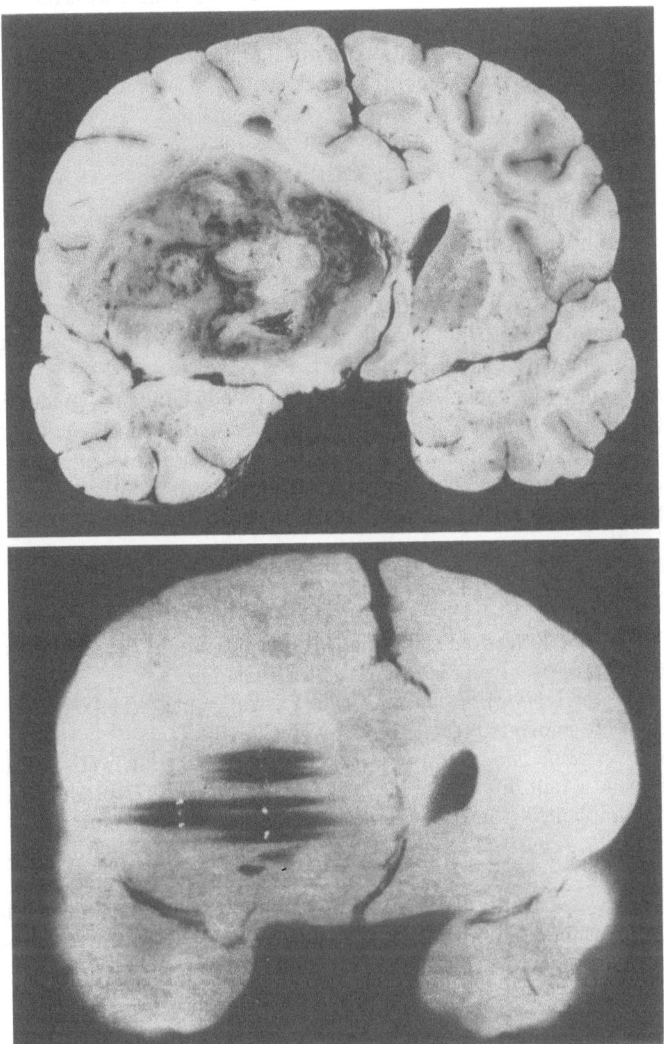

Fig. 1. Anaplastic astrocytoma of the left frontal lobe extending into the corpus striatum. The postmortem autoradiograph (lower) shows three radioactive seeds with inhomogeneous, predominantly lateral radiation distribution[4]. Comparison with the gross morphology (upper) reveals extensive necrotic foci in the vicinity of the implanted ^{125}I seeds (case 2)

walls. Outside the necrotic foci were solid tumour masses, histopathologically classified as anaplastic astrocytoma (WHO Grade III). The tumour extended in dorsolateral direction, including the insular cortex and in these areas the neoplasm showed no necroses and less signs of anaplasia. There was an extensive perifocal edema with transtentorial herniation, midbrain hemorrhages and infarcts in the territory of both posterior cerebral arteries.

Case 3

CT-Scan of the 46 year-old female patient showed a poorly delineated hypodense zone in the fronto-temporal region of the right hemisphere.

Stereotactic biopsy revealed a fibrillary astrocytoma (WHO Grad II). A single ^{125}I seed was implanted (15.4 mCi).

Postoperative course. Initially, the patient recovered well but died 6 months later from pulmonary embolism.

Autopsy showed an anaplastic astrocytoma (WHO Grade III) predominantly located in the right temporal lobe. The radioactive seed was located at the upper margin of the tumour and was surrounded by a focal radionecrosis (8 mm diameter). This necrosis was located in the infiltration zone of the tumour and in this area no clear signs of anaplasia were histopathologically detectable.

Case 4

CT-Scan. The 20 year old female patient showed a poorly demarcated, slightly hyperdense space-occupying lesion in the left thalamus.

1st Stereotactic biopsy revealed a fibrillary astrocytoma (WHO Grade II). Two ^{125}I seeds were implanted (total activity 17 mCi).

2nd Stereotactic biopsy was performed $10^1/_2$ months later. Histopathology showed again a well differentiated fibrillary astrocytoma. Two additional ^{125}I seeds were implanted (total activity 56 mCi).

Postoperative course. The patient recovered well but died approximately one year later from tumour recurrence with increased intracranial pressure.

Autopsy revealed a fibrillary astrocytoma in the left thalamus which extended into the hippocampus and left cerebral peduncle. The ^{125}I seeds were surrounded by extensive radionecroses but in the periphery viable tumour tissue was present.

Case 5

CT-Scan. The 14 year old boy showed a poorly demarcated cystic tumour in the left basal ganglia with extension into the insular region.

Stereotactic biopsy revealed a low grade astrocytoma (WHO Grad II). Three ^{125}I seeds were implanted (total activity 29 mCi), followed by postoperative external radiation (4,500 rads).

Postoperative course was characterized by marked tumour regression with formation of a large central cyst. The patient died two years later from bronchopneumonia.

Autopsy. Examination of the brain revealed large areas of radionecroses which extended into the left temporal lobe and adjacent parts of the hippocampus, fornices, amygdalae and thalamus. The pathological features included radiation damage of the vessels, necrotising demyelination and focal mineralization. The periphery of this lesion showed a marked reactive gliosis but tumour tissue was not identifiable.

Case 6

CT-Scan. The 2 year old girl presented with a well demarcated tumour in the basal midline structures bordering the third ventricle.

1st Open surgery revealed an anaplastic astrocytoma (WHO Grad III). Postoperative treatment consisted of external radiation (5,000 rad) and chemotherapy with CCNU and Vincristine.

2nd Open surgery was performed two years later, with partial tumour resection.

Stereotactic biopsy was performed another $3^1/_2$ months later and confirmed the presence of an anaplastic astrocytoma. A single ^{125}I seed was implanted (16 mCi).

Postoperative course. The girl died approximately three years after the first operation from a viral respiratory infection with pleuritis.

Autopsy. Histological examination of the brain revealed complete tumour regression with extensive hyalinosis and calcification. There were areas with marked vessel fibrosis which enlarged into a dense network of connective tissue (Fig. 2, lower). These changes also extended into adjacent brain structures (thalamus, nucleus lentiformis, tractus opticus). No viable tumour cells were detectable.

Case 7

CT-Scan. The 36 year-old female patient presented with a tumour in the suprasellar region with extension into the third ventricle.

Open surgery. Only a small part of the tumour could be removed, histopathologically classified as craniopharyngioma. Postoperative treatment consisted of external radiation (6,000 rads).

Stereotactic biopsy was performed one year later, with implantation of a single ^{125}I seed (5.9 mCi).

Postoperative course. The patient died $2^1/_2$ years after the first operation with acute hemorrhagic pneumonia.

Autopsy. The remaining tumour mass was located at the bottom of the third ventricle but showed extensive regression with marked hyalinosis and fibrosis. Only a very small focus of identifiable squamous epithelium (craniopharyngeoma) was detectable. In the adjacent brain structures (hypothalamus, chiasma, corpora mamillaria) areas of delayed radiation necrosis were present (Fig. 2, upper).

Case 8

CT-Scan. The 20 year-old male patient presented with a hyperdense tumour in the pineal region extending into the third ventricle.

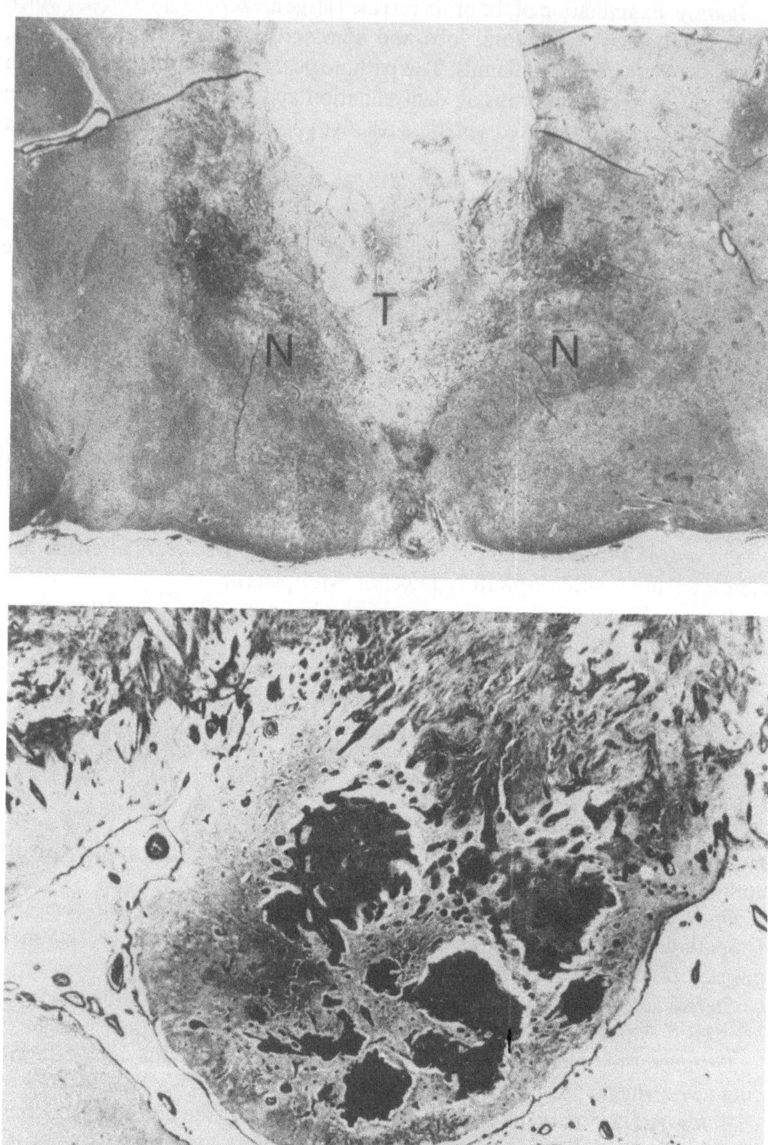

Fig. 2. *Upper:* Craniopharyngioma (*T*) in the third ventricle with extensive regressive tissue changes (hyalinization and fibrosis) following interstitial irradiation with ^{125}I. Delayed radionecroses (*N*) in the adjacent hypothalamus (case 7). PTAH, × 6.9. *Lower:* Extensive reactive fibrosis in the optic tract in the vicinity of an anaplastic astrocytoma interstitially irradiated with ^{125}I (case 6). PTAH, × 11.9

Stereotactic biopsy revealed a germinoma. A single ^{125}I seed was implanted (10 mCi), followed by external radiation (3,000 rads).

Postoperative course. The patient recovered very well and CT follow-up revealed complete tumour regression. Approximately 6 months after the operation the patient developed ocular muscle paralysis, paraparesis and ataxia and died approximately one year after the operation.

Autopsy revealed a focal necrosis with fibrotic tissue changes and mineralization around the radioactive seed which was located in the pineal region. In addition, there was an extensive area of delayed radionecrosis of the midbrain and the rostral portion of the pons. The splenium corporis callosi, although equidistant to the seed, showed no signs of radiation damage. Viable tumour cells were not detectable.

Discussion

The aim of the present study was to seek confirmation that interstitial radiotherapy is capable of causing tumour regression, and to determine whether or not effective treatment is possible without radiation damage to adjacent brain structures. Analysis of the present series of 8 autopsy cases clearly demonstrates that permanent implantation of ^{125}I seeds causes extensive tumour necroses. Complete tumour regression with no identifiable remnants of neoplastic tissue was observed in case 1, *i.e.* a patient with a malignant Non-Hodgkin lymphoma in the left insular region. Only a small central radionecrosis with perifocal demyelination ("early delayed" radionecrosis) was present. In grade II and III astrocytomas of the cerebral hemispheres (cases 2 and 3) and the basal ganglia (case 4) necrotic tumour areas were fairly well delineated and largely restricted to the vicinity (approximately 1 cm diameter) of the implanted radioactive source. The presence of tumour vessels with fibrinoid degeneration indicates that these necrotic areas were indeed produced by irradiation rather than being due to rapid tumour growth with insufficient blood supply. In all of these 3 cases, however, viable tumour masses progressed outside the effective radiation range and ultimately led to the death of the patient. Despite precise positioning of the seeds, incomplete regression resulted in cases 2 and 4. In case 3 the ^{125}I seed was obviously implanted in the tumour periphery (infiltration zone). This also led to a diagnostinc misjudgement of tumour grading, since bioptic samples did not contain the centrally located anaplastic foci. In two other patients with astrocytomas grade II (case 5) and III (case 6), tumour regression was more extensive but radiation effects extended into surrounding normal brain structures. In both of these cases the entire tumour mass was transformed into a cystic (case 5) or highly fibrotic (case 6) lesion, in which viable neoplastic cells were no longer detectable. However, extensive areas of delayed radionecrosis were found in adjacent basal midline structures, *i.e.* hypothalamus, fornices, amygdalae and optic tract. This was similarly true in a patient with craniopharyngioma (case 7). Again, the tumour had completely regressed and presented histologically as a fibrotic mass at the base of the third ventricle (Fig. 2, upper) with only very small nests of viable epithelial structures identifiable as craniopharyngeoma. Delayed radionecrosis with demyelination and fibrinoid vessel degeneration was present in the neighbouring diencephalic structures. In the patient with interstitial radiation of a pineal germinoma (case 8) there was also complete tumour regression but autopsy findings suggest that the postoperative course was adversely affected by delayed radionecrosis which developed in adjacent midbrain structures approximately 6 months following interstitial implantation of a ^{125}I seed.

Morphological analysis of the brains of patients treated with external radiotherapy for intracranial gliomas have shown that radiation damage to the normal brain constitutes a risk which is, to some extent, unpredictable if doses in the range of 5,000–6,000 rads are employed[2,7]. There are indications that peritumoural edema may enhance radiosensitivity of the surrounding white matter and that midbrain structures exhibit an increased tendency for the development of delayed radionecrosis[2]. The present study corroborates these observations. Permanent implantation of ^{125}I seeds caused marked tumour regression and in some cases neoplastic cells were no longer detectable. In the latter cases, however, delayed radionecroses developed in the adjacent normal brain[8] and these were particularly extensive in basal midline structures. It is noteworthy that in all patients with adverse radiation effects (cases 5–8) interstitial ^{125}I implantation was combined with external radiation at doses ranging from 4,500–6,000 rads, suggesting a cumulative radiation damage.

References

1. Bernstein, M., Gutin, P. H., Interstitial irradiation of brain tumors: A review. Neurosurg. *6* (1981), 741—750.
2. Burger, P. C., Mahaley, M. S., jr., Dudka, L., Vogel, F. S., The morphologic effects of radiation administered therapeutically for intracranial gliomas. A postmortem study of 25 cases. Cancer *44* (1979), 1256—1272.

3. Kiessling, M., Anagnostopoulos, J., Lombeck, G., Kleihues, P., Diagnostic potential of stereotactic biopsy of brain tumours. A report of 400 cases. In: Tumours of the Central Nervous System in Infancy and Childhood (Voth, D., Gutjahr, P., Langmaid, C., eds.), Vol. 1, pp. 245—256. Berlin-Heidelberg-New York: Springer. 1982.
4. Ling, C. C., Anderson, L. L., Shipley, W. U., Dose inhomogeneity in interstitial implants using ^{125}I seeds. Int. J. Radiation Oncology Biol. Phys. *5* (1979), 419—425.
5. Mundinger, F., The treatment of brain tumours with interstitially applied radioactive isotopes. In: Radionuclide Applications in Neurology and Neurosurgery (Wang, Y., Paoletti, P., eds.), pp. 199—265. Springfield, Ill.: Ch. C Thomas. 1970.
6. Ostertag, Ch. B., Mundinger, F., Weigel, K., Biopsie stéréotactique et radiothérapie interstitielle des tumeurs cérébrales. Médecine et Hygiène *39* (1981), 1994—2008.
7. Schiffer, D., Giordana, M. T., Soffietti, R., Tarenzi, L., Milani, R., Vasario, E., Paoletti, P., Radio- and chemotherapy of malignant gliomas. Pathological changes in the normal nervous tissue. Acta Neurochir. (Wien) *58* (1981), 37—58.
8. Szikla, G., Constans, J. P., Talairach, J., Correlations of dosage and histological changes following cerebral implantation of gamma emittor isotopes. IInd Int. Congr. Neurolog. Surgery, Washington. Excerpta Medica Int. Congress Series 36, E 145—146, 1961.
9. Szikla, G., Peragut, J. C., Irradiation interstitielle des gliomes. Neurochirurgie *21*, Suppl. 2 (1975), 187—228.
10. Talairach, J., Bonis, A., Szikla, G., Schaub, G., Bancaud, J., Covello, L., Bordas-Ferrer, M., Stereotaxic implantation of radioactive isotopes in functional pituitary surgery: Technique and results. In: Radionuclide Applications in Neurology and Neurosurgery (Wang, Y., Paoletti, P., eds.), pp. 267—299. Springfield, Ill.: Ch. C Thomas. 1970.

Acta Neurochirurgica, Suppl. 33, 291—299 (1984)

Radiolesion versus Recurrence: Bioptic Data in 39 Gliomas After Interstitial, or Combined Interstitial and External Radiation Treatment

C. Daumas-Duport[1], S. Blond[2], Cl. Vedrenne[1], and G. Szikla[2]

With 1 Figure

Summary

Between 1975 and 1982 serial stereotactic control biopsies were performed in a series of 39 patients 0.5 to 7 years after temporary 192 Ir (36 patients) or permanent 198 Au (3 patients) implantation, combined or not to external irradiation. The aim of control biopsies was to establish, whether observed clinical or CT changes were due to post-radiation changes, to tumour growth, or a combination of both.

While density patterns are similar in these conditions, bioptic data might contribute to the choice between surgical removal, reirradiation or medical treatment.

Radionecrosis found in 32 out of 39 patients, was always limited to the heavily irradiated tumoral target volume; obliteration of microvessels appeared to play a major role in necrotic changes and may explain variable and unpredictable delay of late necrotic changes (5 to 39 months).

In cases with sudden clinical deterioration, extensive thrombosis of microvessels was usually found.

While in 10% no conclusion could be reached on the presence or absence of continous tumour growth ("recurrence"), comparison of histology and follow-up shows that information given by control biopsies was reliable in 90%, provided only samples located outside the target volume are considered. Actually, heavily irradiated tumour cells may be difficult to differentiate from reactive gliosis, furthermore typical tumour tissue apparently unchanged at the time of the bioptic control may later become necrotic.

Keywords: Supratentorial gliomas; focal high dose radiotherapy; histological changes; stereotactic biopsies.

---

[1] Department of Pathology and [2] Department of Neurosurgery, C. H. Sainte Anne, 1 rue Cabanis, F-75014 Paris, France.

Introduction

Clinical and or CT worsening following high dose focal radiation therapy (curietherapy or combined curie + ext. radiotherapy) may be due to the late radiation effects, to tumour growth ("recurrence") or a combination of both.

Radionecrosis alone or radionecrosis with tumour growth may have the same CT aspects[5].

Such is the case in particular for the frequently observed ring formation after contrast enhancement.

Considering that histological data might be helpful in differentiating these conditions, postradiation control biopsies were performed at our unit since 1975.

We report here some data from 39 patients in order to appreciate the diagnostic value of such material in the light of the subsequent follow up, and more generally, in order to add some information on focal high dose radiation induced changes of tumour and brain.

Material and Methods

Between 1975 and 1982 a total of 47 post-radiation controls has been performed in 39 patients, with a variable delay, from 4 months to 7 years after irradiation.

18 patients had curietherapy alone (temporary 192 iridium: 15 patients, 198 gold permanent implantation: 3 patients).

Curietherapy with temporary 192 iridium was combined with external radiotherapy in 21 patients.

The dose in the periphery of the target volume was usually 50 Gys in 4–10 days in cases with curietherapy alone; in cases with combined treatment, curietherapy delivered at the estimated outer limit of the tumour was 35 Gys in the same interval, fractionated external high voltage photon therapy added 25 Gys in 10 f/17 d in a field extending 2 cm beyond the curietherapy volume[6]. Our series includes a majority of astrocytomas "B" (~ grade 2) and a majority of infiltrating gliomas (spatial type II).

Malignancy and 3 D configuration are given in Table 1 according to our double codification[2].

1 to 3 tracks per control were performed ($\bar{M}$: 5 samples/tracks) technical aspect are described elsewhere in another presentation in this volume[4].

Results

Histological Changes

Histological changes of tumour and adjacent parenchyma after focal radiotherapy are characterized by their dynamic aspects and their strict relationship to radiation isodose curves.

Table 1. *Case Material (n = 39)*

Histological type		Spatial configuration	
Astrocytomas	28		
A (~ gr. 1)	4		
B (~ gr. 2)	17	Type I	7
C (~ gr. 3)	5	Type II	22
Malignant	2	Type III	1
Pilocytic astrocytomas	4	Type ?	9
Oligodendrocytomas	2		
Ependymomas	2		
Pinealoblastoma	1		
Unclassified gliomas	2		

Elementary lesions are too complex to be detailed here, so we would just mention that:

Gliosis, edema and spongiosis are linked, their aspect and importance depends on delay after irradiation and on radiation dose; they are generally slight or absent in the grey matter.

Inflammatory reactions and macrophagic activity are generally mild or absent.

Complete demyelination appears to be limited to necrotic foci.

Cysts seem to be linked to necrosis; actually cysts walls are often partially necrotic and "coagulum-like" material is frequently observed in necrotic foci.

Necrosis and radiation induced changes of the tumour will be described in detail.

Radionecrosis

Radionecrosis after focal irradiation appeared with a variable delay in 32 out of 39 patients (5 to 39 months, Table 2).

No necrotic changes were found after 5 or more years in 6 patients, 5 of these had a cyst. Long term follow-up without cyst nor apparent radionecrosis is rare in this series (one patient).

No correlation was found between the delay of radionecrosis and the following parameters: target volume, curietherapy alone or combined with external radiotherapy, microscopic vascularity of tumour, malignancy or age of patients.

Appearance of a ring-like enhancement within the target volume coincides in all cases with radionecrosis.

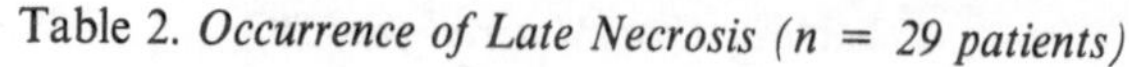
Table 2. *Occurrence of Late Necrosis (n = 29 patients)*

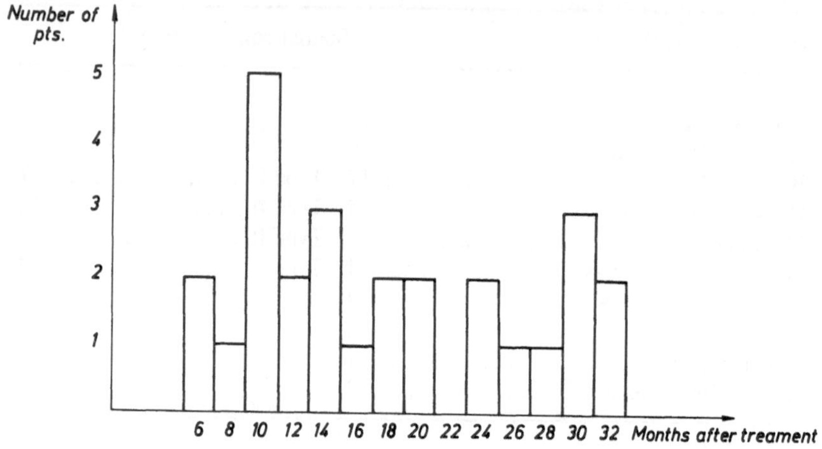

The frequent stereotyped histological sequence corresponding to ring like formations suggests that:

Central low attenuation corresponds to necrosis.

Peripheral contrast enhancement may correspond to new formed and/or telangiectasic vessels as well as to tumour tissue.

Peripheral hypodensity corresponds to edema, spongiosis and gliosis with or without tumour cells (Fig. 1 a and b).

Obliteration of microvessels appears to play a prominent part in late radionecrosis. This may be due to progressive sclerosis, to thrombosis or a combination of both. In case of progressive obliterating sclerosis of microvessels, foci of necrosis and foci of tumour tissue can coexist without transition, foci of residual tumour tissue coincide with still permeable vessels, whereas necrosis coincides with obliterated vessels. Juxtaposition of small necrotic foci of different age giving a histological aspect of mosaic pattern suggests a slow patchy progression of the necrotic process. In other cases, extensive and homogeneous necrosis appears related to an extensive thrombosis of microvessels.

Tumour growth: Identification of infiltration or tumour tissue is more or less difficult according to the location of biopsy samples.

Outside the target volume, where there are no important changes due to radiotherapy, the tumour is easily recognized. Within the target volume tumour tissue or infiltration may be difficult to differentiate from reactive gliosis. Moreover, histological interpretation of radiation induced cytologic changes seems rather subjective.

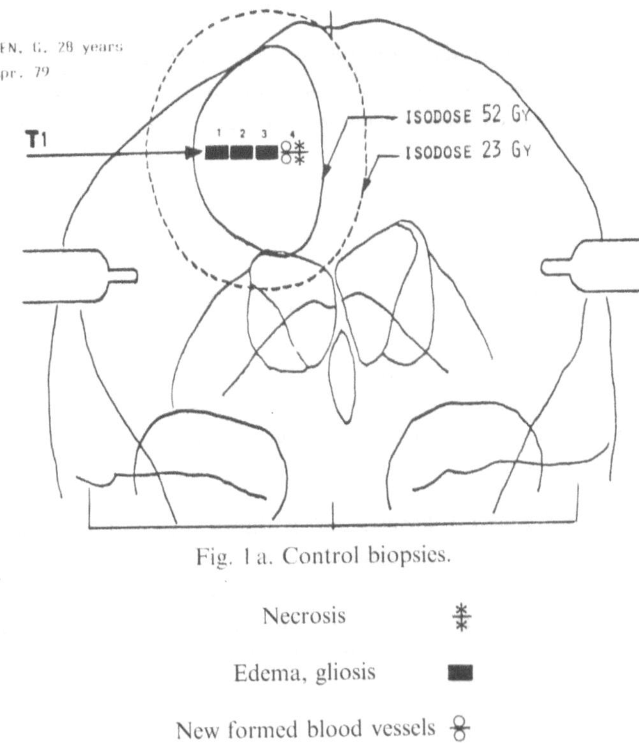

Fig. 1a. Control biopsies.

Fig. 1a and b. Oligo-astrocytoma B (~ gr. 2) control 10 months after curietherapy

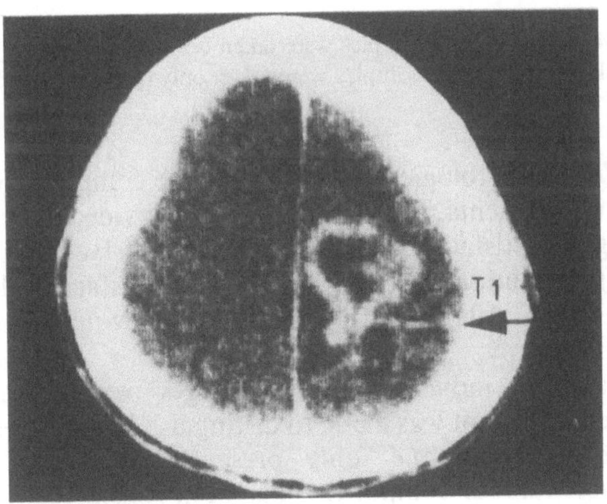

Fig. 1b. Post contrast CT. 10 days after control biopsies (biopsy track is visualized as a rectilinear contrast enhancement)

Table 3. *Control Biopsies.* Improved or stabilized: 12 patients, 13 controls

Biopsy data	N. control	Tumor	No tumor	Tumor?	Necrosis
Overall results	13	5	5	3	11
In target vol.	13	5	6	2	11
Outside target vol.	8*	0	7	1	0

* In 5 controls samples were taken only inside the target-volume.

Table 4. *Control Biopsies.* Progression of disease or death: patients = 21, controls = 34

Biopsy data	N. control	Tumor	No tumor	Tumor?	Necrosis
Overall results	34	32	1	1	19
In target vol.	30*	25	4	1	18
Outside target vol.	23**	20	1	2	1

* In 4 biopsy control, samples were taken only outside the target-volume.
** In 11 biopsy control samples were taken only inside the target-volume.

Reliability: Histological findings could be compared to follow-up data in 32 patients. These 32 patients are divided in two groups according to satisfactory (Table 3) or unsatisfactory evolution (Table 4). Evolution has been considered satisfactory based on clinical and CT criteria, with a minimal follow-up of four years since radiotherapy.

As radiation induced tumour changes seem to us rather subjective no attempt was made to distinguish between residual or proliferative tumour, *i.e.* only presence or absence of still recognizable tumour components has been considered.

Patients improved or stabilized: Table 3: In the 13 controls corresponding to 12 improved or stabilized patients, samples were taken inside the target volume in all cases, samples were taken also outside the target volume in 8 controls. In this group, overall results show that tumour was found in 5 controls, but tumour was never found outside the target volume.

Patients with progression of disease or death: Table 4: In the 34 controls corresponding to 21 patients with progression of disease or death, samples were taken inside the target volume in 30, outside the target volume in 23. Overall results show that tumour was not found in one case only (but in this case the samples were taken only inside the target volume).

Malignant transformation has been observed in half of the patients with tumour growth (11 patients).

Discussion

Only few literature data can be found on histological changes induced by interstitial irradiation of human brain tumours[1-3].

Our material corresponds to control biopsies taken 0.5 to 7 years after temporary 192 Ir or permanent 198 Au implantation, combined or not to external irradiation. The aim of the control biopsies was to establish wether observed clinical and CT changes were due to postradiation processes or to tumour growth. The importance of this distinction seems obvious: a reirradiation of a recurrence might be appropriate but would lead to disastrous worsening in the first alternative.

Obviously, the trajectory along which the samples are taken plays an important role and should be chosen according to previous localizing data such as CT changes. Therefore more attention should be paid to positive findings (tumour or necrosis) than to negative ones (absence of tumour or of necrosis).

Corresponding to the high radiation doses necessary for the destruction of such relatively resistant tumours as astrocytomas etc...., the expected radiation induced necrotic and/or cystic changes of the tumour were found in practically all cases (38 in 39). It should be emphasized however that in this material necrotic changes were always limited to the heavily irradiated target volume *i.e.* the tumour and were never found in samples taken outside of this volume. Similarly complete demyelination has always been limited to necrotic foci. In the exceptional case where extensive necrosis was found beyond the irradiated volume 5 months after treatment, the histological aspect suggests spontaneous necrosis of a rapidly growing malignant pinealoblastoma.

Delay of late radionecrosis is variable and seems unpredictable, as suggested by the lack of correlation between delay and the different parameters studied. This might be related to the prominent role of obliteration of microvessels by sclerosis or thrombosis. Thrombotic vascular changes might well explain the frequently sudden onset of clinical and CT aggravation due to late radionecrosis. Actually, in 9 out of 12 patients with sudden and recent worsening, histology showed extensive and apparently recent thrombosis of microvessels.

Beyond the question wether there is a necrosis or not, the bioptic control has to answer a second question: is there still proliferating tumour or not? Study of the present series shows that histological data can answer this question if the location of the biopsy samples is taken into account. Actually, outside the target volume, where there are no important changes due to radiotherapy, identification of tumour tissue or infiltration is easy; furthermore, follow-up shows progression of disease or death in all cases where tumour was found beyond the limits of the heavily irradiated volume (see Table 4). On the contrary, inside the target volume, tumour tissue or infiltration may be difficult to differentiate from reactive gliosis. Furthermore as necrosis is a delayed phenomenon, even typical tumour tissue apparently unchanged at the time of control biopsy may later become necrotic. This fact has been observed in two interesting cases: a second control performed exactly along the same trajectory showed that tumor previously identified within the target volume at the first control became necrotic at the second, 11 and 13 months after the first.

Incidentally we would like to stress a point of practical interest: in 9 grade 2 astrocytoma cases with tumour recurrence after focal irradiation, reexamination of the initial biopsy material allowed to recognize a posteriori infiltrating tumour cells in the neighbouring brain tissue. The site of the recurrence corresponded to these infiltrated areas, which initially have not been included in the target volume.

These cases illustrate the risk of under-estimation of the target volume which should obviously include peripheral infiltrated areas.

Conclusion

These data suggest, that persistence of tumour tissue within the target volume has no prognostic value, whereas tumour outside of the target volume is doubtlessly a sign of progression of uninhibited tumour growth. Taking into account this essential topographic criterion, stereotactic control biopsy provided reliable information in 90% of our cases.

References

1. Afra, D., Muller, W., Wilcke, O., Spätveränderungen am menschlichen Gehirn nach intraoperativer Einlage von Co^{60}-Perlen. Acta Neuropathologica *4* (1965), 299—311.
2. Daumas-Duport, C., Monsaingeon, V., Szenthe, L., Szikla, G., Serial stereotactic biopsies: a double histological code of gliomas according to malignancy and 3 D-configuration, as an aid to therapeutic decision and assessment of results. Proc. 8th Meeting World Soc. Stereotactic and Functional Neurosurgery, Part III, Zürich 1981. Appl. Neurophysiol. *45* (1982), 431—437.
3. Kiessling, M., Kleihues, P., Mundinger, F., Ostertag, C. B., Weigel, K., Morphologic findings after permanent interstitial Ir-192 and I-125 radiation therapy. In: Advances in Stereotactic and Functional Neurosurgery. 6th Meeting European Soc. Stereotactic and Functional Neurosurgery. Rome 1983 (Gybels, J., *et al.*, eds.), pp. 281—289. Acta Neurochir. (Wien), Suppl. 33. Wien-New York: Springer. 1984.
4. Monsaingeon, V., Daumas-Duport, C., Mann, M., Miyahara, S., Szikla, G., Stereotactic sampling biopsies in a series of 268 consecutive cases—validity and technical aspects. In: Advances in Stereotactic and Functional Neurosurgery. 6th Meeting European Soc. Stereotactic and Functional Neurosurgery. Rome 1983 (Gybels, J., *et al.*, eds.), pp. 195—200. Acta Neurochir. (Wien), Suppl. 33. Wien-New York: Springer. 1984.
5. Ostertag, Chr. B., Weigel, K., Birg, W., CT-changes after long-term interstitial iridium-192-irradiation of cerebral gliomas. In: Stereotactic Cerebral Irradiation. INSERM Symposium No. 12 (Szikla, G., ed.), pp. 149—155. Elsevier/North Holland Biomedical Press. 1979.
6. Schlienger, M., Bouhnik, H., Missir, O., Constans, J. P., Szikla, G., Association of temporary interstitial 192 Ir implantation and external radiotherapy in the management of supratentorial tumours—technique and dosimetry. In: Stereotactic Cerebral Irradiation. INSERM Symposium No. 12 (Szikla, G., ed.), pp. 117—121. Amsterdam: Elsevier/North Holland Biomedical Press. 1979.

Acta Neurochirurgica, Suppl. 33, 301—305 (1984)

Response of Human Malignant Gliomas and CNS Tissue to ^{125}I Brachytherapy: A Study of Seven Autopsy Cases*

R. L. Davis[1], **G. R. Barger**[2], **Ph. H. Gutin**[3], and **Th. L. Phillips**[4]

Summary

The effects of ^{125}I brachytherapy on malignant human gliomas and CNS tissue was studied in seven patients dying after such treatment. All the patients had biopsy proven malignant gliomas and all had failed therapy with external radiation and chemotherapy. Isodose curves of the brachytherapy were superimposed on the sectioned brain and sections prepared to determine the effects of various dose levels on tumor and CNS tissue. Tumor recurred in six of seven patients and was within 2.0 cm of the initial tumor site as determined by computed tomographic (CT) and radionuclide (RN) studies in five of six patients. There were three zones of tissue response: 1. a central zone of complete coagulative necrosis from high radiation doses; 2. an intermediate zone of complete to almost complete demyelination with extensive tissue destruction but preservation of altered vascular and astrocytic elements with a variable inflammatory and reactive response, and, 3. a zone of invomplete and irregular demyelination also with gliosis and inflammatory-reactive response.

---

* Supported in part by the National Cancer Institute Grant, CA 13525 and by BSRG Grant S07RR0355.

[1] R. L. Davis, M.D., Professor of Pathology, Neurology, and Neurological Surgery, School of Medicine, University of California, San Francisco, CA 94143, U.S.A.

[2] G. R. Barger, M.D., Neuro-oncology Fellow, Brain Tumor Research Center, Department of Neurological Surgery, School of Medicine, University of California, San Francisco, CA 94143, U.S.A.

[3] Ph. H. Gutin, M.D., Associate Professor, The Section of Functional and Stereotactic Surgery and The Brain Tumor Research Center, Department of Neurological Surgery, University of California, San Francisco, CA 94143, U.S.A.

[4] Th. L. Phillips, M.D., Professor and Director, Department of Radiation Oncology, School of Medicine, University of California, San Francisco, CA 94143, U.S.A.

In previously radiated brain there appears to be accelerated necrosis of tumor and CNS tissue, but the amount of necrosis and demyelination in lower dose areas was quite variable. Further, though clinical response to this therapy has been encouraging, recurrent tumor was present in the areas given brachytherapy in five six of cases in the present series.

Keywords: Malignant Glioma; brachytherapy; ^{125}I.

Introduction

There has been a revival of interest in the brachytherapy of human malignant glial neoplasms particularly since the development of removable implants which permit delivery of high focal doses of radiation to tumors at high dose rates[3]. Over 50 patients have been treated with removable high activity ^{125}I implants after failure of response to conventional external radiation and chemotherapy. The clinical responses to this therapy have been encouraging[3].

In order to study of the effects of such therapy on brain tumor and CNS tissue, seven patients who died at varying times after brachytherapy were carefully studied neuropathologically.

Materials and Methods

The brains of seven patients who died four to twenty months following ^{125}I brachytherapy were available for study. Each of these patients had biopsy proven malignant glioma (see Table 1). Each had been treated with conventional external radiation and chemotherapy and had failed to responded to that therapy. The ^{125}I brachytherapy was administered with removable implants arranged to deliver a minimum of 6,000 rad to the periphery of the tumor mass as determined by computerized tomographic scans (CT) and radionuclide studies (RN). After routine immersion fixation in 20% buffered formaldehyde, the brains were sectioned so as to permit superimposition of a series of isodose curves on the specimens. The specimens were sectioned so that the approximate radiation dose to various zones of the tissue could be determined and the changes studied. The sections were stained with hematoxylin and eosin but selected sections were also stained with phosphotungstic acid hematoxylin, luxol fast blue, reticulin stains and the Bodian method.

Results

Residual tumor was found at autopsy in 6 of the 7 patients studied. In all but one of these patients the tumor was within 2 cm of the original lesion as determined by the CT and RN studies. In the

Table 1. *Brachytherapy Cases Evaluated at Autopsy*

Case	Age/Sex	Primary diagnosis*	Interval between implant and death (months)	Residual tumor <2 cm	Residual tumor >2 cm
1	50 M	GM	3	+	
2	32 M	GM	5		+
3	50 F	HAA	6	+	
4	53 M	GM	7	+	
5	54 M	GM	8	?	
6	37 F	MMG	15	+	
7	56 M	AA	20	+	

* GM = Glioblastoma Multiforme. HAA = Highly anaplastic astrocytoma. AA = Anaplastic astrocytoma. MMG = Mixed malignant glioma.

single patient whose tumor was outside of the area of therapy, extensive glioblastoma multiforme was found in the opposite centrum semiovale.

Three zones of damage could be distinguished in each of the cases studied. There was a central zone of necrosis in the tissue that received the highest amounts of radiation, but the zone of necrosis was quite variable and extended into lower dose areas with some frequency. In one instance extensive necrosis was present in an area which had received a calculated interstitial dose of less than 2,000 rad. In areas receiving 20,000 rad or more the necrosis was relatively constant. Most of the necrotic tissue could be recognized as tumor but significant areas of white matter were also involved. Grey matter was not usually subject to the higher doses and thus was less frequently affected, but complete destruction of grey areas was occasionally seen.

The second zone consisted of almost complete demyelination with a variable vascular, inflammatory, and phagocytic response. Some gliosis was also occasionally seen. This zone had received between four and 15,000 rad interstitially. The peripheral zone of damage showed gliosis of the white matter with residual myelin and rarely with pools of edema fluid. The vascular, inflammatory, and phagocytic responses were variable. These changes were usually seen in areas receiving two to 4,000 rad interstitially.

Discussion

Considering the variability of the tumor types, the extent of involvement, differences in inherent vascularity and amount of necrosis in individual tumors, and the surrounding edema as well as the fact of previous external radiation and chemotherapy it is not surprising that there is a significant variability in the response to given doses of interstitial radiation.

The presence of tumor in the opposite centrum semiovale, untreated by brachytherapy, was a disappointment in the case in which it occured, but was not a surprise in a tumor which may infiltrate so widely[1]. The presence of recurrent tumor within the field of brachytherapy was even more disappointing since the elimination of tumor from a limited field is the aim of this type of therapy[4]. We have, as a result of this experience, increased the estimated dose of radiation to the periphery of the tumor to 8,000 rad, in the hopes of eliminating residual tumor in these areas.

The response of the non-neoplastic tissue to the radiation conformed to previous experimental experience with the three zones of damage, comparing quite well to those described by Csanda in experimental animals[2]. Though we did not expect to find the complete zone of coagulative necrosis to extend into areas receiving less than 2,000 rad interstitially, considering the other variables this is not so surprising. The surrounding two zones of lesser damage, though also somewhat irregular, were more consistent.

The development of removable high activity ^{125}I implants enables the delivery of high doses of radiation to a limited field and offers the possibility of an effective therapy for malignant brain tumour. Such therapy cannot be expected to cure patients with extensive spread of their disease within the CNS. On the basis of the present study, however, an increased level of radiation to the periphery of the neoplasm as estimated by CT and RN studies appears necessary in order to achieve local control.

References

1. Burger, P. C., Dubois, P. J., Schold, S. C., Smith, K. R., jr., Odom, G. L., Crafts, D. C., Giangaspero, F., Computerized tomographic and pathologic studies of the untreated, quiescent, and recurrent glioblastoma multiforme. J. Neurosurg. *58* (1983), 159—169.
2. Csanda, E., Radiation brain edema. Advances in Neurology, *26* (Cervós-Navarro, J., Ferszt, R., eds.). New York: Raven. 1980.

3. Gutin, P. H., Phillips, T. L., Wara, W. M., Leibel, S. A., Hosobuchi, Y., Levin, V. A., Weaver, K. A., Lamb, S., Removable high activity iodine-125 implants for the brachytherapy of recurrent brain tumors. J. Neurosurg. (in press).
4. Hochberg, F. H., Pruitt, A., Assumptions in the radiotherapy of glioblastoma. Neurol. *30* (1980), 907—911.

Acta Neurochirurgica, Suppl. 33, 307—309 (1984)

Radiation Damage to Normal Canine Brain Induced by Radiation from Interstitially-Implanted ^{125}I Sources

J. R. Fike[1, 2], Ch. E. Cann[2], Ph. H. Gutin[1, 4], Th. L. Phillips[2], R. L. Davis[1,3], and V. Da Silva[1]

Summary

The effects of 10–100 Gy of radiation delivered from interstitially implanted I^{125} sources on canine brain were evaluated using quantitative computed tomographic techniques. Dose related changes in edema and contrast enhancement were observed.

Introduction

Low dose rate interstitial irradiation from ^{125}I sources implanted directly into brain tumors is a promising therapeutic modality. However, clinical experience shows that radiation necrosis can be a serious complication of interstitial brachytherapy. In the studies reported here, dogs were used as a model to assess the effects on the brain of radiation from ^{125}I sources. Quantitative computed tomography (QCT) was used to measure radiation induced changes that were correlated with histopathologic findings.

Materials and Methods

Model and procedure. Single removable ^{125}I sources (specific activities of 30–40 m Ci) were implanted for periods of 1–10 days into the right frontal/parietal lobes of eight dogs. Calculated doses that were delivered to tissue 1 cm from the source ranged from 10–100 Gy.

[1] Brain Tumor Research Center of the Department of Neurological Surgery, and the [2] Departments of Radiation Oncology, and [3] Pathology (Neuropathology), School of Medicine, University of California, San Francisco, CA 94143, U.S.A.

CT measurements. Quantitative measurements used included precontrast CT number and contrast enhancement. Details of scanning techniques and data analysis have been reported[1]. In surviving dogs, quantitative CT measurement were performed 2, 3, 4, 8, 12, and 16 weeks after implantation, and were assessed as a function of dose and distance from the source. Special computer software made it possible to evalute adjacent 2.7 mm diameter "rings" of tissue centered on the site of implantation. Repositioning for serial determinations was accurate to within 0.3 mm.

Histopathology. Moribund dogs were sacrificed after a final CT measurement. Dogs surviving to 16 weeks were sacrificed at that time. All brains were processed and examined as described[1].

Results

Survival. In this model, 100 Gy of radiation killed dogs within 2 weeks of implantation; dogs irradiated with 50 Gy survived an average of 8 weeks after implantation, and half the dogs irradiated with 30 Gy died within 8 weeks of implantation. However, dogs irradiated with 10 Gy survived for long periods with minimal neurologic dysfunction.

CT Findings. Precontrast CT numbers were significantly reduced near the source and remained low. In tissues that were more distant from the source and, because of the inverse square law, received lower doses (less than 70 Gy), CT number was inversely related to dose; in distant tissues that received less than 10 Gy, CT numbers were normal. By 2 months after implantation, CT numbers for regions that had received 10–40 Gy had returned to normal values.

After administration of contrast medium, there was a characteristic ring enhancement (RE) surrounding the central necrotic area. Location and magnitude of the RE were apparently dose-related. In dogs that survived for more than 2–3 months, the size of the RE and the amount of enhancement appeared to reduce gradually, presumably because the permeability defect resolved.

Histopathology. Brain tissue near the site of implantation showed extensive coagulation necrosis. Pronounced edematous changes were observed throughout the irradiated hemisphere. The RE was characterized by pronounced vascular changes associated with areas of coagulation necrosis. Fibrinoid necrosis of vessel walls, endothelial proliferation, and petechial hemorrhage were observed.

Discussion

Changes in preconstrast CT numbers reflect changes in brain tissue density such as edema and/or necrosis. The reduced CT number at the implantation site reflected changes characteristic of radiation necrosis[2], and, in tissue distant from the implantation site, reduction in CT number suggest the transient nature of edematous changes. Contrast enhancement reflected a dose-related breakdown of the blood-brain barrier. After lower total doses, a gradual resolution of the RE occurred. The quantitative relationship between the resolution of edema and change in contrast enhancement is unclear.

The study of the morphologic and physiologic changes in the brain that can be conducted with QCT will provide valuable information of the effects of low dose rate radiation.

Acknowledgements

This research was supported in part by NIH Program Project Grant CA 13525, and the Andres Soriano Fund. We thank Neil Buckley for editorial assistance.

References

1. Fike, J. R., Cann, C. E., Berninger, W. H., Quantitative evaluation of the canine brain using computed tomography. J. Comput. Assist. Tomogr. *6* (1982), 325—333.
2. Fike, J. R., Cann, C. E., Davis, R. L., Phillips, T. L., Radiation effects in the canine brain evaluated by quantitative computer tomography. Radiology *144* (1982), 603—608.

Acta Neurochirurgica, Suppl. 33, 311—315 (1984)

An Animal Tumor Model for the Study of the Radiation Biology of ^{125}I Interstitial Brachytherapy

V. Da Silva[1], Ph. H. Gutin[1,2], M. Bernstein[1], K. Weaver[2], and D. F. Deen[1,2]

With 4 Figures

Summary

A model for the study of the radiation biology of interstitial brachytherapy that uses the RIF-1 murine tumor implanted with removable high activity ^{125}I sources is described. Results of experiments that studied the relative biological effectiveness of interstitial ^{125}I sources, the effects of an hypoxic cell sensitizer, and the effects of drugs and radiation used in combination are discussed.

Introduction

A suitable animal model for brachytherapy has not been developed because it is difficult both to protect investigators from radiation exposure and to calculate dosimetry reliably in a small tumor mass. We have developed an animal model based on the RIF-1 murine flank tumor implanted with ^{125}I sources[1]. Because of the low energy of its radiation compared to other isotopes used for brachytherapy, ^{125}I is a relatively safe isotope for experimental and clinical use. Special sampling techniques have been developed to determine dosimetry, and a cell survival assay is used as the experimental endpoint.

---

[1] Brain Tumor Research Center of the Department of Neurological Surgery, and the [2] Department of Radiation Oncology, School of Medicine, University of California, San Francisco, CA 94143, U.S.A.

Materials and Methods

RIF-1 tumors cells were inoculated into the flanks of C3H mice; solid tumors grew at the innoculation site. Removable ^{125}I sources were implanted into the centers of tumors. After irradiation, tumors were excised and isodosed annuli about the source axis were sampled with a special circular, concentric cutting tool. Single cell suspensions were prepared from the annuli and a cell survival assay was performed.

Because results of *in vitro* experiments suggested that the relative biologic effectiveness (RBE) of ^{125}I is greater than 1.0, we compared the effects of ^{125}I and ^{192}Ir sources at dose rates of 40 rad/hr. The effects of the radiosensitizing agent desmethylmisionidazole (DMM) on irradiation with ^{125}I was examined; DMM administered by continuous intraperitoneal (i.p.) infusion at a rate of 2.7 mg/gm of body weight/24 hours consistently achieved tumor levels of 40–100 μgm/gm tumor tissue. cis-Platinum (3 mg/kg) was administered i.p. at various times before and after ^{125}I interstitial irradiation, and the effects of the two agents used in combination were assessed using the cell survival assay.

Results

The radiation survival curve for the RIF-1 tumor irradiated with ^{125}I sources, characterized by an initial shoulder followed by an exponential portion, is shown in Fig. 1. The D_0 is approximately 1,000 rad. Survival curves for ^{125}I and ^{192}Ir are superimposable (Fig. 2), which suggests that for these two isotopes, there is no detectable RBE. Use of DMM shifted the radiation survival curve downwards (dose modifying factor of 1.6) (Fig. 3)[2]. No synergism was found for treatment with cis-platinum and ^{125}I radiation; survival curves obtained were essentially the curves that would be expected for merely additive cytotoxic effects (Fig. 4).

Discussion

The RIF-1 flank tumor is a suitable model for brachytherapy because it is easily reproducible, does not metastasize, has an hypoxic fraction, and is nonimmunogenic. In this model, the D_0 of the interstitial irradiation survival curve is almost identical to survival curves for irradiation from an external source. The findings that the *in vivo* RBE of ^{125}I, compared with ^{192}Ir, is merely 1.0, and that DMM sensitizes tumor cells irradiated at low dose rates, were unexpected and could not have been predicted from data obtained in other systems.

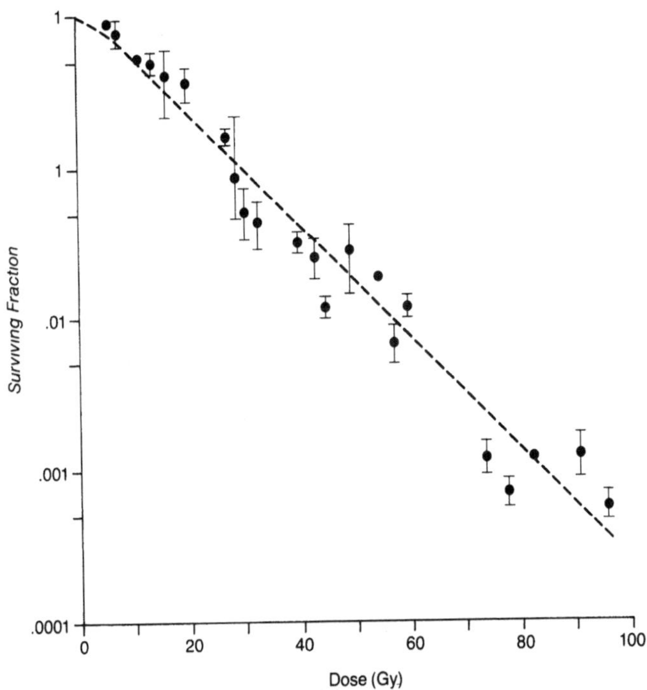

Fig. 1. Radiation survival curve for the RIF-1 tumor irradiated interstitially with ^{125}I sources

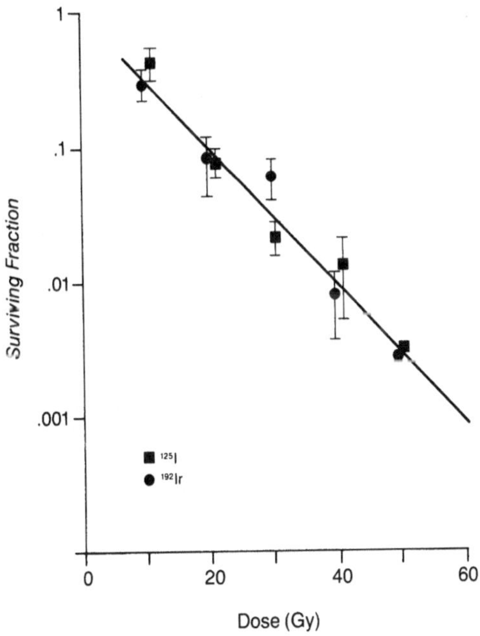

Fig. 2. Superimposed radiation survival curves for RIF-1 tumor irradiated with ^{125}I and ^{192}Ir

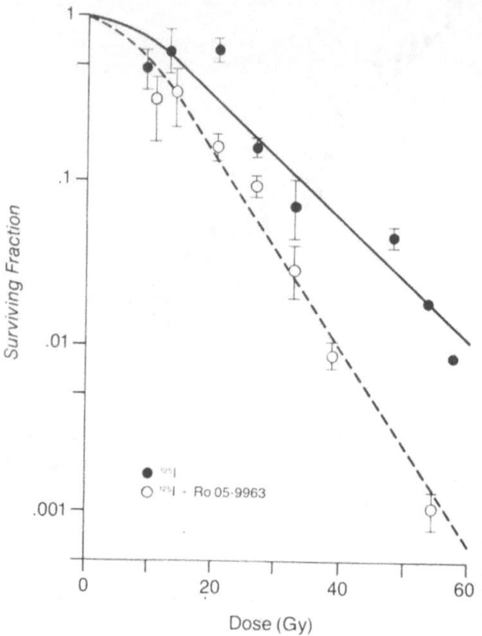

Fig. 3. Effect of DMM on ^{125}I interstitial irradiation

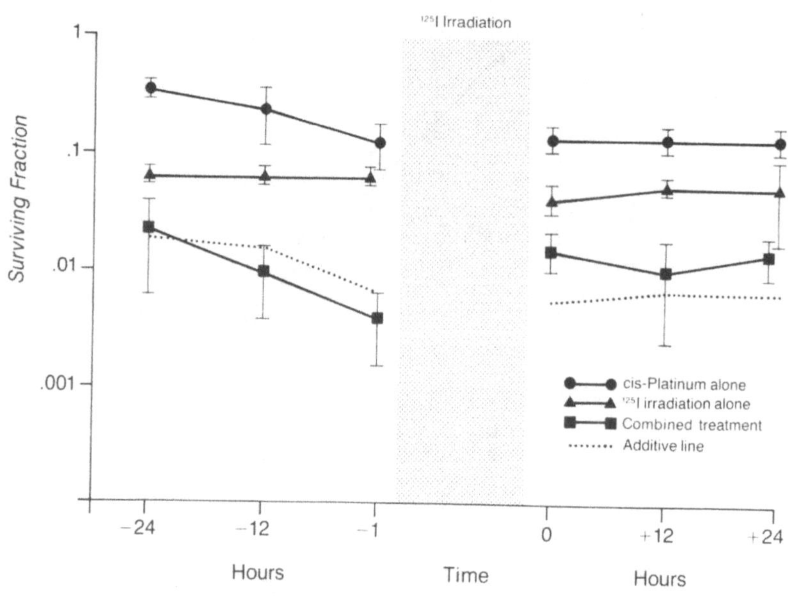

Fig. 4. Survival curves for the effects of combination treatment with cis-platinum and ^{125}I sources

Acknowledgments

This research was supported in part by National Cancer Institute Grant CA 13525 and the Andres Soriano Cancer Research Fund. Dr. Gutin is the recipient of an American Cancer Society Junior Faculty Clinical Fellowship (557) and a New Investigator Research Award (CA 30024) from the National Cancer Institute. We thank Neil Buckley for editorial assistance.

References

1. Bernstein, M., Gutin, P. H., Weaver, K., Deen, D. F., Barcellos, M. H., ^{125}I interstitial implants in the RIF-1 murine flank tumor: an animal model for brachytherapy. Radiat. Res. *91* (1982), 624—637.
2. Bernstein, M., Gutin, P. H., Deen, D. F., Weaver, K., Levin, V., Barcellos, M. H., Radiosensitiziation of the RIF-1 murine flank tumor by demethylmisonidazole (Ro 059963) during interstitial brachytherapy. Int. J. Radiat. Oncol. Biol. Phys. *8* (1982), 487—490.

Acta Neurochirurgica, Suppl. 33, 317—321 (1984)

Pathological Findings in Acoustic Neurinoma After Stereotactic Irradiation

J. L. Barcia-Salorio[1], M. Cerda, G. Hernandez, V. Bordes, J. Beraha, C. Calabuig, and J. Broseta

With 5 Figures

Although with some experience in the radiosurgical treatment of acoustic neurinomas, the minimal dose required to cause necrosis or arrest of growth of the tumour, in a single session, is not yet known.

Leksell[3] (1971), assuming that the minimal lethal dose for growing tumour cells would be lower than that necessary for the production of a therapeutic thalamic lesion, has calculated a dose from 50 to 70 Gy for the treatment of acoustic tumours.

With the CT scanner this assumption was confirmed. A hypodensity in the central core of the tumour without contrast enhancement was seen[1,4].

The anatomical examination of an irradiated tumour removed by open surgery showed that this zone corresponds to a necrosis[2].

Kjellberg (1979)[2] however has calculated a lower dose (35 Gy) to produce necrosis in acoustic neurinomas. The irradiated volume (30 mm) and proton beam (22 mm) were greater than those of other authors.

The authors have had the opportunity to study an irradiated neurinoma in order to estimate the minimal dose required to produce necrosis in this class of tumours.

Material and Method

A 30 year old woman with a seven months history of headache, tinnitus, and vomiting presented a left deafness, palsy of the fifth and sixth craneal nerve, ataxia and nystagmus.

[1] Departments of Neurosurgery, Pathology and Physic Radiation, Hospital Clinico Universitario, Valencia, Spain.

Skull radiogram, vertebral angiography and CT revealed a large neurinoma of 50 mm diameter on the left side.

With a collimator of 5 mm and a maximum target dose of 90 Gy, the tumour was irradiated on July, 26th, 1977.

The clinical improvement began two months after radiosurgery and two years later all symptoms had disappeared. A control CT showed a central tumour necrosis; with contrast enhancement only a light blush of the tumour capsule appeared.

Nevertheless, 6 months later the symptoms appeared again and a clear worsening of the clinical condition was seen.

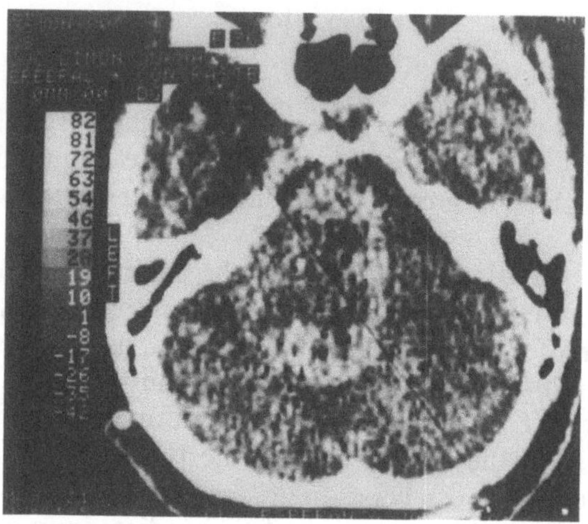

Fig. 1. Tumour CT scan

A new CT revealed a decrease in the size of the hypodense zone and a internal growth of the tumour, although its diameter was the same size.

A new irradiation on 20th, December, 1979 was therefore done with 90 Gy and the symptoms disappeared once more. The last CT showed a great hypodense area in the centre of the tumour and only a light ring form delimited the capsula in enhanced CT images (Fig. 1).

The patient died on October, 21st, 1980 with peritonitis. In the postmortem examination the tumour was cut in the same plane as the CT. Gross view showed a grey, smooth central area of the tumour, 8 × 16 mm of size, surrounded by a reddish-blue of 2–3 mm with dark spots and hemorrhages. More peripherally the mass had the same aspect and colour as that of a normal tumour (Fig. 2).

Histological sections were stained by H and E, Masson's trichrome and Gomori reticuline stain. Microscopically, one observes that the central area corresponds to a coagulation necrosis, with a lack of staining affinity (Fig. 3). The

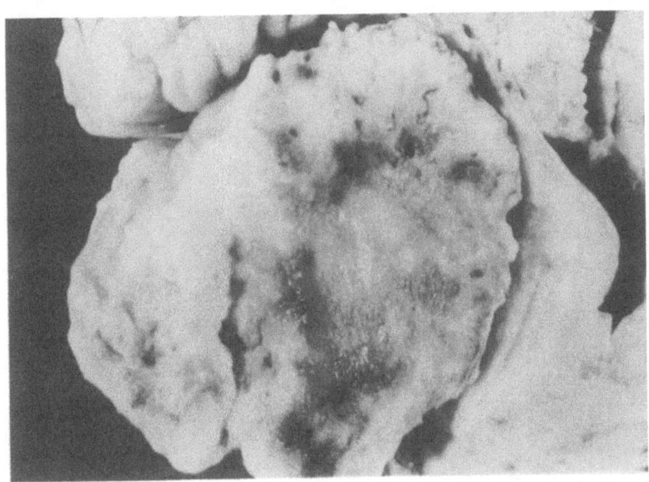

Fig. 2. Post-mortem specimen

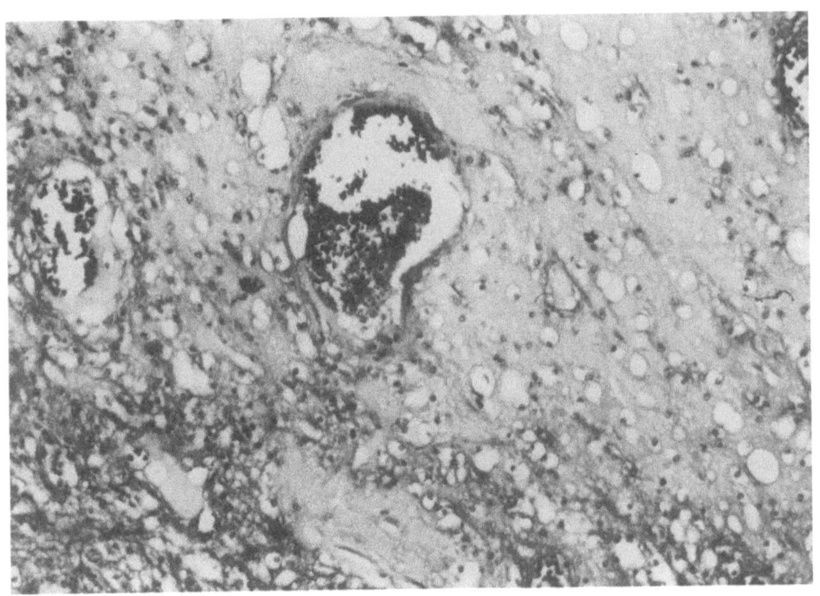

Fig. 3. Central area of tumour. H. & E. × 16

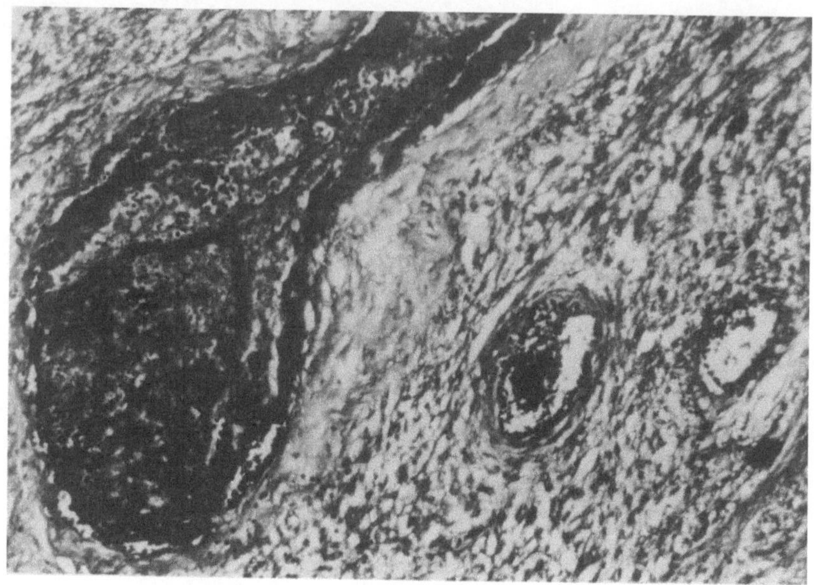

Fig. 4. Peripheral zone of tumour. H. & E. × 25

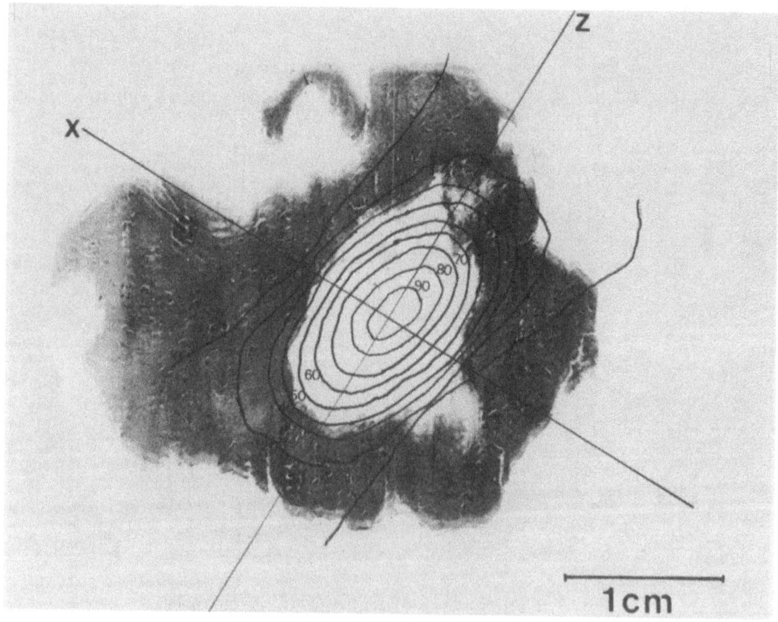

Fig. 5. Isodose diagram over a tumour section of 0.1 mm thickness. The white central area corresponds to coagulation necrosis

peripheral zone corresponds to vascular changes, and fibrinoid necrosis of the blood vessel walls.

Allmost all of the vessels were occluded by endothelial proliferation. There were also different degrees of periadventitial fibroblastic proliferation spreading from the vessels walls to the centre of necrosis (Fig. 4). The peripheral part of the tumour has the characteristics of neurinoma tissue.

Putting the isodose diagram over a tumour section of 0.1 mm thickness one can observe that the necrotic area corresponds to the isodose of 50 Gy and the thrombotic area to the 25 Gy isodose (Fig. 5).

Conclusions

It is difficult to calculate precisely the minimal dose required to produce necrosis or vascular thrombosis because both types of lesions extend irregulary out of the isodose curve because of secondary necrosis by vascular ischemia.

Nevertheless we estimate that the approximate necrosis dose is about 50 Gy and vascular thrombosis about roughly 25 Gy.

References

1. Barcia-Salorio, J. L., Broseta, J., Hernandez, G., Barbera, J., Bordes, V., Ballester, B., Radiosurgical treatment in huge acoustic neurinomas. In: Stereotactic Cerebral Irradiation. INSERM Symposium No. 12 (Szikla, G., ed.), pp. 245—249. Amsterdam: Elsevier/North Holland. 1979.
2. Kjellberg, R. N., Stereotactic Bragg Peak proton radiosurgery. In: Stereotactic Cerebral Irradiation. INSERM Symposium No. 12 (Szikla, G., ed.), pp. 233—240. Amsterdam: Elsevier/North Holland. 1979.
3. Leksell, L., A note on the treatment of acoustic tumours. Acta Chir. Scand. *137* (1975), 763—765.
4. Norën, G., Leksell, L., Stereotactic treatment of acoustic tumours. In: Stereotactic Cerebral Irradiation. INSERM Symposium No. 12 (Szikla, G., ed.), pp. 241—244. Amsterdam: Elsevier/North Holland. 1979.

[illegible] due to vascular changes, and fibrinoid necrosis of the blood vessel walls.

Almost all the vessels were occluded by endothelial proliferation. There were [illegible] different degrees of partially [illegible] fibrinoid [illegible] spreading [illegible] vessel walls to the centre of necrosis (Fig. 4). The peripheral part of the [illegible] has the characteristics of [illegible] tissue.

[illegible] diagram over [illegible] section [illegible] that the necrotic area corresponds to the isodose of 50 Gy and the thrombosis [illegible] to the 75 Gy isodose (Fig. 4).

Conclusions

It is difficult to state [illegible] the minimum dose required to produce necrosis or vascular thrombosis because [illegible] irregularity [illegible] of the isodoses [illegible] necrosis by vascular ischemia.

Nevertheless we estimate that the approximate necrosis dose is about 50 Gy and vascular thrombosis about roughly 75 Gy.

References

1. [illegible]
2. Kolleck [illegible] stereotactic Bragg Peak proton radiosurgery [illegible]
3. [illegible]
4. [illegible] Symposium [illegible]

Acta Neurochirurgica, Suppl. 33, 323—330 (1984)

II. Clinical Results

Indication and Results of Stereotactic Curietherapy with Iridium-192 and Iodine-125 for Non-resectable Tumours of the Hypothalamic Region

F. Mundinger[1] and K. Weigel

With 4 Figures

Introductory Remarks

Therapeutic approaches to tumours of the hypothalamic region vary primarily depending on the degree to which the tumour can be surgically resected. However, residual portions of the tumour following surgery or recurrent tumours present special problems. In the case of hypothalamic gliomas, severe clinical deficits, significant postoperative neurologic morbidity and mortality are expected after attempts at open resection. Therefore at many institutions nothing is done after the clinical or CT diagnosis of a hypothalamic process, or at most, "ut aliquid fiat", external irradiation might be carried out. Today this mode of procedure is highly unsatisfying and the situation calls for an effective therapy concept. Knowledge of the type of tumour and its grading is prerequisite for selecting the therapeutic procedure. CT-stereotactic biopsy is the most reliable and least dangerous method of obtaining this information[1,4,6,7]. Based on the findings from the intraoperative smear preparation, the form of therapy can be immediately decided upon. Interstitial curietherapy, for example, can be initiated right away[2,5].

---

[1] Abteilung Stereotaxie und Neuronuklearmedizin, Neurochirurgische Universitätsklinik, Hugstetter Strasse 55, D-7800 Freiburg im Breisgau, Federal Republic of Germany.

Medical ethics dictates, however, that we not justify creating an iatrogenic clinical cripple just to be able to show a good palliative effect. Only by keeping this in mind will we be able to prevent the inappropriate use of the increasingly popular CT-stereotactic curietherapy technique. If this is not done, this promising form of therapy develop the poor reputation attributed to other methods which were effective but nevertheless were applied indiscriminately. The results of such indiscriminate application not only do not meet therapeutic expectations but sometimes result in postoperative complications worse than the natural history of the disease. This should be kept in mind in evaluating the results presented in the following report.

Results

From 1965 to 1982, we evaluated 902 intracranial tumors out of a total number of 1,306 stereotactically operated intracranial tumours. Of these 902 122 (= 14%) were tumours of the hypothalamic region (Table 1). 62 were only biopsied, of which 2 astrocytomas were externally irradiated later. Iridium-192 permanent implantation was carried out on 32, 11 of which were additionally irradiated later. Since 1979, we have implanted Iodine-125 in 28 cases. All cases were confirmed in a smear preparation and using conventional biopsy procedures. Table 2 lists the preoperative neurological deficits in this group of patients. In Table 3 a pre-implantation therapy is summarized; additive treatment is given in Table 3 b. Consecutive treatment as well as the mortality and morbidity rates are given in Tables 3 c and 3 d respectively.

Survival Times and Their Dependence on the Treatment Methods:

Craniopharyngioma (Fig. 1): twenty-three (23) cases of CT-established cystic craniopharyngiomas underwent cyst aspiration and lavage. Rickham catheters were placed in the cysts in 16 of these cases. The catheters passed through the lateral ventricle in order to allow drainage of the cyst contents into the ventricle. Alternately the contents could be withdrawn by percutaneous puncture of the Rickham reservoir. Patients having solid craniopharyngiomas implanted with Iodine-125 did not survive as long as those implanted with Iridium-192.

Table 1. *Bioptic Diagnosis of 122 Tumours of the Hypothalamic Region (1965–1982)*

Astrocytoma I	36 (30%)
Astrocytoma II	7 (6%)
Astrocytoma III	4
Glioblastoma IV	3
Ependymoma	4
Medulloblastoma	1
Papilloma	3
Meningioma	2
Craniopharyngioma	37 (30%)
Epidermoid	2
Teratoma	3
PNET	4
Colloid cyst	5
Metastasis	5
Neuroblastoma	2
Gliosis	4

Table 2. *Neurological Deficits (before treatment)*

Visual acuity impaired	55 (45%)
Visual field defect	37 (30%)
Oculomot. paresis	25 (20%)
Extremity paresis	13 (10%)
Increased intracranial pressure	86 (70%)

Table 3 a. *Pre-treatment*

Shunt	55 (45%)
Partial resection	17 (14%)
External irradiation (without histology 4)	7 (5%)

Table 3 b. *Additive Treatment*

Tumor cyst evacuation	28 (23%)
Catheter implantation into cysts	16 (13%)
Shunt implantation (ventricle)	9 (7%)

Table 3c. *Consecutive Treatment*

		n	dead
Biopsy	and external radiation	7	4
	and curietherapy combined with external irradiation	5	2
	in this second group:		
	and GammaMed®-Brachy Curietherapy	1	1
	and I-125-permanent implantation with external irradiation	2	1
	and Ir-192 permanent implantation with external irradiation	2	0

Table 3d. *Surgical Mortality and Morbidity After 122 Stereotactic Operations on Tumours of the Hypothalamic Region (1965–1982)*

Mortality (hemorrhage)	1 (0.8%)
Morbidity:	
transient:	
small hemorrhage (CT only)	2 (1.6%)
extremity paresis	1 (0.8%)
seizures	2 (1.6%)

Pituitary adenoma: the good long-term results of interstitial curietherapy have already been reported[8].

Fig. 2 shows the length of survival in *25 diverse processes and tumours*.

Glioma: the combination of interstitial and external irradiation is the most favorable method for malignant gliomas, grade III and IV (Fig. 3).

The pilocytic astrocytomas (I) (Fig. 4), 12 of which are optic gliomas with hypothalamic invasion, show similar survival times for the 3 groups including those with only biopsy, those treated with I-125 and those treated with Ir-192. For pilocytic astrocytomas, we recommend biopsy and observation. Iodine-125 is not implanted unless the tumour grows further.

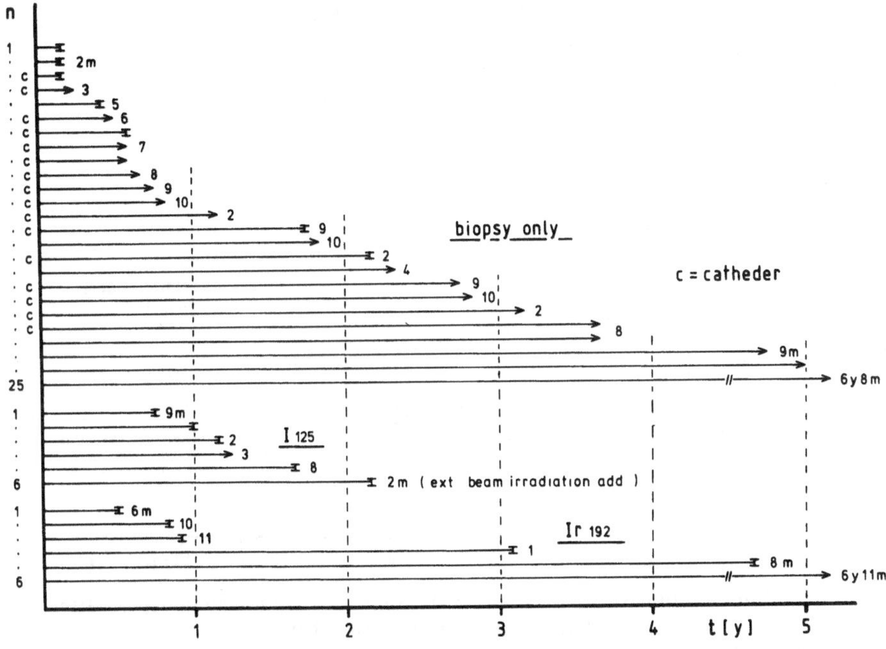

Fig. 1. Survival time of *craniopharyngiomas* of the hypothalamic region after stereotactic operations (n = 37)

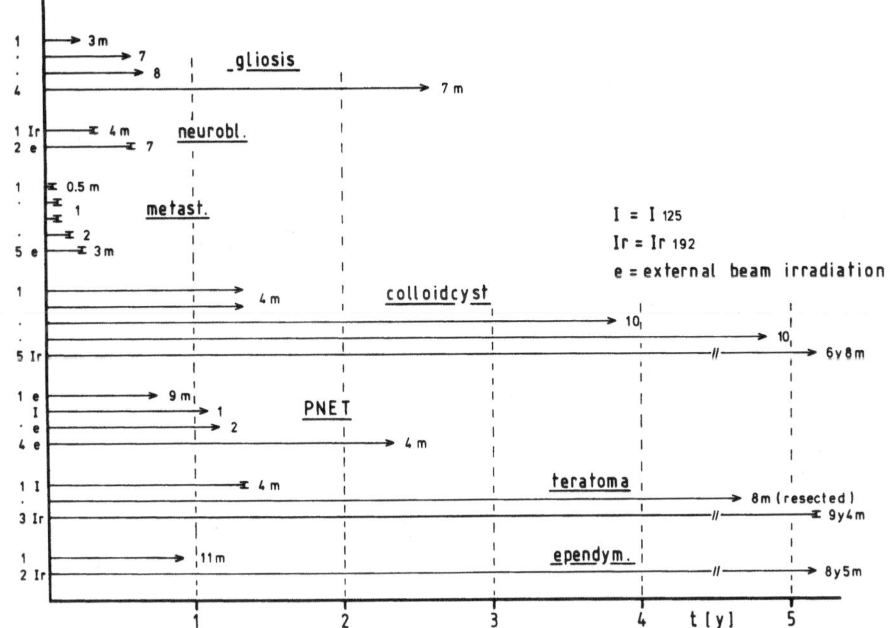

Fig. 2. Survival time of *diverse tumours* of the hypothalamic region after stereotactic operations (n = 25)

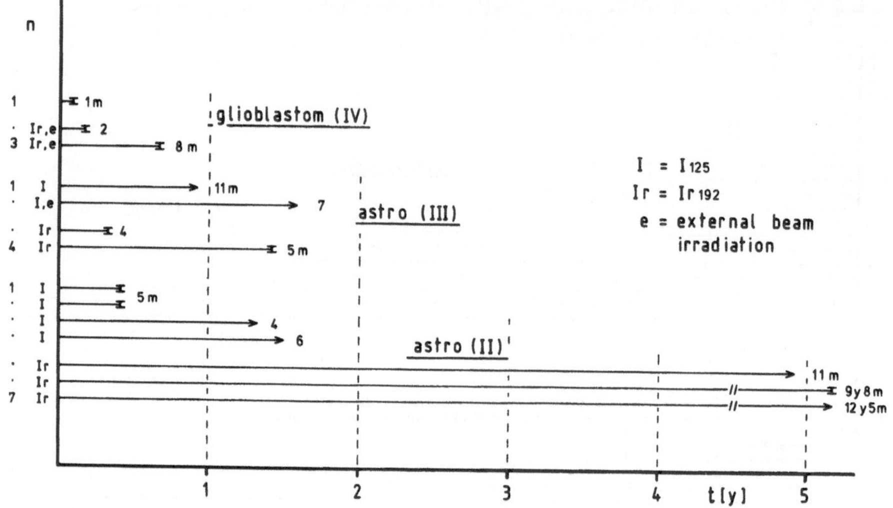

Fig. 3. Survival time of *gliomas* (grade II–IV) of the hypothalamic region after stereotactic operations (n = 14)

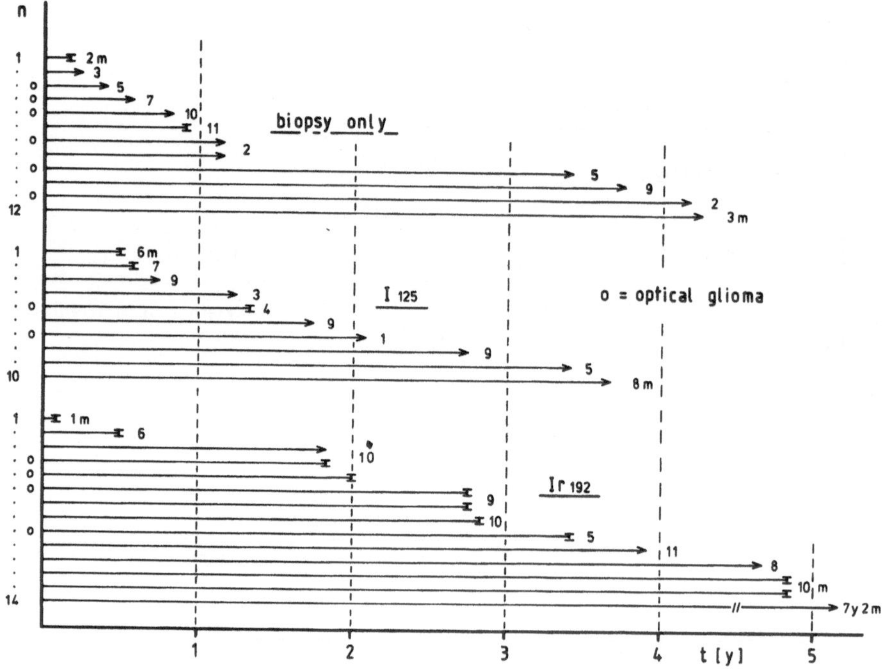

Fig. 4. Survival time of *pilocytic astrocytomas* (gr. I WHO) of the hypothalamic region after stereotactic operations (n = 36)

Summary and Indications for Curietherapy

An evaluation of our results from 122 tumours shows that curietherapy is indicated for unresectable intra- and extracerebral tumours of the hypothalamic region of the following histologic types:

For craniopharyngiomas, CT-stereotactic cyst puncture with installation of radionuclide colloids is indicated[3] if the cyst cannot be sufficiently drained by simple catheter implantation, if the catheter has to be removed because of ependymitis, or in the case of a recurrence.

Pituitary adenomas: for recurrent or functionally hyperactive tumour, refractory to medication, we consider the interstitial implantation of Iridium-192 or Iodine-125 to be more effective than external irradiation, and with respect to late recurrent tumours, more appropriate with less morbidity. Our opinion is based on our own experience with several hundred cases and on the cases reported in the literature (cf. Ref. 8 for a compiled presentation).

Optic glioma: these should be implanted with Iodine-125 if growth is demonstrated, or if they have already filled the basal cisterns. Tumours having attachment to or effacement of the third ventricle or inoperable tumors are also candidates for this procedure. In addition, we feel that residual tumor following open resection should be implanted with Iodine-125.

Intracerebral glioma: Iodine-125 is indicated when the central-hypothalamic glioma is sharply demarcated and when the tumors invades diencephalic and mesencephalic structures. Iridium-192 is indicated in poorly demarcated tumours. We consider Brachy-curietherapy (GammaMed) to be absolutely contraindicated in these cases. Interstitial curietherapy is not indicated if severe endocrine deficiency symptoms are present and if the tumour volume cannot be accurately determined. In these cases, if the tumours are low-grade (I and II), particularly pilocytic astrocytomas (I), one has to wait and see. For malignant astrocytomas grades III and IV, external irradiation—if anything—is indicated. External radiation therapy can be augmented by the permanent implantation of Iridium-192 or Iodine-125, which can be done immediately following the biopsy procedure.

With the availability and precision provided by modern CT-stereotactic techniques physicians are more apt to recommend aggressive interventional therapy in any case. We have to guard against considering every documented tumour an implantable object for radioisotopes, just to be able to proudly apply this technique. The patient's entire situation as well as his chances for a "useful life" should be the decisive criteria for therapeutic action.

References

1. Birg, W., Mundinger, F., Direct target point determination for stereotactic brain operations from CT data and the calculation of setting parameters for polar-coordinate stereotactic devices. Appl. Neurophysiol. *45* (1982), 387—395.
2. Mundinger, F., Treatment of brain tumors with radioisotopes. In: Progress of Neurological Surgery, Bd. I (Krayenbühl, H., Maspes, M., Sweet, Ch., eds.), pp. 202—257. Basel: Karger. 1966.
3. Mundinger, F., The treatment of brain tumors with interstitially applied radioactive isotopes. In: Radionuclide Applications in Neurology and Neurosurgery (Wang, Y., Paoletti, P., eds.), pp. 199—265. Springfield, Ill.: Ch. C Thomas. 1970.
4. Mundinger, F., CT-Stereotactic biopsy of brain tumours. In: Tumours of the Central Nervous System in Infancy and Childhood (Voth, D., Gutjahr, P., Langmaid, C., eds.), pp. 234—246. Berlin-Heidelberg-New York: Springer. 1982.
5. Mundinger, F., Implantation of radioisotopes (Curietherapy). In: Stereotaxy of the Human Brain, 2nd ed. (Schaltenbrand, G., Walker, W., eds.), pp. 410—435. Stuttgart: Thieme. 1982.
6. Mundinger, F., Birg, W., Stereotactic brain surgery with the aid of computed tomography (CT-stereotaxy). In: Computerized Tomography, Brain Metabolism, Spinal Injuries (Driesen, W., Brock, M., Klinger, M., eds.), pp. 17—24. Advanc. Neurosurg. 10. Berlin-Heidelberg-New York: Springer. 1982.
7. Mundinger, F., Metzel, E., Interstitial radioisotope therapy of intractable diencephalic tumors by the stereotaxic permanent implantation of Iridium-192, including bioptic control. Confin. neurol. *32* (1970), 195—202.
8. Mundinger, F., Riechert, T., Hypophysentumoren — Hypophysektomie. Klinik-Therapie-Ergebnisse. Stuttgart: Thieme. 1967.

Acta Neurochirurgica, Suppl. 33, 331—339 (1984)

Colloidal Rhenium-186 in Endocavitary Beta Irradiation of Cystic Craniopharyngiomas and Active Glioma Cysts. Long Term Results, Side Effects and Clinical Dosimetry

G. Szikla[1], **A. Musolino**[1], **S. Miyahara**[1], **C. Schaub**[1], and **S. Askienazy**[2]

With 3 Figures

Summary

Intracystic injection of colloidal Rhenium-186 has been introduced at our unit for endocavitary irradiation of cystic craniopharyngiomas and actively expanding glioma cysts in 1973. Follow-up of 13 craniopharyngioma and 29 glioma cysts treated with Re-186 till July 1982 shows that fluid formation has been consistently stopped in all craniopharyngiomas and low grade gliomas with progressive shrinkage of the formerly expansive cysts. In high grade gliomas progression of tumour-growth usually rapidly compensated inactivation or shrinkage of cyst. No early or late side-effects were observed in craniopharyngiomas. In glioma-cysts dose dependent regressive perifocal edema appeared 1–2 months after injection in 5 cases. No clinical complications were noted after leakage to CSF spaces observed more frequently with craniopharyngiomas (15%) than gliomas (1.6%). Late reexpansion of cyst observed at 1 to 4.5 years in 8–10% was treated successfully in all cases by a second injection. Long term follow up data seem to warrant further use of intracystic injection of colloidal Re-186 as this treatment appears to achieve consistently satisfactory results with minimal risks in the treatment of cystic craniopharyngiomas and expanding cyst of low grade gliomas.

Keywords: Stereotactic cyst treatment; intracystic Rhenium-186; cystic craniopharyngioma; expanding glioma-cysts.

---

[1] Department of Neurosurgery B and [2] Department of Nuclear Medicine, C. H. Sainte Anne, 1 rue Cabanis, F-75014 Paris, France.

Introduction

Since the first publication by Leksell and Liden [5] in 1952, several authors reported good results of intracystic injection of colloidal P-32, Au-198, and Y-90 preparations in cystic craniopharyngiomas [1,2,5–7]. Because of its advantageous physical properties, we introduced the use of colloidal Rhenium-186 in 1973 for cystic craniopharyngiomas and rapidly recurring hyperactive glioma cysts. Restricted soft tissue penetration of the relatively low energy ($\bar{m}$: 358 KeV) beta radiation of Re-186 limits the depth of cyst wall necrosis to 1–1.5 mm instead of 3–4 mm with Y-90. This might reduce the risk of both late radiation damage of adjacent structures (optic chiasma, hypothalamus) and of radiation edema induced in the white matter by Y-90 [3,4,9]. Furthermore the soft gamma emission (138 KeV) of Re-186 allows for easy scintigraphic control of a possible leakage of radioactivity to CSF spaces. We assumed therefore that the safety of the endocavitary irradiation might be increased by the use of Re-186. Long term follow-up data were collected in order to assess the validity of our initial assumptions in terms of effectiveness and side effects *i.e.* early or late radiation damage.

Material and Methods

44 cysts were treated in 38 patients between July 1973 and July 1982: cystic craniopharyngioma: 15 cysts/13 patients, expansive glioma cysts recurring after evacuation: 29 cysts/25 patients.

Stereotactic localization of the cyst was performed with the Talairach system in the usual way. Volume detetermination was based on radiographic and isotope dilution data. Imperviousness of the cyst-wall was checked with tracer doses of Re-186. The therapeutic dose of Re-186 delivered more than 200 Gys to the cyst wall. Intraoperative and then daily scintigraphic control of leakage was performed during the treatment. After 10–14 days, or in case of major leakage to CSF spaces (Table 1) the cyst was evacuated.

Follow-up studies included systematic clinical, paraclinical, and CT controls every 6 months in the first two years, then yearly.

Results

Data on treated cysts and long term follow-up treatment are summarized in Tables 2–4 for craniopharyngiomas, in Tables 5 and 6 for respectively low and high grade glioma cysts.

Table 1. *Intracystic Injection of Colloidal Rhenium-186*

Leakage to CSF spaces

(1) *Type:*

(A) rupture at injection
(B) progressive contamination of CSF spaces
(C) minor contamination on withdrawal of needle, decreasing after first day: not considered

(2) *Frequency*

Craniopharyngiomas
6/39 inj. (test: 3. ther.: 3) 15%
Gliomas 1/64 inj. (ther.) 1.6%

(3) *Follow-up after leakage*

After aspiration of cyst content no untoward reactions observed (meningeal s., blood cell count)
(4) therapeutic inj.: 5, 12, 40, 72 mCi)

Table 2. *Intracystic Colloidal Rhenium-186*

Craniopharyngioma 13 patients—15 cysts

Type I (solitary cyst)	2 patients
I–II (cyst ≫ solid tumor)	5 patients
II (cyst = solid tumor)	6 patients

Cyst volume: $\bar{m}$ 45 cm^3 (8–270)

Previous treatment:

Radical surgery	11 patients
Radiotherapy	3 patients

Follow up > 9 months: 11 patients—13 cysts
Lost at 3 m: 1
Dead 5th day: 1
(Vol. irradiated recurrence, poor condition)
Follow up (9 m—5.5 years): $\bar{m}$ 33 months.

Table 3. *Intracystic Injection of Colloidal Rhenium-186*

Craniopharyngiomas: Results in 13 cysts

Satisfactory anatomical result	13
–cyst < retracted + + (at 9–11 months)	3
–cyst < disappeared (CT) (at 2 months – 2 years)	10
Reexpansion at 11 months, 2nd treatment → retracted, stable since 29 months	1

Table 4. *Intracystic Injection of Colloidal Rhenium-186*

Craniopharyngiomas: Results in 11 patients

Vision

- improved: 7 eyes (4.1/10 → 7.7/10)
- unchanged: 12 eyes (blind or < 1/20: 9)
- worse: 3 eyes (6/10 → 3.5/10)

Previous optic atrophy 18/22 eyes

Memory

- severe impairment in 2 patients × normal
- normal, unchanged 9 patients

Endocrine insufficiency:

- Moderate or severe 9 patients
  partial recocery 3 patients
  unchanged 6 patients
- prevously normal, unchanged 2 patients

Table 5. *Intracystic Injection of Colloidal Rhenium-186*

Low grade gliomas – "active cysts": 17 patients, 21 cysts.
Volume 20–240 cm^3, $\bar{m}$ 90 cm^3.
Follow up $\bar{m}$: 34.5 months (min. > 10 months).

stabilized (obs. $\bar{m}$ 18 months)	10 cysts
retracted (obs. $\bar{m}$ 38.5 months)	5 cysts
disappeared (obs. $\bar{m}$ 36.5 months)	6 cysts
	21 cysts
Late recurrence (at 1, 2 and 4.5 years) 2nd treatment: good result	3 cysts

Edema (white matter)

major (hemispheric, mass effect + +)	0
minor (perifocal, mass effect ±, transitory aggrauation neurol. signs) 1–2 months after treatment.	2/24 treatments

Table 6. *Intracystic Injection of Colloidal Rhenium-186*

High grade gliomas: 8 patients – 8 cysts

cyst	disappeared	1 cyst
	retracted + +	3 cysts
	stable	2 cysts
	no appreciable effect	2 cysts

Survival after treatment m̄: 5 month
dead < 1 m – 21 m 6 pt.
alive at 3 and 5 m 2 pt.

Tumor progression compensated rapidly the clinical improvement due to inactivation of cyst.

Overall benefit estimated appreciable in 2/8 patients.

Table 7. *Clinical Dosimetry of Colloidal Rhenium-186*

Craniopharyngioma

Injected doses: m̄ 21.5 mCi (5–70)
Dose/cyst wall*: m̄ 430 Gy (160–830)
Retraction of cyst: all cyst (13/13)
(1 recurrence at 12 months, 2nd inj. → retracted since 29 months)
no early or late side effects

Glioma

Injected doses: m̄ 40 mCi (10–85)
Dose cyst wall*: m̄ 580 Gy (160–1910)
retraction of stabilization of cyst
– low grade: all cysts (21/21)
(2nd treatment necessary at 1.2 and 4.5 years)
– high grade: less constant (6/8)
(benefit compensated by tumour progression)
Side effect: dose related minor white matter edema at 1–2 months
(dose* < 400 Gy: 1 ed./20 inj. significant
> 400 Gy: 4 ed./12 inj. ($p < 0.05$)

* Theoretical values assuming homogeneous distribution of Re-186 in cystic fluid.

Rhenium 186: β DOSIMETRY

$$D'_{(rad.h^{-1})} = 2\,130 \times C \times \overline{T\beta} \times 0.5$$

$$D_{rad} = \frac{D'}{\frac{0.693}{90.6}} \left(1 - e^{-\frac{0.693}{90.6} \times T}\right)$$

C : radioactive concentration in the cystic fluid $mCi_{Re\,186}/ml_{cystic\ fluid}$

D′: dose rate rad h^{-1}

$\overline{T\beta}$: mean energy of β radiation [MeV]

D: total dose delivered to cyst wall [rad]

T: time of application [hours]

Fig. 1. Dosimetry of Re-186

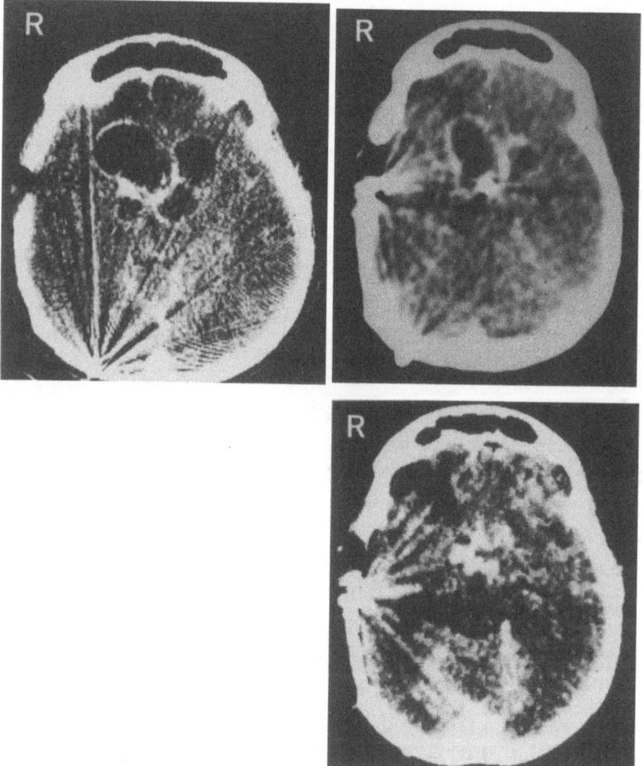

Fig. 2a. L. D. 23 years. Polycystic recurrence of an operated craniopharyngioma. Left: before cyst treatment, Middle: at 19 m, right: at 44 m after treatment

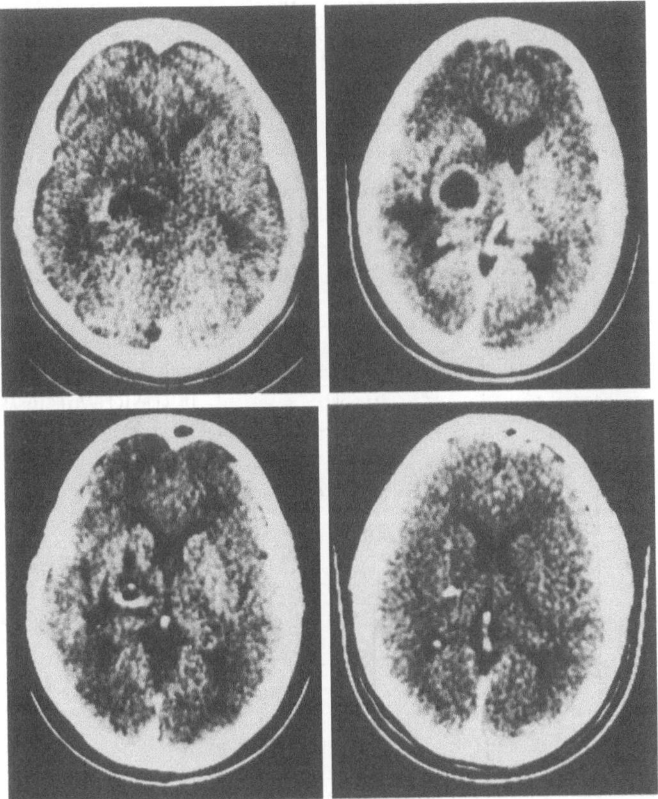

Fig. 2 b. C. A. 15 years. Pilocytic astrocytoma. Upper left: 1 m before treatment. Upper right: at 1 m. Lower left: at 8 m. Lower right: at 12 m after treatment

Migration of Re-186 to Cyst Wall—Clinical Dosimetry

Radioactivity removed by aspiration + lavage at the end of treatment proved to be considerably lower than expected according to physical decay (without leakage, Fig. 3). Preliminary data suggest that the injected radiocolloid progressively migrates to the cyst wall during treatment (upper left in Fig. 3), possibly increasing the delivered dose. Considering this finding together with other factors like irregular shape of cysts, difficulties of volume-estimation etc., the dose calculated according to the formula of Fig. 1 is only an approximate indication of the dose actually delivered to the cyst wall. However, equally good results were observed in lower

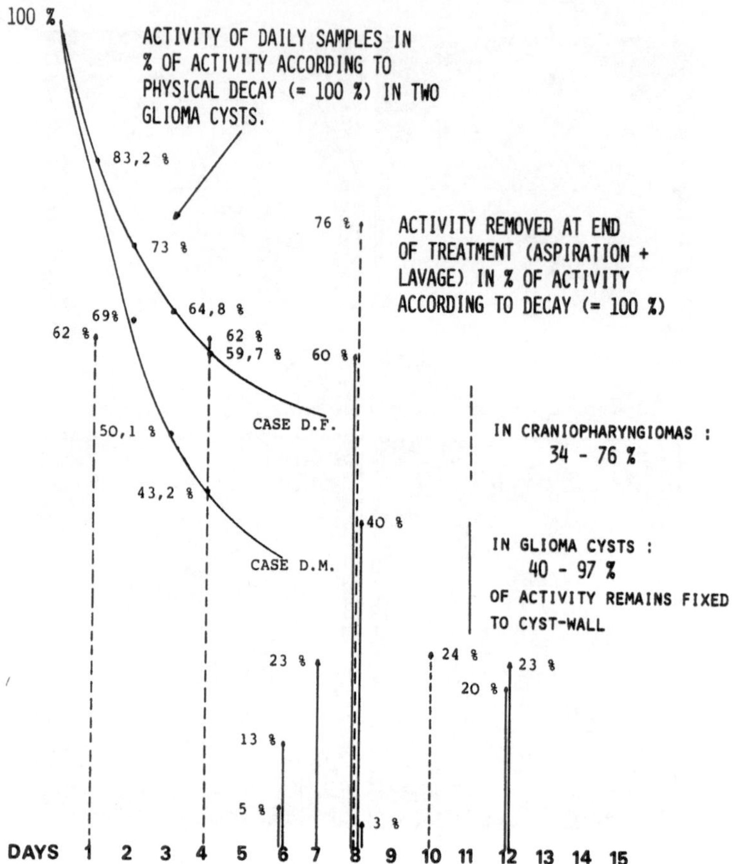

Fig. 3. Radioactivity of daily samples (upper left) and activity removed at end of treatment expressed in % of expected values according to decay suggest migration of colloidal Re-186 to cyst wall during treatment

as in higher dose ranges (Table 7). Therefore, in our present practice, we inject doses corresponding to 2–300 Gys/cyst wall, as calculated according to the formula of Fig. 1.

References

1. Backlund, E. O., Studies on craniopharyngiomas. III. Stereotaxic treatment with intracystic Yttrium 90. Acta Chir. Scand. *139* (1973), 237—247.
2. Backlund, E. O., Stereotactic radiosurgery in intracranial tumours and vascular malformations. In: Advances and Technical Standards in Neurosurgery, Vol. 6 (Krayenbühl, H., *et al.*, eds.), pp. 1—37. Wien-New York: Springer. 1979.

3. Csanda, E., Szikla, G., Vedrenne, C., Étude expérimentale des modifications de la barrière hémoencéphalique sous l'effet du rayonnement bêta. 7th Int. Congr. Neuropath. Excerpta Med. Int. Congr. Series. 1970.
4. Csanda, E., Radiation brain edema. In: Advances in Neurology, Vol. 28 (Cervós-Navarro, J., Ferszt, R., eds.), pp. 125—146. New York: Raven Press. 1980.
5. Leksell, L., Lidén, K., A therapeutic trial with radioactive isotope techniques, Vol. 1. Oxford: H. M. Stationery Office. 1952.
6. Mundinger, F., Brain tumour therapy by interstitial application of radioactive isotopes. In: Radionuclide Applications in Neurosurgery and Neurology (Paoletti and Yen Wang, eds.), pp. 199—265. Springfield, Ill.: Ch. C Thomas. 1970.
7. Overton, M. C., Scheffel, D. D., Recurrent cystic formation in craniopharyngioma treated with radioactive chromic phosphate. J. Neurosurg. *20* (1963), 707—710.
8. Szikla, G., Peragut, J. Cl., Irradiation interstitielle des gliomes. In: Radiothérapie des tumeurs du système nerveux central (Constans, J. P., Schlienger, M., eds.), Neurochirurgie (Paris), *21,* Suppl. 2 (1975), 187—228.
9. Schaub, C., Bluet-Pajot, M. T., Videau-Lornet, C., Askienazy, S., Szikla, G., Endocavitary beta irradiation of glioma cysts with colloidal 186 Rhenium. In: Stereotactic Cerebral Irradiation, INSERM Symposium No. 12 (Szikla, G., ed.), pp. 293—302. Amsterdam-New York-Oxford: Elsevier/North Holland Biomedical Press. 1979.

Acta Neurochirurgica, Suppl. 33, 341—344 (1984)

Results of Stereotactic Intracavitary Irradiation of Cystic Craniopharyngiomas. Comparison of the Effects of Yttrium-90 and Rhenium-186*

G. Netzeband[1], V. Sturm[1], P. Georgi[2], H. Sinn[2], K. Schnabel[2], W. Schlegel[2], S. Schabbert[2], M. Marin-Grez[2], and H. Gahbauer[2]

Summary

From May 1979 through October 1982, 33 patients with predominantly cystic craniopharyngiomas have been treated by intracavitary irradiation with stereotactically injected Yttrium-90 (n = 32) and Rhenium-186 (n = 6) using the technique of Leksell and Backlund. In 5 patients both radiocolloids have been used.

Since the β-irradiation of Yttrium-90 caused radiation-damage of the optic nerves in 5% of the cases, we replaced this radiocolloid by Rhenium-186 in patients with marked visual disturbances. Rhenium-186 has a lower β-energy and thus a smaller depth of penetration than Yttrium-90. In the patients, treated with Rhenium-186, no radiation-damage of the optic nerves was observed. On the other hand, the incidence of leakage to internal and external CSF-spaces and also the rate of cyst-refilling was much higher than in the Yttrium cases, in most of which good clinical results could be achieved so far.

Keywords: Cystic craniopharyngiomas; intracavitary irradiation; stereotactic treatment.

Introduction

The intracavitary contact-irradiation of cystic craniopharyngiomas, introduced by Leksell[6] and standardized by Backlund[1,2], has proved to be safe and effective. According to Backlund[3] and in our

---

* Dedicated to Prof. Dr. med. H. Penzholz on the occasion of his 70th birthday.

[1] Neurosurgical Department, Surgical Center, University of Heidelberg, Im Neuenheimer Feld 110, D-6900 Heidelberg 1, Federal Republic of Germany.

[2] Tumour-Center Heidelberg-Mannheim. Federal Republic of Germany.

own experience radiation-damage to the optic nerves occurs in about 5% of the cases, if colloidal Yttrium-90 is used as radiating agent. In patients with marked visual deficits due to mechanical lesions of the optic nerves by tumour-pressure, the incidence of additional radiation-damage seems to be higher than in patients with no or mild visual disturbances[3]. This prompted us to use Rhenium-186 in a pilot study comprising 6 consecutive patients with cystic craniopharyngiomas and severe visual deficits. The β-irradiation of this isotope has a shorter range than that of Yttrium-90. It was introduced by Szikla[9] for the intracavitary irradiation of cystic brain tumours. In this paper the results of the Yttrium-90 and Rhenium-186 irradiation of cystic craniopharyngiomas are analysed.

Material and Methods

Yttrium-90 is a pure $\bar{\beta}$-emitter (mean $\bar{\beta}$-energy 0.93 MeV, half life 64.1 h, half value layer in soft tissue 1.1 mm). It is available as colloidal silicate. Rhenium-186 is a $\bar{\beta}$- and γ-emitter (mean $\bar{\beta}$-energy 036 MeV, half life 90.6 h, half value layer in soft tissue ~0.4 mm). It is available as sulfide.

The application of the radionuclides was performed stereotactically using the technique of Backlund[1,2] with a Riechert-Mundinger device, modified by our group for the use within the CT-scanner[8]. The therapeutic β-dose for both Yttrium-90 and Rhenium-186 was 200 Gy to the inner surface of the cyst-wall. It was calculated according to Loevinger[7] from the volume of the cysts, which was assessed by both CT-measurements and radiodilution (Technetium-99)[4]. The implantation of the radionuclides was performed under intraoperative Gamma-camera control. Additional Gamma-camera investigations were performed 2 h after operation and later on in daily intervals through the first half life of the therapeutic agent. The effect of the treatment was assessed by regular clinical and CT-investigations.

Results

From May 1979 through October 1982, 33 patients with predominantly cystic craniopharyngiomas were treated with Yttrium-90 (n = 32) and Rhenium-186 (n = 6). The time of follow-up is 7 months up to 4 years. In 3 patients, in the first place Rhenium-186 was used, some months later an additional treatment with Yttrium-90 was necessary because of cyst-recurrence. This was effective in only 1 case. The therapeutic effects as well as the side effects, gained with Yttrium-90 and Rhenium-186 are listed in Table 1.

Table 1

	Treatment by Yttrium-90	Treatment by Rhenium-186
Number of treated cysts	33	7
Number of well responding cysts (reduction of volume up to disappearance)	30	3
Number of recurring cysts	3*	4
Side effects due to irradiation damage (number of patients)	2**	0
Deaths due to mechanical pressure from recurring cysts	2*	4
Operative deaths	0	0
Deaths for reasons, not related to treatment or cyst-recurrence	4	0
Leakage to CSF	2	7

* Two patients were treated with Yttrium-90 after ineffective treatment with Rhenium-186.

** In 1 patient, radiation damage to the optic nerves caused blindness. In 1 patient radiation damage to the hypothalamus is held to be the cause of a lethal hyperosmolar state. No verification by autopsy.

Discussion

The high incidence of cyst-recurrence and of leakage to CSF prompted us to stop the pilot study with Rhenium-186, although the number of treatments is too small for a statistical analysis. In 2 out of 3 recurrences after initial treatment with Rhenium-186, who were later on treated with Yttrium-90, both radionuclides have been ineffective. This could be due to an accidentally high proportion of "non-responders" in the small Rhenium series, but also to induction of radioresistance after ineffective initial irradiation[5].

The high rate of recurrences after initial Rhenium-treatment, if compared with those cases, initially treated with Yttrium, could be explained by a too short range of the β-irradiation of Rhenium-186. The higher tendency of Rhenium-186 to leak to CSF, may be due to the chemical compound. Rhenium-186 is a sulfide which tends to convert to water-soluble perrhenate, whereas Yttrium-90 is a stable silicate.

The good results, gained with Yttrium-90, are in accordance with the results of Backlund[2,3] and indicate the value of intracavitary β-irradiation of cystic craniopharyngiomas.

References

1. Backlund, E. O., Johansson, L., Sarby, B., Studies on craniopharyngiomas. II. Treatment by stereotaxis and radiosurgery. Acta Chir. Scand. *138* (1972), 749—759.
2. Backlund, E. O., Studies on craniopharyngiomas. III Stereotaxic treatment with intracystic Yttrium-90. Acta Chir. Scand. *139* (1973), 237—247.
3. Backlund, E. O., Pers. communication 1981.
4. Georgi, P., Strauss, L., Sturm, V., Ostertag, H., Sinn, H., Rommel, T., Prä- und intraoperative Volumenbestimmung bei Kraniopharyngiomzysten. Nucl. Med. *14* (4) (1980), 187—190.
5. Schmitt, H. P., Physikalische Schäden des ZNS und seiner Hüllen. In: Spezielle pathologische Anatomie, Vol. 13/II (Doerr, W., Seifert, G., Uehlinger, E., eds.), p. 777. Berlin-Heidelberg-New York: Springer. 1983.
6. Leksell, L., Backlund, E. O., Johansson, L., Treatment of Craniopharyngiomas. Acta Chir. Scand. *133* (1967), 345—350.
7. Loevinger, R., Japha, E. M., Brownell, G. C., In: Radiation Dosimetry (Hine and Brownell, eds.). New York: Academic Press. 1959.
8. Sturm, V., Pastyr, O., Schlegel, W., Scharfenberg, H., Zabel, H.-J., Netzeband, G., Schabbert, S., Berberich, W., Stereotactic computer tomography with a modified Riechert-Mundinger device as the basis for integrated stereotactic neuroradiological investigations. Acta Neurochir. (Wien) *68* (1983), 11—17.
9. Szikla, G., Peragut, J. C., Irradiation interstitielle des Gliomas. Neurochirurgie *21*, Suppl. 2 (1975), 187—228.

Acta Neurochirurgica, Suppl. 33, 345—353 (1984)

Combined Interstitial and External Irradiation of Gliomas

A. Rougier[1], **J. Pigneux**[2], and **F. Cohadon**[1]

With 4 Figures

Summary

The results of 43 small gliomas grade I to IV that were considered inoperable and treated with combined interstitial and external radiotherapy are reported. The full tumor dose was not less than 70 Gy. On a second target volume 2 cm around the tumor, the delivered dose was not less than 40 Gy at the outer limits. Tolerance can be considered acceptable given the location of these tumors in highly functional areas with long-term deficit in 13% of the cases. The results of combined irradiation of glioblastomas in its present form are considered deficient. On the other hand, this technique seems to be as effective as surgery plus radiotherapy for anaplastic and grade I astrocytomas.

Keywords: Gliomas; interstitial irradiation; tolerance; therapeutic results.

Introduction

For inoperable brain tumors, radiotherapy seems to be the only possible treatment, and interstitial irradiation would appear to be a technique especially suitable for small gliomas located in highly functional areas[13].

In addition to the concentration of irradiation, interstitial radiotherapy provides a low dose rate irradiation. Bernstein[2] has discussed the theoretical radiobiological advantages of this method. The delivered dose, however, is inhomogeneous in relation to the distance from the source, with overdose and risk of radionecrosis near the source and underdose at the outer limit with the risk of tumor regrowth[7]. Various solutions have been proposed by different teams. Mundinger uses a temporary implantation of a

[1] Service de Neuro-chirurgie A, CHU Pellegrin Tripode, Bordeaux, France.

[2] Centre anti-cancéreux Fondation Bergonié 33, Bordeaux, France.

high activity ^{192}Ir wire in malignant gliomas, and permanent implantation (^{192}Ir, ^{125}I) in low-grade brain tumors[4]. Our tentative solution for tumors with diameters less than 35 mm is to increase the radio-activity of the sources and to combine interstitial with external radiotherapy. This protocol proposed by the Sainte Anne Hospital team[11] is based on their experience of interstitial gamma irradiation. This report deals with results of small gliomas grade I to IV that were considered inoperable and treated with combined interstitial and external radiotherapy.

Patients and Method

When the CT scan revealed a space-occupying lesion in a highly functional area or in a deep-seated zone which was particularly difficult to reach surgically, a stereotaxic exploration was performed. A radiological morphogram was obtained and CT slices were transposed in the stereotactic space with the help of the scoutview mode[8]. When necessary, stereo-EEG with multilead electrodes provided a reliable means of assessing the tumoral volume[9]. One to five biopsies were performed. When the glioma was considered to be well delineated, inoperable and less than 35 mm in diameter, interstitial irradiation was performed.

To date, 43 patients have been treated (Table 1). The previously mentioned tumor volume parameters were not considered in 18% of the cases (Table 2) and, a posteriori, four cases (9%) could have been operated upon. The number, the spacing (10 to 15 mm) and the length of the ^{192}Ir wires was decided on after discussion between the neurosurgeon and the radiotherapist. These decisions were taken according to the size and the volume of the tumor and implantation possibilities. The implants were left for 2 to 10 days to deliver about 35 Gy at the external limit of the tumor with a dose rate varying between 0.10 Gy/hour and

Table 1. *Combined Interstitial and External Irradiation.* 43 cases

	Mean age	Performance status (Karnofsky scale) mean
Glioblastomas 13	58	60%
Anaplastic astrocytomas 12	40	70%
Grade I astrocytomas 18	36	80%

Table 2

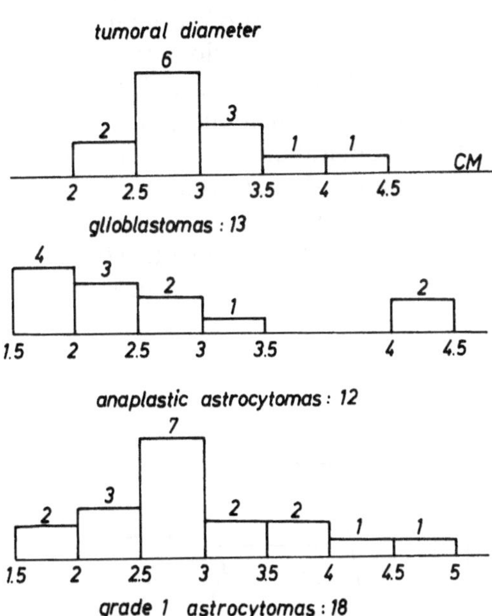

0.60 Gy/hour. External irradiation was based on a second target volume extending 2 cm beyond the outer limit of the tumor. According to the location of the tumor, Co^{60} for cortico-subcortical or 18–25 MEV X-rays for deep-seated tumors were chosen in an arrangement of 2 to 4 beams. Owing to energy and dose rate differences between interstitial gamma irradiation and external irradiation, the radiobiological effects are not the same. Nevertheless, the doses delivered by each method were added together. The full tumoral dose had to be at least 70 Gy. External radiotherapy complements interstitial irradiation thereby giving about 35 Gy. The dose at the outer limit of the second target volume around the tumor is about 40 Gy when the two types of irradiation are added together.

For glioblastomas the first course of chemotherapy is scheduled after the interstitial irradiation. Teniposide (60 mg/m^2) on 2 successive days and C.C.N.U. (60 mg/m^2) for the next two days are repeated once every 5 weeks.

Results

Tolerance: The operative mortality was 4.5%. One death resulted from the implantation of a tumor located in the wall of the third ventricle. The second death was probably due to a massive pulmonary embolism.

No alteration was noted in 34 cases (70%). Six cases with temporary deterioration were observed (13.5%). About 15 to 20 days of corticotherapy were necessary to bring the patients back to their original state. In four cases of permanent deterioration was observed immediately after the radio-active implantation (9.5%) and a new deficit appeared in one case (2.5%).

Late complication: When the patients were seizure free, interstitial irradiation did not provoke epilepsy. An anticonvulsant treatment, however, was administered in every case. The seizure frequency increased in two-thirds of the cases and these seizures were very resistant to medical treatment. About 10 months after irradiation, seizure frequency decreased to less than the previous level (Fig. 1).

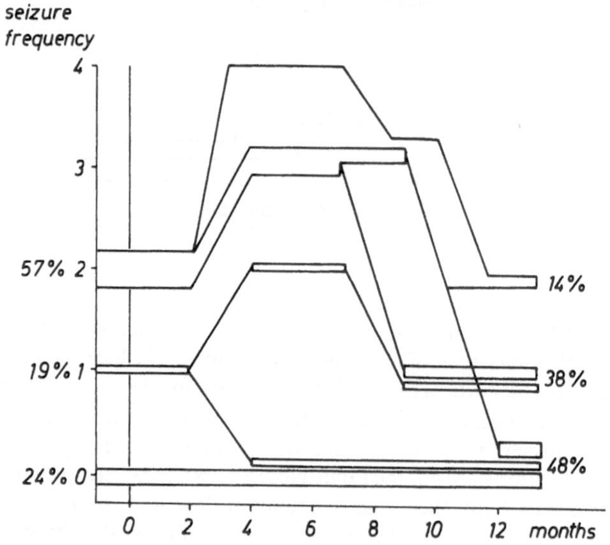

Fig. 1. Evolution of seizure frequency after interstitial and external irradiation

Radionecrosis: Of the 43 patients, 5 presented successive CT changes. After progressive enlargement, the contrast-enhanced zone decreased after 6–8 months. In three patients the outcome was poor with frequent seizures. Two cases had no clinical consequences.

Survival data: The median survival time for glioblastomas does not exceed 7 months (Fig. 2). None out of thirteen patients presented both incomplete remission with slight clinical improvement under corticoids, and a persisting enhancing lesion in CT. In the other cases, the clinical deterioration was progressive

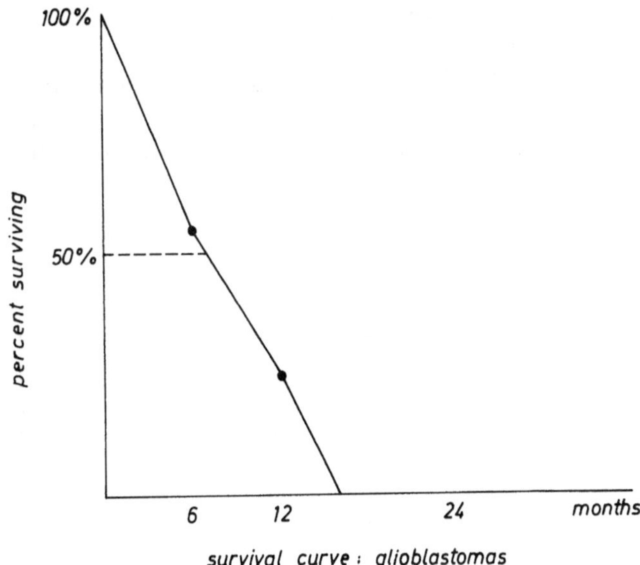

Fig. 2

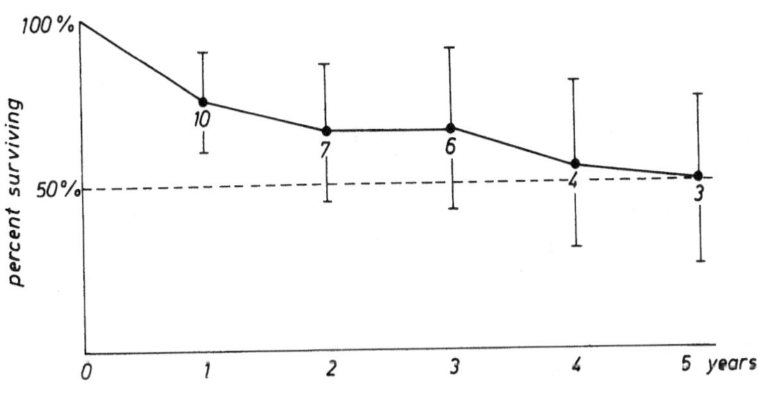

Fig. 3

after a short steady state, during which anti-edematous treatment was administered. Tumor recurrence always appeared near the irradiated zone.

In twelve cases of anaplastic astrocytomas one suffered progressive deterioration (Fig. 3). Three focal tumor recurrences are known to date. The median survival time is about 5 years, given the limited number of cases, the 95% confidence limits are very wide at this point of time.

In eighteen cases of grade I astrocytomas 5 tumor recurrences have appeared to date (Fig. 4). An insufficient tumor volume measurement was encountered in one case. In the other cases,

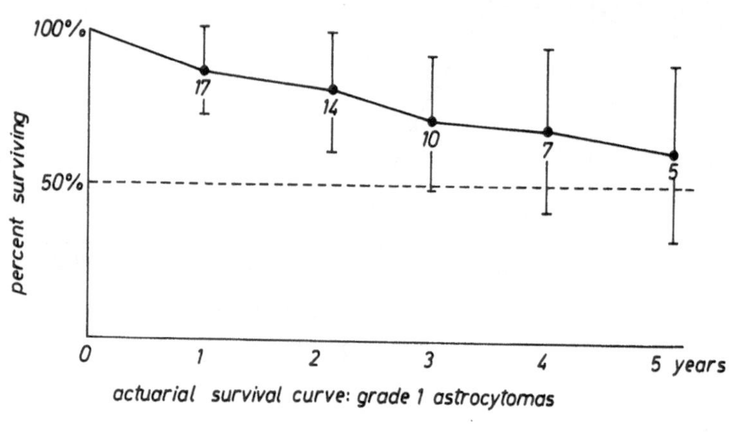

Fig. 4

tumor recurrence (11th, 31th, 39th, 47th months) was related to ana-plastic transformation which was indicated in CT by enhancing lesions and confirmed in 3 cases by biopsy or surgery. At present 2 enhancing lesions are either recurrence or radionecrosis. Tumor remission is currently ranges from 7 to 63 months. A hypodense area is still present with focal atrophy and ventricular widening.

Discussion

Experience with interstitial irradiation of brain gliomas is currently limited to a few departments. Since 1954, interstitial gamma irradiation has been used by the stereotactic team of Talairach and Szikla. Their findings have shown that tumors of more than 5 cm in diameter must not be treated by this technique because of intolerance and poor results. Taking into consideration that tumor growth is found beyond the outer limits of the target volume has led Szikla to propose combined interstitial and external irradiation[13]. The first results of the combined treatment by a multicenter study were reported in 1981: "The present experience seems to warrant further study of the value of this therapeutic association in selected cases"[1]. Present results vary according to histological types. With regard to glioblastomas, results seem to be obvious: no survival beyond 15 months with 7 months mean survival time. These results must be compared with those of patients treated by surgical resection plus radiation and chemotherapy. Salcman[10] quotes data taken from the most well-known reports, the median survival time being 10 months. Consequently we now are abandoning combined irradiation of glioblastomas in its present form. The possible explanation is that the field of irradiation is too confined and the dose rate too low for this type of tumor. Brachycurie-therapy as proposed by Mundinger[5], delivering high dose rate irradiation, seems to be more adapted to malignant tumors. It is administered only to tumors previously operated on. As regards anaplastic astrocytomas and grade I astrocytomas, results of combined irradiation can be compared with those obtained by permanent implantation. The dose rate, however, and histological criteria are different. Tolerance must be evaluated according to the inoperable nature of these tumors. Mortality and morbidity in the immediate follow-up are 4.5 and 12% respectively, whereas in the progress report of the cooperative study no significant morbidity was noted[1]. For Mundinger[6] complete or partial remissions are not uncommon, which is in contrast to our experience. No late deficit is reported and 40% are free of seizures. In our series radionecrosis, epilepsy and late brain swelling are the cause of transitory or permanent deficits in 13% of the cases. The pre-existent deficit persisted without significant improvement. Nevertheless, in our opinion, the tolerance can be considered acceptable for these tumors in highly functional areas. The survival data of anaplastic astrocytomas treated by combined irradiation and of gliomas (grade I–III) treated by ^{192}Ir permanent implantation are similar with 50% and 48.5% survival probability after 5 years.

These results can be considered better than those obtained using resection and radiotherapy. Kuhlendahl[3] gives a survival probability after 5 years of 30% for grade II astrocytomas. Sheline[12] gives 25% after 5 years for grade II and 18% for grade III. These results must be interpreted with respect to the relatively young age and good neurological status of our patients.

In astrocytomas grade I few differences are noteworthy when comparing the various methods of treatments. The mean survival time is about 4 years as reported by Kuhlendahl[3] and Sheline[12].

Mundinger reported survival rates of 63.4% after 5 years in spongioblastomas and pilocytic astrocytomas and 36.9% in fibrillary astrocytomas. These results seem to indicate that combined interstitial and external irradiation is at least as effective as surgery plus radiotherapy for low-grade astrocytomas.

References

1. A cooperative study. Combined interstitial and external irradiation of gliomas. In: Stereotactic Cerebral Irradiation. INSERM Symposium No. 12 (Szikla, G., ed.), pp. 329—338. Amsterdam-New York-Oxford: Elsevier/North Holland Biomedical Press. 1979.
2. Bernstein, M., Gutin, P. H., Interstitial irradiation of brain tumors: a review. Neurosurgery *9* (1981), 741—750.
3. Kuhlendahl, H., Miltz, H., Wüllenweber, R., Die Astrozytome des Großhirns: Untersuchung zur Gruppierung und Prognose. Acta Neurochir. (Wien) *29* (1973), 151—162.
4. Mundinger, F., Rationale and methods of interstitial iridium 192 brachycurie therapy and iridium 192 or iodine 125 protacted long term irradiation. In: Stereotactic Cerebral Irradiation. INSERM Symposium No. 12 (Szikla, G., ed.), pp. 101—115. Amsterdam-New York-Oxford: Elsevier/North Holland Biomedical Press. 1979.
5. Mundinger, F., Ostertag, C., Post operative stereotactic curie therapy using the iridium 192 gamma Med contact irradiation apparatus combined with radio-sensitizers in treating of multiform glioblastomas. Acta Neurochir. (Wien) *42* (1978), 73—77.
6. Mundinger, F., Busam, B., Birg, W., Schildge, J., Results of interstitial iridium 192 brachycurie therapy and iridium 192 protracted long term irradiation. In: Stereotactic Cerebral Irradiation. INSERM Symposium No. 12 (Szikla, G., ed.), pp. 303—319. Amsterdam-New York-Oxford: Elsevier/North Holland Biomedical Press. 1979.
7. Pierquin, B., Précis de curie-thérapie. Paris: Masson et Cie. 1964.
8. Rougier, A., Pigneux, J., Richaud, P., Cohadon, F., La prise en charge diagnostique et thérapeutique des gliomes malins. Neurochirurgie *27* (1981), 315—320.
9. Rougier, A., Sajeaux, J. C., Certain, O., Cohadon, F., Stereoelectroencephalography in cerebral tumors. Appl. neurophysiol. *45* (1982), 413—418.
10. Salcman, M., Survival in glioblastoma: historical perspective. Neurosurgery *7* (1980), 435—439.
11. Schlienger, M., Bouhnik, H., Missir, O., Constans, J. J., Szikla, G., Association of temporary insterstitial 192 Ir implantation and external radiotherapy in the management of supratentorial tumors. Technique and dosimetry. In: Stereotactic Cerebral Irradiation. INSERM Symposium No. 12 (Szikla, G., ed.), pp. 117—122. Amsterdam-New York-Oxford: Elsevier/North Holland Biomedical Press. 1979.

12. Sheline, G. E., Radiation therapy of brain tumors. Cancer *39* (1977), 873—881.
13. Szikla, G., Peragut, J. C., Irradiation interstitielle des gliomes. In: Radiothérapie des tumeurs du système nerveux central de l'adulte (Constans, J. P., Schlienger, M., eds.), pp. 197—228. Neurochir. 21, Suppl. 2. Paris: Masson et Cie. 1975.
14. Talairach, J., Ruggiero, G., Aboulker, J., David, M., A new method of treatment of inoperable brain tumors by stereotaxic implantation of radioactive gold: a preliminary report. Br. J. Radiol. *28* (1955), 62—74.

Acta Neurochirurgica, Suppl. 33, 355—362 (1984)

Interstitial and Combined Interstitial and External Irradiation of Supratentorial Gliomas. Results in 61 Cases Treated 1973–1981

G. Szikla[1], M. Schlienger[4], S. Blond[1], C. Daumas-Duport[2], O. Missir[3], S. Miyahara[1], A. Musolino[1], and C. Schaub[1]

With 4 Figures

Summary

Follow-up data of 61 small (d ⩽ 5 cm) unresectable supratentorial gliomas grade 1 to 4, treated at our unit 1973–1981 by stereotactic temporary 192 Iridium implantation, either alone (n = 34) or combined with external radiotherapy (n = 27) are presented in order to assess results and indications of the method: Life table curves show a 5 year survival of 78% in 25 grade 1 gliomas, 69% in 20 grade 2 astrocytomas, 55% in 7 grade 3 astrocytomas. Malignant grade 4 gliomas (n = 9) survive at 1 year in 44%, at 2 years in 19%. Functional loss probably related to late radiation effects was observed in about 25% of cases. Seizure tendency disappeared or was markedly reduced after the first year. Our data compare favourably with other surgical and/or radiotherapeutic series and warrant further application of this treatment to unresectable supratentorial gliomas within the indicated volume limits.

Keywords: Neurosurgical curietherapy; brain tumour therapy; supratentorial gliomas; combined interstitial and external irradiation.

Introduction

Permanent intratumoral implantation of radioactive isotopes (Au 198 and later Ir 192) has been performed at our unit since 1954[8,11]. Better localization by CT and biopsies gave a new

Departments of [1] Neurosurgery, [2] Pathology and [3] Radiology, C. H. Sainte Anne, 1 rue Cabanis, F-75014 Paris; [4] Department of Radiotherapy, Hôpital Tenon, F-75019 Paris, France.

impetus to cerebral curietherapy with temporary Ir 192 application. A dosimetric protocol associating curietherapy and external radiotherapy has been formulated in 1975[7]. First results have been published in 1979 and 1981[9,10]. The aim of this presentation is to assess results and indications of this treatment in the light of presently available follow-up data.

Material and Methods

61 small (diameter ≤ 5 cm) supratentorial gliomas of all grades were treated 1973 through 1981. Tumour location was hemispheric in the majority of cases (43) many of them in rolandic or speech areas, 18 were deep seated (basal ganglia, third ventricle).

Target volume was established by stereotactic X-ray studies, serial biopsies and since 1976 by CT data. Grading of biopsies was evaluated according to C. Daumas[5]. Double plastic catheters were used for temporary Ir 192 application (afterloading).

Smaller, 2–3 cm gliomas were usually irradiated by Ir 192 alone, the 50 Gy isodose encircling the lesion in 4–7 days. Greater and more infiltrating lesions had interstitial therapy with a peripheral dose of 35 Gy associated to fractionated external high voltage photon therapy delivering 25 Gy/10 f/14 d on a bigger volume with a safety margin of 2 cm beyond the stereotactic target. Lesions above 5 cm (not included in this presentation) were treated with external radiation only. Clinical follow-up was regularly documented at our unit, with CT controls performed by one of us (O. M.): Data derived from control biopsies are presented in another study of our group[6].

Results

Life table curves and relevant data corresponding to each group are presented separately according to malignancy grade. Tumour volume includes the central bulk of the tumour (T) together with the infiltrated brain parenchyma (inf.) where isolated tumour cells can be recognized in biopsy specimens. Tumour-index corresponds to maximal length (l) × width (w) × height (h) of the tumour in cm.

Crude survival figures do not show significant differences between subgroups according to age (children below 16 years: 9), to hemispheric versus deep location or to diameter below or above 4 cm. In infiltrating grade II astrocytomas, survival is better with combined treatment than with curietherapy alone.

Comments

a) Best possible *delimitation of the target* including peripheral infiltrated areas is obviously crucial for focal irradiation. Under-

Table 1

Slowly evolutive grade I gliomas; biopsy grade: "A" (n = 25),
(astrocytoma "A": 7, pilocytic: 10, oligodendroglioma: 4,
ependymoma: 1, not classified: 3).
Age: • 16 years: 7, 16–40 years: 18.
Anamnesis (years): m̄: 3.2 (0.1–17, median: 1.5).
Clinical condition at beginning of treatment:
No neurol. deficit 15, slight 9, major 1.
Tumour vol. diam. m̄ ~ 3.6 cm.
(Index T. + Inf.: 1 × h × w, cm: m̄ 48, 13.1–125).
Location: hemispheric 14 (central-paracentral 10).
deep 11.
Type of irradiation: interstitial 16.
combined 9.
Follow-up (years) m̄ 4.25 (0.9–8, median 3.75).
Recurrence free interval m̄ 4 years (0.9–7, median 3.6).

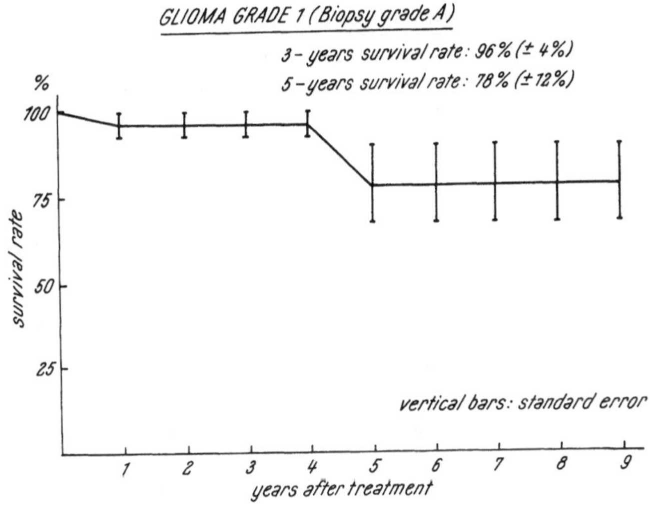

Fig. 1. Glioma grade 1 (biopsy grade A). 3-years survival rate 96% (± 4%), 5-years survival rate 78% (± 12%)

estimation of the target volume seems to be a major factor in recurrencies: in 9 out of 12 recurrent grade II astrocytomas (75%), reexamination of the initial biopsies found scattered tumour cells in peripheral samples, beyond the limits of the estimated target. Careful cytological study of the tumour periphery might differentiate isolated tumour cells from reactive gliosis and

Table 2

Gliomas grade 2 (biopsy Gr. "B"). n = 20 astrocytomas B. Age: 24–54 years. Anamnesis (years) m̄ 3.2 (0.25–11, median 1.5). Clinical condition at beginning of treatment: No neurol. deficit 11, slight 8, major 1. Tumour vol. diam. m̄: 3.8 cm. (Index T. + Inf.: m̄ 53, 24.5–90). Location: hemispheric 18 (central paracentral 12). deep 2. Type of irradiation: interstitial 11. combined 9. Follow-up (years) m̄ 4.4 (1.6–8.5, median 4.25). Recurrence free interval (years) m̄ 3.8 (0–8.5, median 3.9).

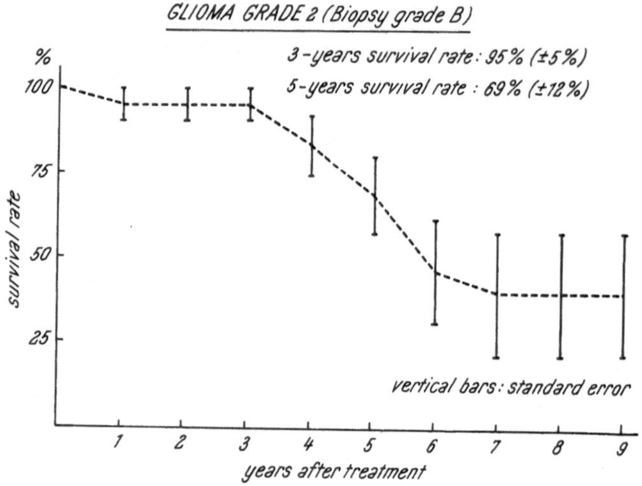

Fig. 2. Glioma grade 2 (biopsy grade B). 3-years survival rate 95% (± 5%), 5-years survival rate 69% (± 12%)

contribute in an important manner to establish the boundaries of the treatment volume[4, 5].

b) *Tolerance of treatment: Late radiation damage*

After the usually uneventful treatment and a first silent period, volume dependent late brain swelling requiring steroid treatment

Table 3

Gliomas grade 3 (biopsy grade: "C").
n = 7 astrocytomas "C".
Age: 22–51 years.
Anamnesis (years) m̄ 4.8 (0.4–17, median 2.5).
Clinical condition at beginning of treatment:
No neurol. deficit 1, slight 6.
Tumour vol. diam. m̄: 3.9 cm.
(Index T. + Inf.: m̄ 59.5, 42–72).
Location: hemispheric 6 (central-paracentral 4).
deep 1.
Type of irradiation: interstitial 3.
combined 4.
Follow-up (years) m̄ 3.7 (0.5–5.7, median 3.75).
Recurrence free interval (years) m̄: 2.7 (0–5.7, median 3).

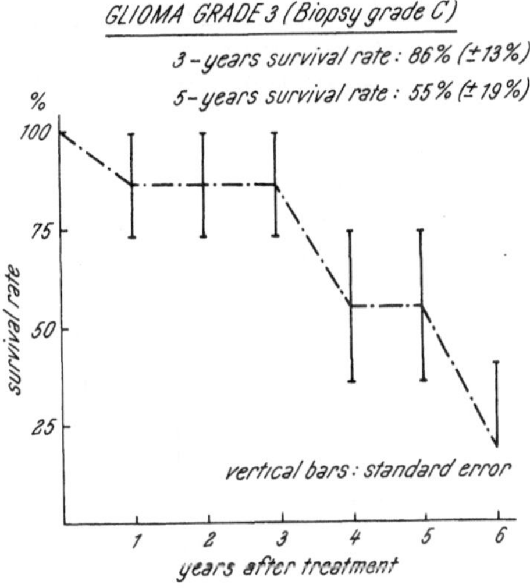

Fig. 3. Gioma grade 3 (biopsy grade C). 3-years survival rate 86% (± 13%), 5-years survival rate 55% (± 19%)

appears usually at 6–16 months after irradiation[9]. Only partially regressive clinical worsening (*e.g.* hemiparesis → hemiplegia) probably related to late radiation effects on neighbourhood structures has been observed in 20–25%. As expected, necrotic changes of the heavily irradiated target were found in the majority of these cases at bioptic controls, surrounded by a 1–2 cm halo of

Table 4

Gliomas grade 4 (biopsy grade: "malignant").
n = 9 (malignant astrocytoma 4, glioblastoma 5).
Age (years) 16: 1, 20–58: 8.
Anamnesis (months) m̄ 2.9 (0.3–15, median 1).
Clinical condition at beginning of treatment:
No neurol. deficit 1, slight 8.
Tumour vol. diam. m̄: 3.8 cm.
(Index T. + Inf.: m̄ 57, 27–87).
Location: hemispheric 4 (central paracentral 2).
deep 5.
Type of irradiation: interstitial 4.
combined 5.
Follow-up (months) m̄ 10.3 (2–18, median 10).

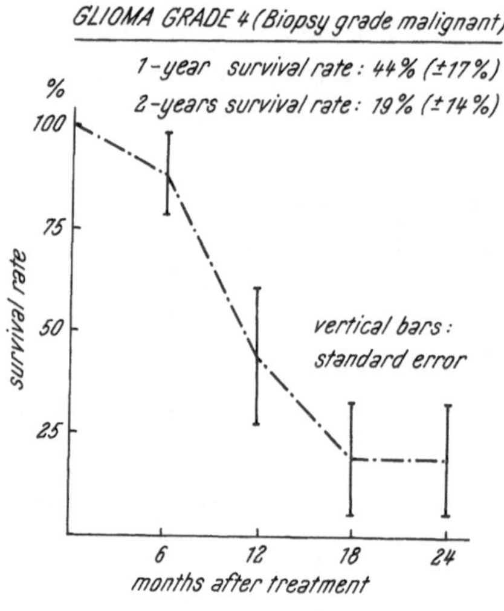

Fig. 4. Glioma grade 4 (biopsy grade malignant). 1-year survival rate: 44% (± 17%), 2-years survival rate: 19% (± 14%)

rapidly decreasing edema-gliosis, corresponding closely to the dosimetric curves[6]. The risk of functional loss induced by late radionecrosis seems to us an acceptable price for the cure of an otherwise fatal glioma located in the hemispheres or the basal ganglia. We would however not advocate this type of treatment for slowly evolutive grade I lesions in hypothalamic or brain stem location, especially in children with only slight endocrine and/or neurological impairment, as late radionecrotic changes imply not only increased functional but also vital risks in these areas of the brain.

Conclusion

In the light of long term follow-up data, focal high dose irradiation with temporary 192 Iridium implantation associated or not to external photon therapy appears to be an efficient treatment of small unresectable gliomas with an acceptable risk/benefit ratio both in hemispheric and basal ganglia location. Treatment of grade I to III lesions seems to be particularly rewarding.

References

1. Bancaud, J., Talairach, J., Szikla, G., Stereo-EEG exploration in interstitial irradiation of gliomas. In: Stereotactic Cerebral Irradiation, INSERM symposium no. 12 (Szikla, G., ed.), pp. 57—62. Amsterdam-New York-Oxford: Elsevier/North Holland Biomedical Press. 1979.
2. Betti, O., *et al.*, Combined interstitial and external irradiation of gliomas. A progress report. In: Stereotactic Cerebral Irradiation, INSERM Symposium no. 12 (Szikla, G., ed.), pp. 329—338. Amsterdam-New York-Oxford: Elsevier/North Holland Biomedical Press. 1979.
3. Chavaudra, J., Schlienger, M., Szikla, G., Some considerations on the physical and clinical aspects of stereotactic cerebral irradiation. In: Stereotactic Cerebral Irradiation, INSERM Symposium no. 12 (Szikla, G., ed.), pp. 177—184. Amsterdam-New York-Oxford: Elsevier/North-Holland Biomedical Press. 1979.
4. Cohadon, F., Rougier, A., Da Silva Nuñez Neto, D., Sageaux, J. C., Billeret, J., Caille, J. M., Imbernon, A., CT scan as an aid to the assessment of tumoral volume. In: Stereotactic Cerebral Irradiation, INSERM Symposium No. 12 (Szikla, G., ed.), pp. 11—23. Amsterdam-New York-Oxford: Elsevier/North Holland Biomedical Press. 1979.
5. Daumas-Duport, C., Monsaingcon, V., Szenthe, L., Szikla, G., Serial stereotactic biopsies: a double histological code of gliomas according to malignancy and 3 D configuration, as an aid to therapeutic decision and assessment of results. J. Appl. Neurophysiol. *45* (1982), 431—437.
6. Daumas-Duport, C., Blond, S., Vedrenne, C., Szikla, G., Radiolesion versus recurrence: bioptic data in 39 gliomas after interstitial or combined interstitial and external radiation. 6th Meeting of the European Society of Stereotactic and Functional Neurosurgery, Rome, June 2–4, 1983. Acta Neurochir. (Wien) Suppl. 33, pp. 291—299. Wien-New York: Springer. 1984.
7. Schlienger, M., Bouhnik, H., Missir, O., Constans, J. P., Szikla, G., Association of temporary interstitial 192 Ir implantation and external radiotherapy in the management of supratentorial tumours. Technique and

dosimetry. In: Stereotactic Cerebral Irradiation, INSERM Symposium No. 12 (Szikla, G., ed.), pp. 117—121. Amsterdam-New York-Oxford: Elsevier/North Holland Biomedical Press. 1979.

8. Szikla, G., Peragut, J. Cl., Irradiation interstitielle des gliomes. In: Radiothérapie des tumeurs du système nerveux central de l'adulte (Constans, J. P., Schlienger, M., eds.), pp. 187—228. Neurochir. *21*, Suppl, 2. 1975.
9. Szikla, G., Betti, O., Blond, S., Data on late reactions following stereotactic irradiation of gliomas. In: Stereotactic Cerebral Irradiation, INSERM Symposium No. 12 (Szikla, G., ed.), pp. 167—174. Amsterdam-New York-Oxford: Elsevier/North Holland Biomedical Press. 1979.
10. Szikla, G., Betti, O., Szenthe, L., Schlienger, M., L'expérience actuelle des irradiations stéréotaxiques dans le traitement des gliomes hémisphériques. Neurochir. *27* (1981), 295—298.
11. Talairach, J., Aboulker, J., Ruggiero, G., David, M., Utilisation de la méthode radiostéréotaxique pour le traitement radioactif i *in situ* des tumeurs cérébrales. Rev. Neurol. (Paris) *90* (1954), 656—657.

Acta Neurochirurgica, Suppl. 33, 363—366 (1984)

Brachytherapy with Removable Iodine-125 Sources for the Treatment of Recurrent Malignant Brain Tumors

Ph. H. Gutin[1,2,3], **Th. L. Phillips**[3], **W. M. Wara**[3], **St. A. Leibel**[3], **Y. Hosobuchi**[2], **V. A. Levin**[1], **K. A. Weaver**[3], and **Sh. Lamb**[2]

With 1 Figure

Summary

Thirty-seven patients harboring recurrent malignant primary or metastatic brain tumors were treated by 40 implantations of high activity iodine-125 (^{125}I) sources. All patients had been treated with radiation and most had been treated with chemotherapeutic agents, primarily nitrosoureas. Implantations were performed using computed tomography-directed stereotaxy; ^{125}I sources were held in one or more afterloaded catheters that were removed after the desired dose (minimum tumor dose of 3,000–12,000 rad) had been delivered. Results of 34 implantation procedures are evaluable, and are discussed here.

Introduction

Many solid systemic tumors that are localized when they are detected can be cured by surgery and radiation therapy. Most malignant gliomas are localized to a single area of the brain[4]; however, radiation toxicity to surrounding normal brain precludes delivery, by external beam irradiation, of doses that control (cure) local disease. The implantation of radioactive isotopes interstitially (brachytherapy) permits delivery of high total doses of radiation to localized tumor volumes.

---

[1] Brain Tumor Research Center and the [2] Section of Functional and Stereotactic Surgery of the Department of Neurological Surgery, and the [3] Department of Radiation Oncology, School of Medicine, University of California, San Francisco, CA 94143, U.S.A.

Materials and Methods

Patients: From December 3, 1979, to October 1, 1982, 37 patients ranging in age from 3 to 68 years who harbored recurrent malignant brain tumors were implanted 40 times with high activity ^{125}I sources. All tumors had recurred after surgery and irradiation (3,600–6,700 rad). Eighteen patients harbored primary anaplastic astrocytomas, 13 glioblastomas, three solitary cerebral metastases from carcinoma of the breast or lung, one a metastasis from melanoma, one a recurrent choroid plexus carcinoma, and a one recurrent malignant meningioma.

Implantation technique: Implantation of sources, held in an afterloaded coaxial silicone catheter system [1], was performed under local anesthesia—except in children—using the Leksell stereotactic system modified for use with the CT scanner [2,3,6]. ^{125}I sources (30–50 mCi) were supplied by special order from the manufacturer. A CT scan was performed to confirm accurate placement of sources, and orthogonal radiographs were taken to determine source relationships. A computer program converted position data and source strengths into dose rate contours in any plane. The implantation time for the desired dose was calculated, and sources were removed in a simple procedure under local anesthesia on the appropriate day.

Evaluation of patients: Patients were evaluated by neurological examinations and CT scans at intervals of 8 weeks, when possible, and graded on a scale of —2 to + 2 (deterioration or improvement); this a modification of published criteria [5]. Time to progression was measured from the day of implantation until progression was documented.

Results

Thirty-four implantations in 31 patients are evaluable. Minimum (peripheral) tumor doses of 3,000–12,000 were delivered to these patients from 44–282 mCi of ^{125}I divided among 1–3 implanted catheters; typically dose rates were 20–100 rad/hr. Eighteen of. 34 evaluable implantations produced clearcut responses for 4— 13 + months (Fig. 1) and five others produced disease stabilization (4–12 months) for an overall response rate of 68%. Eleven patients continued to progress, but among this group were three patients who developed multifocal disease, three who had probable radiation necrosis, and three who were explored surgically and found to have radiation necrosis. These three patients (glioblastoma) and two others (anaplastic astrocytoma, glioblastoma) who intitially responded, then deteriorated, and had focal necrotic tissue resected, form a group of our longest survivors. All were improved by surgery and remain alive 10, 15, 19, 24, and 25 months after implantation. Currently, only one of these patients is deteriorating from the continued growth of recurrent tumor. Initial progression is by no means an indicator of lack of effect of treatment because the evaluation criteria cannot be used to

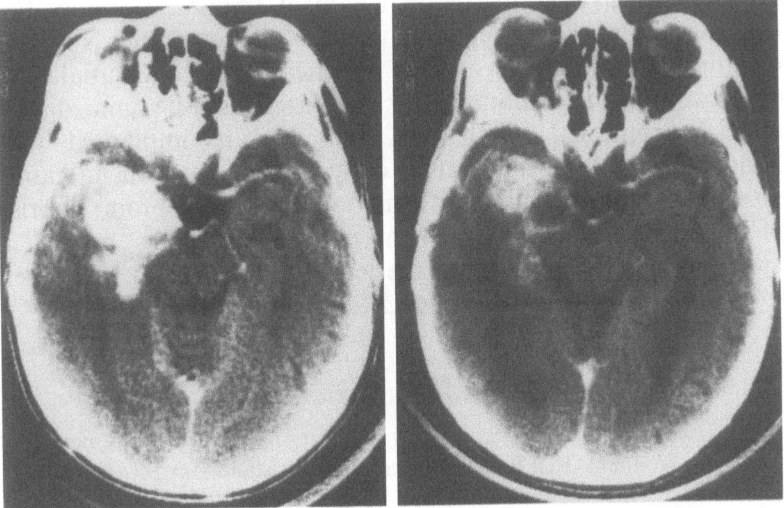

Fig. 1. CT scans showing a recurrent right temporal anaplastic astrocytoma before (left) and two months after (right) brachytherapy. The patient continues to do well four months after the implantation procedure

distinguish focal radiation necrosis from recurrent tumor. It is probable that aggressive interstitial brachytherapy in previously-irradiated patients with tumor recurrences will cause radiation necrosis, and that exploratory craniotomy for resection of a necrotic mass should be a planned sequel to implantation.

Because surviving patients are censored from consideration, survival plots are meaningless in a patient group such as this in which 48% are still surviving. One measure of the success of ^{125}I brachytherapy is the median follow-up time from implantation, which is 9 months for the glioblastoma group and 10 months for the anaplastic astrocytoma group. For the malignant glioma group as a whole, the median follow-up is nine months. These are not overall survival times, which in all instances are much longer, but only the follow-up time after implantation for recurrence. Because 48% of these patients are surviving at the time of this report, survival results will progressively improve.

Discussion

From the results of this series, it is clear that removable ^{125}I sources have definite activity against recurrent malignant brain tumors. The cure of any *recurrent* tumor is enormously difficult to accomplish; it is of course better to control the disease initially. For this reason we have begun a protocol through the Northern California Oncology Group; in an attempt to gain initial local control of what is predominantly a localized disease[4], immediately after conventional teletherapy, patients are implanted with removable ^{125}I "boosts" that are designed to increase the radiation dose to the tumor while sparing surrounding normal brain. The risk of focal radiation necrosis in the patients receiving "boosts" is unknown, but, based on our experience with patients in this series, this complication should be surgically manageable.

Acknowledgments

This work was supported in part by National Cancer Institute Grant CA 13525. We thank Neil Buckley for editional assistance

References

1. Gutin, P. H., Dormandy, R. H., A coaxial catheter system for afterloading radioactive sources for the interstitial irradiation of brain tumors. J. Neurosurg. *56* (1982), 734—735.
2. Gutin, P. H., Phillips, T. L., Hosobuchi, Y., Wara, W. M., Mackay, A. M., Weaver, K. A., Lamb, S., Hurst, S., Local treatment of malignant brain tumors by removable stereotactically implanted radioactive isotopes. In: Progress in Radio-Oncology, Vol. 2 (Karscher, K. H., Kogelnik, K. D., Reinartz, G., eds.), pp. 363—369. New York: Raven Press. 1982.
3. Gutin, P. H., Phillips, T. L., Hosobuchi, Y., Wara, W. M., MacKay, A. M., Weaver, K. A., Lamb, S., Hurst, S., Permanent and removable implants for the brachytherapy of brain tumors. Int. J. Radiat. Oncol. Biol. Phys. *7* (1981), 1371—1381.
4. Hochberg, F. H., Pruitt, A., Assumptions in the radiotherapy of glioblastoma. Neurology *30* (1980), 907—911.
5. Levin, V. A., Crafts, D., Norman, D. M., Hoffer, P. B., Spire, J. P., Wilson, C. B., Criteria for evaluating malignant brain tumor patients undergoing chemotherapy. J. Neurosurg. *47* (1977), 329—335.
6. MacKay, A. M., Gutin, P. H., Hosobuchi, Y., Norman, D. M., Computed tomography-directed stereotaxy for biopsy and interstitial irradiation of brain tumors: Technical note. Neurosurgery *11* (1982), 38—42.
7. Walker, M. D., Strike, T. A., Sheline, G. E., An analysis of dose-effect relationship in the radiotherapy of malignant gliomas. Int. J. Radiat. Oncol. Biol. Phys. *5* (1979), 1733—1740.

Acta Neurochirurgica, Suppl. 33, 367—371 (1984)

Long-term Results of Stereotactic Interstitial Curietherapy

F. Mundinger[1] and **K. Weigel**[1]

With 3 Figures

Of the 7,587 stereotactic operations that we have carried out in our department as of May 19, 1983 using the stereotactic device developed by Riechert and Mundinger, the non-resectable deep-seated tumours of the midline or hemispheres treated with Curietherapy and Brachy-Curietherapy (GammaMed) in 1,445 radiation operations, make up the second most frequent indication after extrapyramidal-motor disturbances.

The clinical data of 904 patients with intracranial tumours among whom 472 had permanent Iridium-192 or Iodine-125

Table 1 a. *Stereotactically Operated Cerebral Gliomas* (n = 639, 1965–1982)

	N. of cases	Alive
Astrocytoma I	144	88
Astrocytoma II	218	146
Astrocytoma III	124	47
Oligodendroglioma II	41	23
Oligodendroglioma III	11	3
Glioblastoma IV	101	18
Total	639	325

[1] Abteilung Stereotaxie und Neuronuklearmedizin, Neurochirurgische Universitätsklinik, Hugstetter Strasse 55, D-7800 Freiburg im Breisgau, Federal Republic of Germany.

Table 1 b. *Stereotactically Operated Extracerebral Lesions* (n = 265, 1965–1982)

	N. of cases	Alive
Ependymoma	15	8
Papilloma	7	5
Meningeoma	10	8
Colloid cyst	5	5
Epidermoid	7	5
Teratoma	10	4
Germinoma	24	13
Medulloblastoma	5	5
Primitive neuroektoderm. tumor (PNET)	11	8
Craniopharyngeoma	43	22
Metastatic tumor	47	13
Unclassified tumor	8	2
Abscess	6	4
Gliosis	55	47
Other	12	12
Total	265	161

Table 2 a. *Stereotactic Curietherapy of 198 Gliomas with Iridium-192 (1965–1982)*

	N. of cases	Alive
Astrocytoma I	58	27
Astrocytoma II	75	34
Astrocytoma III	22	1
Oligodendroglioma II	21	10
Oligodendroglioma III	8	1
Glioblastoma IV	14	2
Total	198	75

Table 2 b. *Stereotactic Curietherapy of 38 Extracerebral Tumors with Iridium-192 (1965–1982)*

	N. of cases	Alive
Ependymoma	5	1
Papilloma	3	1
Meningeoma	2	1
Epidermoid	3	1
Teratoma	3	0
Germinoma	6	3
Primitive neuroektoderm. tumor (PNET)	1	1
Craniopharyngeoma	8	1
Colloid cyst	1	1
Metastatic tumor	2	2
Unclassified tumor	2	0
Gliosis	1	0
Other	1	1
Total	38	13

Table 3 a. *Stereotactic Curietherapy of 186 Gliomas with Iodine-125 (1979–1982)*

	N. of cases	Alive
Astrocytoma I	44	34
Astrocytoma II	69	56
Astrocytoma III	41	19
Oligodendroglioma II	9	6
Oligodendroglioma III	1	0
Glioblastoma IV	22	1
Total	186	116

Table 3 b. *Stereotactic Curietherapy of 50 Extracerebral Tumors with Iodine-125 (1979–1982)*

	N. of cases	Alive
Ependymoma	7	4
Meningeoma	4	4
Teratoma	1	0
Germinoma	10	4
Primitive neuroektoderm. tumor (PNET)	4	2
Craniopharyngeoma	6	1
Medulloblastoma	2	2
Metastatic tumor	13	7
Unclassified tumor	1	0
Gliosis	1	1
Other	1	1
Total	50	26

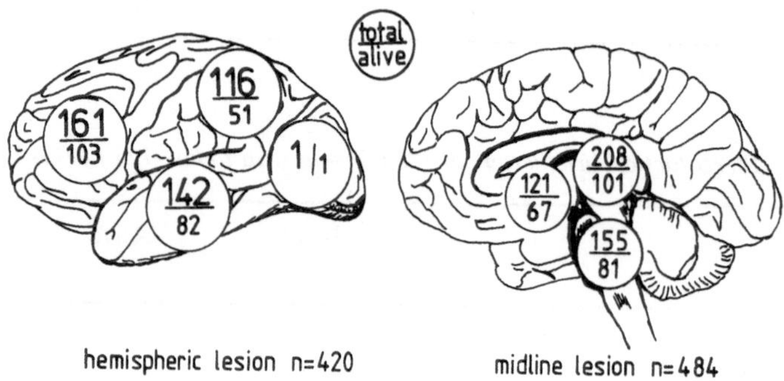

Fig. 1. Total of the stereotactically operated intracranial lesions (n = 904/1965–1982)

implantations between 1965 and 1983, were compiled and evaluated. The location of the tumours, the bioptic diagnosis, the implanted radionuclide and the frequency percentages of the patients still alive are given in figures and tables.

Detailed evaluations are given elsewhere.

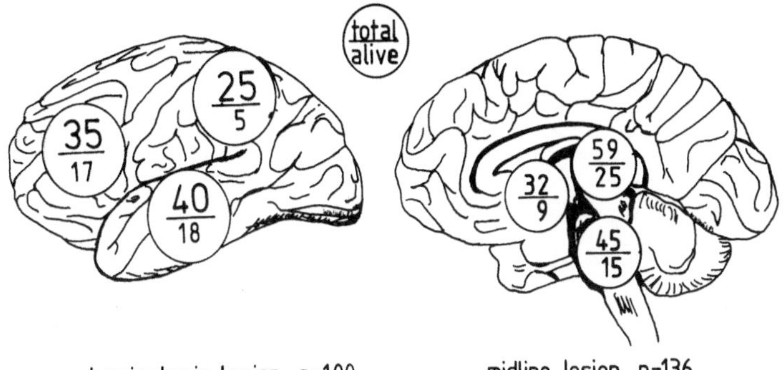

Fig. 2. Stereotactic Curietherapy with Iridium-192 (n = 236/1965–1982)

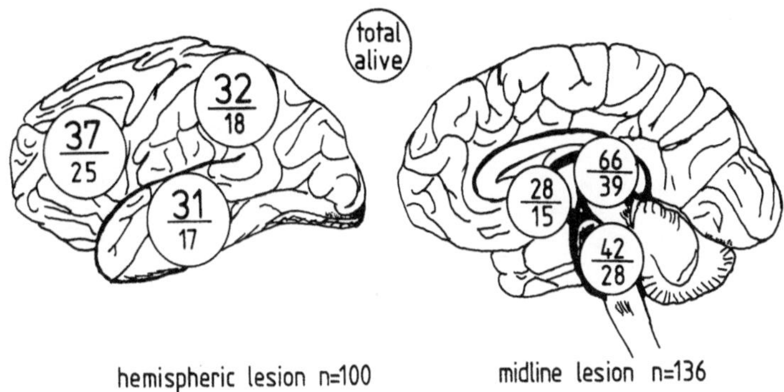

Fig. 3. Stereotactic Curietherapy with Iodine-125 (n = 236/1979–1982)

References

Mundinger, F., The treatment of brain tumors with interstitially applied radioactive isotopes. In: Radionuclide Applications in Neurology and Neurosurgery (Wang, Y., Paoletti, P., eds.), pp. 199—265. Springfield, Ill.: Ch. C Thomas. 1970.

Mundinger, F., CT-stereotactic biopsy of brain tumours. In: Tumours of the Central Nervous System in Infancy and Childhood (Voth, D., Gutjahr, P., Langmaid, C., eds.), pp. 234—246. Berlin-Heidelberg-New York: Springer. 1982.

Mundinger, F., Birg, W., Stereotactic brain surgery with the aid of computed tomography (CT-stereotaxy). In: Computerized Tomography, Brain Metabolism, Spinal Injuries. Advances in Neurosurgery, Vol. 10 (Driesen, W., Brock, M., Klinger, M., eds.), pp. 17—24. Berlin-Heidelberg-New York: Springer. 1983.

Acta Neurochirurgica, Suppl. 33, 373—376 (1984)

Stereotactic Radiosurgery in Acoustic Neurinoma

J. L. Barcia-Salorio[1], **G. Hernandez**[2], **J. Ciudad**[2], **V. Bordes**[1], and **J. Broseta**[1]

Between 1977 and 1982, 16 patients with acoustic neurinomas were treated by stereotactic radiosurgery.

Despite the shortness of this series we can draw several conclusions about the results of this new method in the treatment of these tumours.

Material and Method

The method consists of the attachment of a stereoguide to a conventional ^{60}Co gamma source unit (Theratron)[1].

The target coordinates were calculated by CT scanner[1]. A 5 mm collimator which gives a target volume of 3 × 5 mm in the 90% isodose and 5 × 8 mm in the 50% isodose was used. The maximum target dose was 70–90 Gy.

According to the tumour size and the results we can constitute two homogenous groups.

The first is composed of 8 patients with small and medium sized tumours (from 20 to 30 mm diameter, excepting No. 3, with 36 mm).

The results regarding tumour size and follow-up are shown in Table 1.

All tumours, excepting three, showed central necroses and decrease in size after treatment. In the clinical evolution an improvement of the symptoms was seen and in case No. 3, a 14 year old girl, the postoperative high tone threshold values were better than the preoperative ones.

Cases No. 16 and No. 12, mother and daughther, suffered from bilateral acoustic neurinoma due to a hereditary von Recklinghausen's disease. After a previous unilateral open surgery in another hospital, resulting in deafness and facial palsy, the contralateral tumour was irradiated in case No. 12. One year later the woman was pregnant, and the tumour size increased from 16 to 20 mm and was therefore re-irradiated with a maximum dose of only 54 Gy. Up to date, two year later, the tumour size did not change.

Departments of [1] Neurosurgery and [2] Physic Radiation, Hospital Clinico Universitario, Valencia, Spain.

Table 1

	Case No.	Sex.	Age	Dose (Gy)	Tumour size mm Pre-	Post-	Follow-up Years (months)	Side effects
1	3	F	51	90	36	17	5	—
2	7	F	36	90	26	18	2 (7)	—
3	9	F	14	89	22	22	3	Trigeminal neuralgia
4	10	F	56	90	23	18	3	—
5	11	F	73	90	22	—	3	—
6	12*,**	F	29	90 54	16	20	20	—
7	15	F	66	90	25	20	1 (4)	—
8	16*	F	56	72	9	9	1	—

* Mother (case 16), and daughter (case 12) presenting hereditary Recklinghausen diseaese with bilateral acoustic neurinoma. See text.

** Re-irradiation 1 year after initial treatment because of tumour growth to 20 mm.

Table 2

	Case No.	Sex.	Age	Dose (Gy)	Tumour size mm Pre-	Post-	Follow-up Years (months)	Evolution
1	1	F	30	90	50	50	3	**,*
2	2	F	59	90	35	36	(3)	*
3	4	F	59	90	36	37	1 (1)	open surgery
4	5	M	28	90	40	36	(4)	open surgery
5	6	F	56	90	35	21	(6)	open surgery
6	8	F	34	89	50	70	2 (7)	open surgery
7	13	F	67	76	40	—	—	—
8	14	M	44	90	36	—	—	—

* Reirradiated 2 years after treatment because clinical worsening.
** Dead, respectively 2 years and 3 months after treatment, not related with original process or irradiation.

In case No. 16 (the mother) a tumour relapse after translabyrinthine surgery, was irradiated. This tumour was very small (9 mm diameter) and at the last control (1 year and 3 months after irradiation) the CT tumour image had disappeared.

The second group is formed of 8 patients with large tumours, more than 30 mm 30 mm diameter (case No. 1 and No. 6 with 50 mm, No. 4 and No. 7 with 40 mm diameter). The results are summarized in Table 2.

An initial improvement in the clinical evolution was seen for one or two years in three cases (No. 1, No. 4, and No. 6), but in all cases a worsening forced us to re-irradiate (case No. 1) or to remove the tumour by open surgery.

Two patient died, No. 1 one year after re-irradiation because of peritonitis and No. 2 to respiratory insufficiency.

Discussion and Conclusions

Based on these results one can assume that the acoustic neurinomas smaller than 30 mm diameter have a good response to the irradiation of 70–90 Gy with collimators of 5 mm.

There is a central necrosis, approximately at the level of the 65 Gy isodose which produces tumour shrinkage or arrest of growth.

The greatest decrease in tumour size was observed in case No. 3 (from 36 to 17 mm, that is 50%) due to perhaps the fact that this case has the longest follow-up.

The only side-effect was a trigeminal neuralgia cured by medical treatment. On the contrary, tumours bigger than 30 mm continue to grow after irradiation with the aforementioned parameters due to the peripheral tissue of tumour receiving a dose bellow 25 Gy. The convenience of using wider collimators in acoustic neurinomas over 30 mm diamter can be concluded.

On the other hand, our data confirm the results published by Noren and Leksell in 1979[2].

References

1. Barcia-Salorio, J. L., Broseta, J., Hernandez, G., Barbera, J., Bordes, V., Ballester, B., Radiosurgical treatment in huge acoustic neurinomas. In: Stereotactic Cerebral Irradiation. INSERM Symposium No. 12 (Szikla, G., ed.), pp. 245—249. Amsterdam: Elsevier/North Holland Biomedical Press. 1979.
2. Noren, G., Leksell, L., Stereotactic treatment of acoustic tumours. In: Stereotactic Cerebral Irradiation. INSERM Symposium No. 12 (Szikla, G., ed.), pp. 241—244. Amsterdam: Elsevier/North Holland Biomedical Press. 1979.

Acta Neurochirurgica, Suppl. 33, 377—383 (1984)

III. Technical Aspects

Preoperative Computer Determination of Interstitial Iridium-192 Source Placement into CNS Tumor Volumes

P. J. Kelly[1], **B. Kall**[2], and **S. Goerss**[2]

With 6 Figures

Summary

This report describes a method for preoperative computer simulation for the stereotactic placement of interstitial Iridium-192 sources into CNS tumor volumes. The tumor volume interpolated from stereotactic CT scanning data and stereotactic serial biopsies is suspended in a three dimensional computer matrix. The tumor is sliced by computer orthogonal to an intended implantation angle. Simulated sources can be placed within successive tumor slices so that the resultant isodose contours can best fit the shape of each slice. The computer then calculates the stereotactic target points and length of each source. The technique allows preoperative evaluation of isodose configurations to determine optimal source placement within a tumor volume.

Keywords: Stereotactic techniques; interstitial irradiation; cerebral neoplasm; computed tomography.

Introduction

In the ideal situation, the cumulative isodose configuration produced by multiple stereotactically implanted radioisotope sources should conform to the three dimensional shape of an intracranial tumor[3,6]. Unfortunately, a three dimensional volume may not be accurately represented by two dimensional X-ray

[1] Department of Neurosurgery, State University of New York at Buffalo, 2121 Main Street, Buffalo, NY 14214, U.S.A.

[2] Sisters of Clarity Hospital, Buffalo, New York, U.S.A.

pictures or CT reconstructions. This becomes more apparent when the three dimensional shape of the tumor is complex and/or the angle of source implantation is not orthogonal to the plane of the X-ray pictures or CT slices.

In recent publications we described a system for the interpolation of CT data into stereotactic space[4,5]. A tumor volume is derived from CT data and suspended within a three dimensional computer matrix which corresponds to the stereotactic coordinate system. The volumetric data may be reformatted into a series of two dimensional slices along a surgical viewline. Computer simulated isotope source placements and isodose configurations can be inspected on sequential contiguous slices through the tumor volume as described below.

Method and Material

A stereotactic CT scan is performed. The patient's head is fixed in a CT compatible stereotactic head holder as described previously[2,4,6].

A CT localization system is attached to the head holder (Fig. 1). This creates a series of reference marks on each CT slice. The data tape from the CT scan is input to an operating room computer system*. Utilizing a cursor and trackball, the surgeon digitizes the outline of the tumor on the contiguous CT slices (Fig. 2). An interpolation program suspends the slices in a three dimensional computer matrix, interpolates the slices at one millimeter intervals and creates a three dimensional volume in space (Fig. 3). In order to have the CT derived tumor boundaries better conform to the histologic limits of the tumor, the tumor volume with the computer matrix may be stretched or contracted in the plane of a biopsy trajectory depending on histologic information accumulated during a stereotactic biopsy procedure.

A surgical viewline for proposed source implantations is selected which depends on the spatial orientation of the tumor volume and intracranial vascular structures. The tumor volume is sliced by the computer in planes orthogonal to the viewline (Fig. 4).

A computer program allows placement of simulated sources within the reformatted slices. The surgeon is able to view the resultant isodose configurations in relationship to the outline of the tumor slice. Simulated sources may be added, deleted or moved on each slice. The simulated sources are arranged within each tumor slice so that the resultant isodose contour fits the configuration of the slice (Fig. 5). The aggregate isodose curves produced by the sources are displayed as a percentage of the total dose or rads per hour if the specific activity of the source is known.

---

* Independent Physicians Diagnostic Console (IPDC) for GE 8800 CT scanner (Data General Eclipse S 140 and Ramtek raster display terminal).

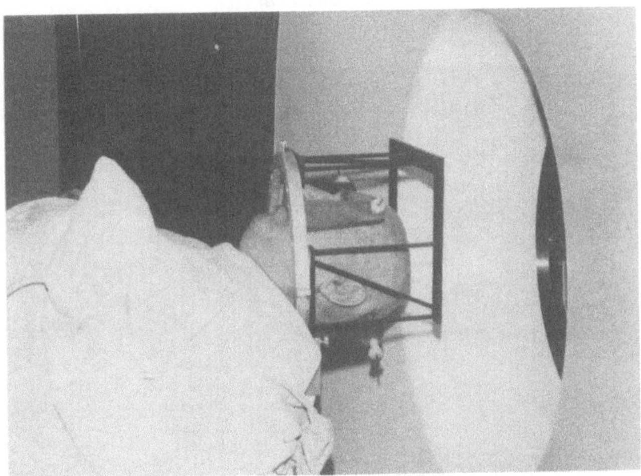

Fig. 1. The patient's head is fixed in a CT compatible stereotactic head frame with a reference localization system attached. The localization system contains three sets of carbon fiber bars resembling the letter "N"

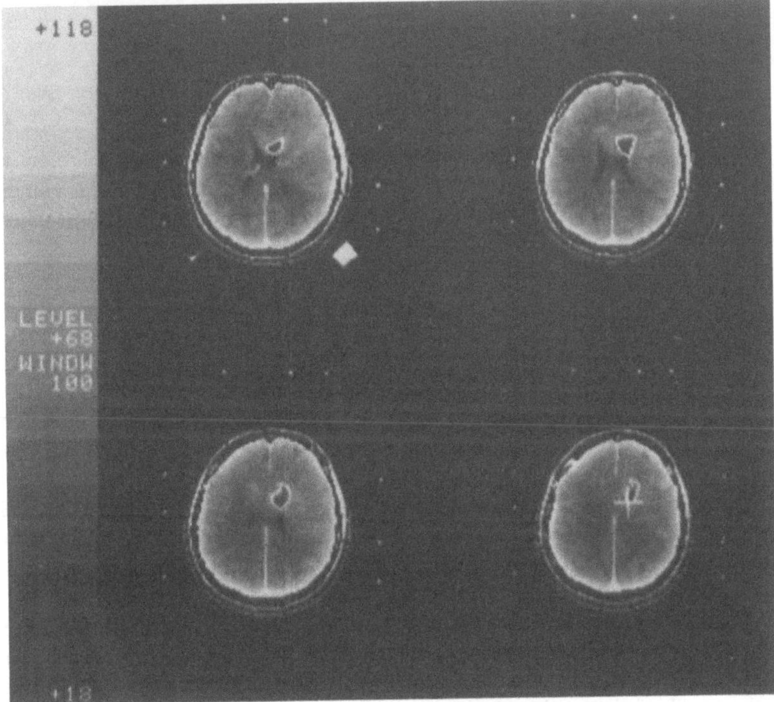

Fig. 2. The nine reference marks on each CT slice are digitized automatically, by an intensity detection program. The surgeon digitizes the outline of the tumor on contiguous CT slices utilizing cursor and trackball

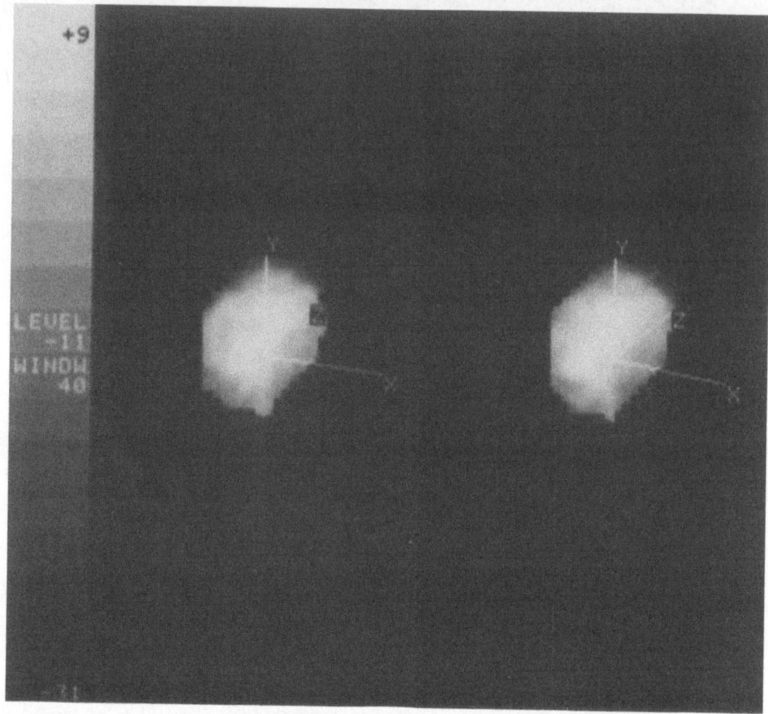

Fig. 3. A three dimensional volume is created in a computer matrix. This volume may be displayed, shaded and rotated or presented as a stereo pair as shown here

After completing the simulation the three dimensional position of the beginning and end of each source is registered within the computer matrix and the length of each source calculated. In addition, the three dimensional positions for the deepest end of each source is calculated in relationship to the stereotactic frame (Fig. 6).

A custom arc-quadrant stereotactic instrument has been developed in which the head moves with three degrees of freedom within a fixed sphere. Movements are performed by servo-motors and positions in X, Y and Z are instantaneously displayed on an optical digital calibration device.

Temporary Iridium-192 sources are implanted utilizing a double catheter after-loading technique similar to that described in previous publications. The outer catheter carrier consists of a hollow teflon button attached to a silicone catheter. This is inserted to the intracranial target point utilizing the stereotactic instrument. All of the carriers are implanted before insertion of inner catheters containing pre-cut lengths of Iridium-192 wire. The length of the Iridium-192 sources are also obtained from the computer program.

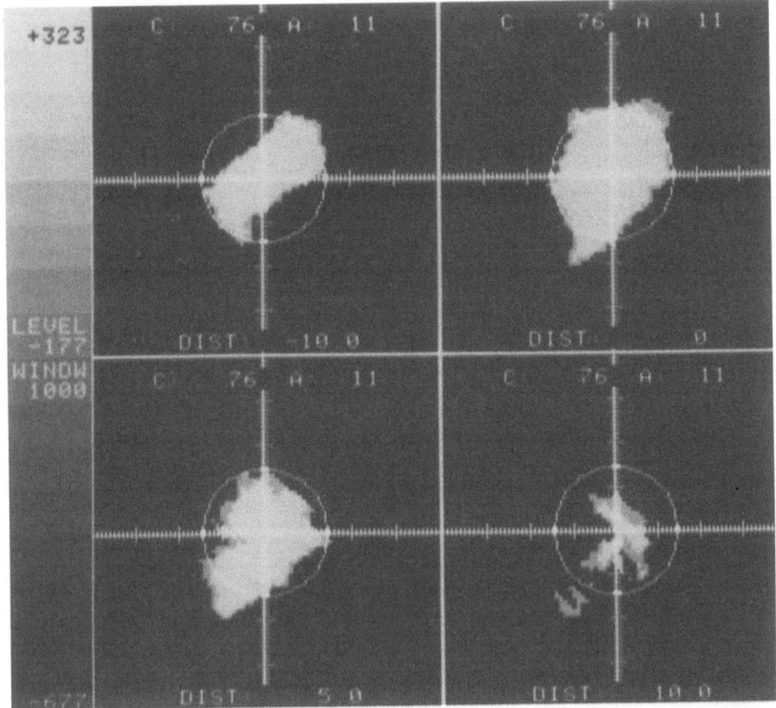

Fig. 4. The tumor volume may be sliced orthogonal to the stereotactic viewline and displayed

Discussion

The system described allows preoperative treatment planning for tumors having a complex three dimensional shape. The volume is displayed as a series of two dimensional slices along a plane perpendicular to the proposed angle of insertion. Thus, the isodoses produced by a series of radioactive sources can be viewed against the tumor volume slice by slice.

It is important to corroborate CT information with data from stereotactic serial biopsies. The boundaries of the tumor may not necessarily correspond to the limits suggested by CT scanning[1,5]. Therefore, an additional advantage of the computer program described in this report is that the volume of the tumor may be expanded or contracted depending on the histologic limits of the tumor suggested by stereotactic serial biopsies.

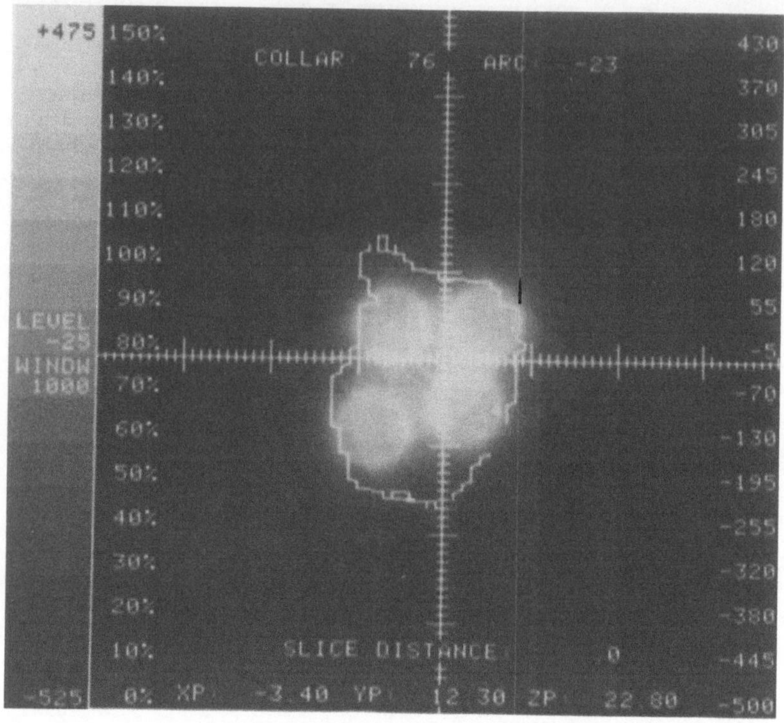

Fig. 5. Simulated sources are deposited in each tumor slice and the isodose configurations resulting from the sources viewed

References

1. Daumas-Duport, C., Monsaingeon, V., Szenthe, L., Szikla, G., Serial stereotactic biopsies a double histologic code of gliomas according to malignancy and 3-D configuration as an aid to therapeutic decision and assessment of results. J. Appl. Neurophysiol. *45* (1982), 431—437.
2. Goerss, S., Kelly, P. J., Kall, B., Alker, G. J., A computed tomographic stereotactic adaptation system. Neurosurgery *10* (1982), 375—379.
3. Kelly, P. J., Olsen, M. H., Wright, A. E., Giorgi, C., CT localization and stereotactic implantation of Iridium 192 into CNS neoplasms. INSERM Symposium No. 12 (Szikla, G., ed.), pp. 123—128. Amsterdam: Elsevier/North Holland Biomedical Press. 1979.
4. Kelly, P. J., Alker, G. J., Goerss, S., Computer-assisted stereotactic laser microsurgery for the treatment of intracranial neoplasms. Neurosurgery *10* (1982), 324—331.
5. Kelly, P. J., Alker, G. J., Kall, B., Goerss, S., Precision resection of intra-axial CNS lesions by CT-based stereotactic craniotomy and computer monitored CO_2 laser. Acta Neurochir. (Wien) *68* (1983), 1—9.

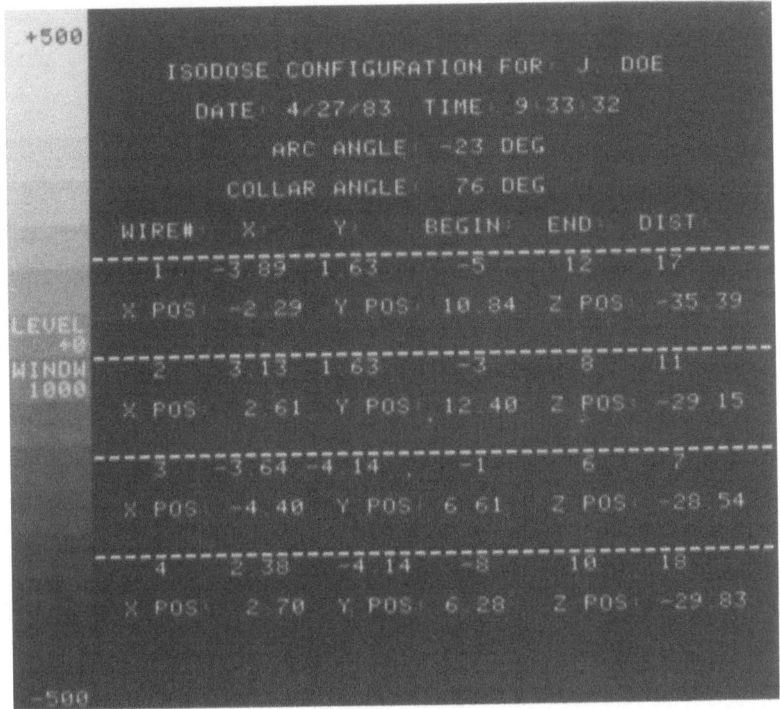

Fig. 6. The computer outputs the X, Y and Z adjustments on a custom stereotactic frame to place the deepest end of the source into the focal point of the frame. The length of the source is also given

6. Schlienger, M., Bouhnik, H., Missir, O., Constans, J. P., Szikla, G., Association of temporary interstitial ^{192}Ir implantation and external radiotherapy in the management of supratentorial tumors. INSERM Symposium NN. 12 (Szikla, G., ed.), pp. 117—121. Amsterdam: Elsevier/North Holland Biomedical Press. 1979.

Acta Neurochirurgica, Suppl. 33, 385—390 (1984)

Hyperselective Encephalic Irradiation with Linear Accelerator

O. O. Betti[1] and **V. E. Derechinsky**[2]

With 3 Figures

Summary

A new development of the Talairach stereotactic system is presented: an external irradiation system based on a principle similar to that of Leksell's Gamma Unit produces an intense cross-firing of the target structure through an infinite number of portals of entry of a collimated high energy beam.

Talairach's stereotactic frame is the nucleus of the system. It permits a threedimensional synthesis of diagnostic data including computerized tomography and stereoscopic stereotactic neuroradiology and ensures precise localization of the radiation fields.

Supplementary collimators adequated individually to volume, shape and pathology of the lesion provide a great versatility. The use of an infinite number of portals of entry instead of a fixed number reduces the irradiation of the neighbouring brain.

Keywords: Stereotactic irradiation; cerebral irradiation with linear accelerator; multibeam unit for convergent irradiation; radiosurgery with linear accelerator.

Based on the principle proposed by Leksell[4], that is, cross-firing irradiation of a cerebral target with multiple portals of entry, a technically different system was developed[2].

The frame of our device makes it possible to place the centre of a target volume in the isocentre of a linear accelerator. The frame can also rotate around a transverse axis. The combination of both movements: a) rotation of the accelerator and b) rotation of the

[1] Departamento de Neurocirugía Tridimensional y Radiocirugía de Institutos Médicos Antártida Rosario 437, (1424) Buenos Aires, Argentina, y [2] Departamento de Radiocirugía del Centro de Radioterapia del Hospital Español, Buenos Aires, Argentina.

stereotactic frame, covers a spherical sector. This spherical sector represents the surface of possible portals of entry, included in a 140° angle on the coronal plane and 120° on the sagittal plane. Using successive portals of entry every 5°, 725 of them will be obtained. In practice, 200 or 300 proved to be sufficient.

Making use of the pendular movement of the accelerator, the whole dose is distributed on a coronal diadem through infinite points of a 140° arc. This results in a reduction of both irradiation time and radiation dose, outside the target.

A device to position the stereotactic frame with an adjustable contention was designed. It allows the placement of the target in the isocentre of the accelerator. The frame can slip on a plate and leaves free the access to the whole grid, that is, the whole brain, from the posterior fossa to the orbites. In this way, a point determined by Talairach's cartesian coordinates[7] becomes the centre of an angular movement.

After placing the target in the isocentre of the mechanical system, we bring it to coincidence with the centre of rotation of the accelerator. With this alignment verified, the conjunction of both systems is obtained.

A special seat movable on a curved axis was designed so that the patient's body accompanies the movements of the frame and is held in a confortable position.

The use of external irradiation through the intact skull for treatment of usually deep lying brain tumours requires a geometrically well-defined beam so as to avoid damaging the surrounding structures while delivering high radiation doses to a small volume of tissue[1,3,5].

To the standard collimation of the accelerator we have added another collimation modifying shape ans size of the beam between 5 and 20 mm according to the diameter of the lesion. In this way geometrical penumbra is drastically reduced.

The penumbra curves of these collimators were established by distributing LiF dosimeters (T.L.D.) in a hemispheric 8 cm radius phantom built in lucite and filled with water. The combination of the described phantom and detectors allows to obtain a penumbra curve of fairly good resolution since the size of the T.L.D. allows to determine experimentally the dose distribution at 1 mm intervals.

The simulation of the therapeutical irradiation was carried out with a Rando anthropomorphic tissue equivalent phantom. 350 detectors were distributed both in depth and on the surface so as to assess the mean absorbed dose for several organs and tissues

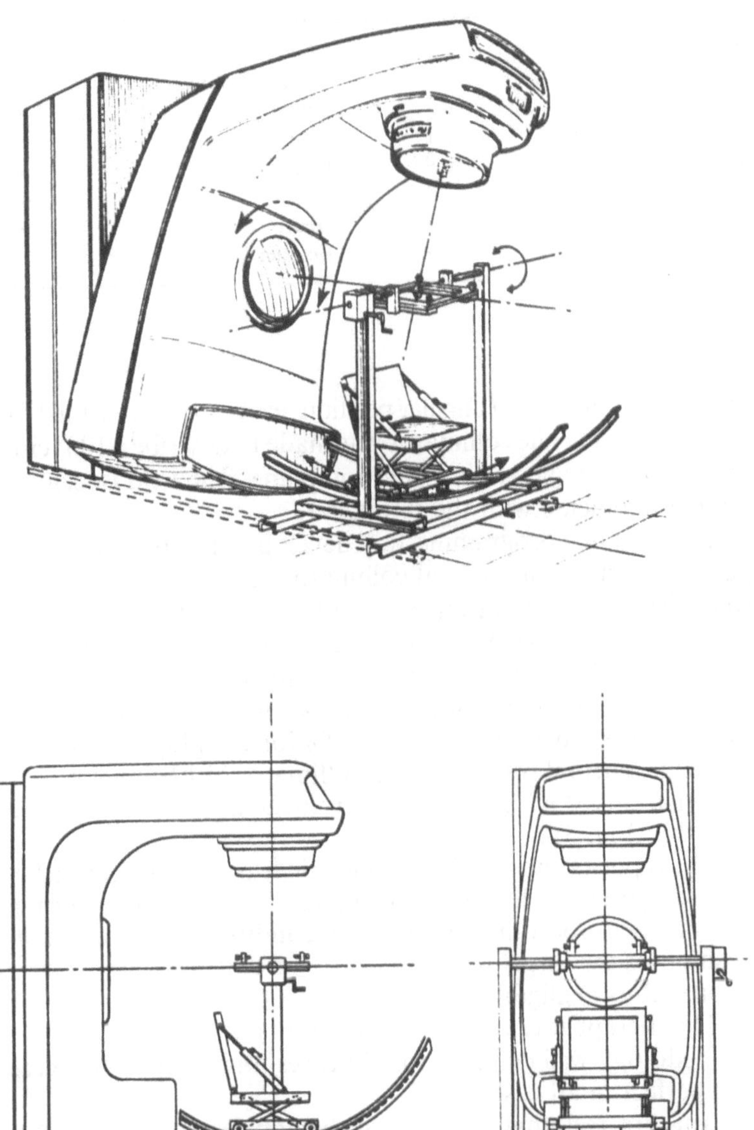

Figs. 1 and 2. Schemes showing the combination of Talairach's stereotactic system with a 10 MeV Linear Accelerator

Table 1. *Mean Organ Absorbed Doses for 10 Krad to the Hypophysis*

Testes	1.2 rad	Brain	149.3
Ovaries	1.7	Small intestine	3.0
Breast	18.7	Kidney	6.7
Red bone marrow	15.1	Liver	5.3
Lungs	10.9	Pancreas	3.8
Thyroid	23.3	Spleen	4.0
Lens	10.4	Heart	9.5
Stomach	3.9	Bladder	1.3

(Table 1). In this case, 7 angular positions every 10° were selected for the phantom head. The collimator was made to describe a 100° circular arc within a single vertical rotation plane. The field isocentre was made to coincide with the pituitary[8].

A computer programme was developed in order to assess the penumbra curve of an ideal collimator in which boundary effects were disregarded. The transport of photons inside the phantom was simulated by applying the Montecarlo method. The results shown in curve "a" have been normalized by referring them to the energy delivered at the centre of the phantom using an ideal collimator. The variation coefficient is below 6% for 10^6 photons introduced. The experimental results using a collimator of 12 mm diameter are shown in curve "b". There is a good correlation between curves "a" and "b" (Fig. 3).

The repositioning of the stereotactic frame at irradiation is very precise. The head is held by metallic fixation as it is during the stereotactic procedure. These two conditions ensure the exact position of the target in the isocentre of both systems. Calculated error is thus negligible[6].

The therapeutical dose is delivered in a single irradiation. This methodology was employed in 20 cases and immediate tolerance was perfect in all cases.

Authors feel that besides the benign lesions treated by the swedish group, the multibeam irradiation can be applied to the treatment of gliomas, especially for only slightly infiltrating gliomas with diameters not exceeding 3 cm.

It may be concluded that the Multibeam Unit for Convergent Irradiation is a promising technique for the treatment of certain inoperable lesions. Longterm follow-up will determine preferential indications.

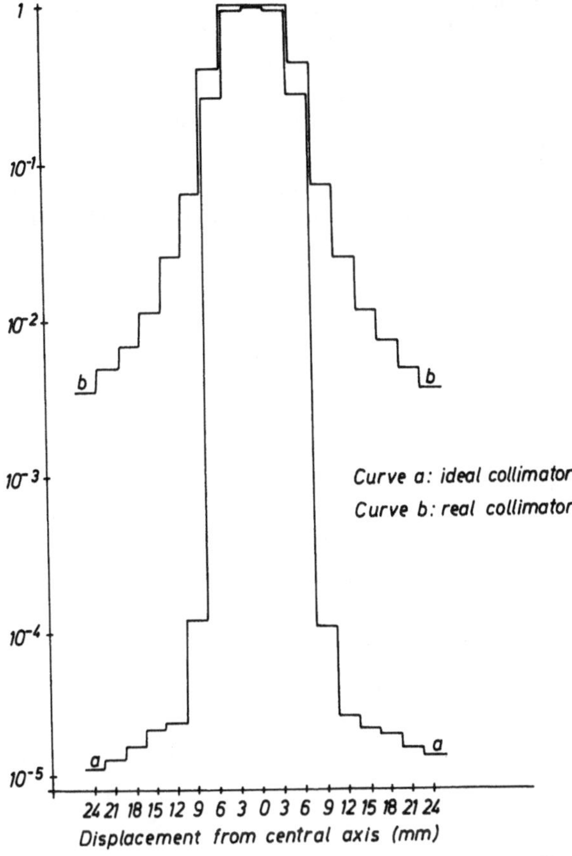

Fig. 3. Isodose curves obtained with a 12 mm diameter collimator

References

1. Arndt, J., Backlund, E. O., Larsson, B., Leksell, L., Noren, G., Rosander, K., Rahn, T., Sarby, B., Steiner, L., Wennestrand, J., Stereotactic irradiation of intracranial structures: physical and biological considerations. In: Stereotactic Cerebral Irradiations, INSERM Symposium No. 12 (Szikla, G., ed.), pp. 81—92. Amsterdam: Elsevier/North Holland Biomedical Press. 1979.
2. Betti, O. O., Derechinsky, V. E., Irradiation stéréotaxique multifaisceau. Neurochirurgie, in press. 1983.
3. Larsson, B., Liden, K., Sarby, B., Irradiation of small structures through the intact skull. Acta Radiol. Ther. Phys. Biol. *13* (1974), 512—534.
4. Leksell, L., Stereotaxis and Radiosurgery. Springfield, Ill., U.S.A.: Ch. C Thomas. 1971.
5. Sarby, B., Cerebral radiation surgery with narrow gamma beams. Physical experiments. Acta Radiol. Ther. Phys. Biol. *13* (1974), 425—445.

6. Szikla, G., Schlienger, M., Askienazy, S., Techniques "classiques" et modalités nouvelles des irradiations stéréotaxiques. Curiethérapie à faible débit et irradiation stéréotaxique multifaisceaux. Abstract, Meeting of the Soc. Neurochir. de Langue Française, Paris, 30. 11. 1981.
7. Talairach, J., Szikla, G., Atlas d'anatomie stéréotaxique du télencéphale. Paris: Masson. 1967.
8. Thomasz, E., Spano, F., Massera, G., Distribution of absorbed doses in brain irradiations with an X-ray beam of 9,1 MeV (to be published).

Acta Neurochirurgica, Suppl. 33, 391—394 (1984)

Concluding Remarks of the Moderator

Progress and Problems in Tumour Stereotaxis

G. Szikla

Stereotactic methods are more and more widely used in the management of intracranial tumours. As at our 4th Meeting in Paris a full day has been devoted to both diagnostic and therapeutic aspects of tumour stereotaxis. Significant progress achieved in the past four years will be commented here.

A. Stereotactic Biopsy

In the light of greater series of several hundred cases presented by Kleihues, Scerrati, Sedan, Monsaingeon and others, CT oriented sampling biopsies appear to give as reliable information on pathology as craniotomy material and can be used to establish with precision location and volume of the lesion. Surgical risks, choice of trajectories according to prebioptic localization by CT and other methods like depth recording etc., together with optimal histological techniques were discussed. Stereotactic biopsies allow one to avoid diagnostic craniotomies and useless irradiations, contributing to the choice of the most adequate therapeutic procedure in problematic cases. Biopsy modified the diagnosis, changing the type of treatment in 25% out of 318 biopsied patients (Sedan).

B. Stereotactic Focal Irradiation of Brain Tumours

Inspite of considerable technical progress achieved in the past few years, many questions are yet waiting for a clear answer, in particular concerning the biology of brain tumours (*e.g.* evolutivity of small grade 1 tumours largely unrecognized before the CT era) and the response of both the different tumour types and the surrounding brain to focal high dose irradiations.

1. *Tumour Volume and "CT-stereotaxis"*

Exactly as ventriculography became "stereotactice" in the old days, CT examination performed with the head fixed in a frame can be called "stereotactic", as the attenuation values will be localized in a coordinate system related to the stereotactic instrument. A target point for biopsy trajectories or isotope implantation can be chosen on the CT images. Several computerized methods of stereotactic localization are currently available. Compared to the current use of bidimensional images, the introduction of computer generated 3 D volume reconstructions as presented by Suetens and by Kelly seems to be a promising step forward, as they allow for a synthetic representation of tomographic information integrated with angiographic, bioptic and other localizing data in a three dimensional computer matrix.

2. *Delineation of the target volume* in infiltrating growths like gliomas is a particularly delicate and at the same time crucial point. Let us emphasize once more that CT data give only partial information on tumour volume. Cytological study of the peripheral biopsy samples may allow one to distinguish to some extent reactive gliosis and tumour cells, estimate the extent of infiltration and thus contribute to approximate more closely the volume to be treated.

3. *Physical Versus Clinical Dosimetry*

Computerized physical dosimetry programs are available for interstitial irradiations and allow one to superimpose isodose curves on CT or other X-ray pictures. This impressive precision should however not occult the fact that the clinical dosimetry of focal high dose irradiations *i.e.* tissue reactions and dose threshold levels of late postradiation changes taking into account volume/dose/time factors of the different types of irradiation are only partially documented. Important and new experimental, autoptic and bioptic data on morphologic radiation effects presented at the meeting (Ostertag, Kleihues, Daumas-Duport, Davis) should be carefully analyzed and taken into account for therapy planning.

4. *Long term results* of Iridium 192 implantations and of intracystic radiocolloidal injections were assessed in several presentations.

Data on 236 intracranial tumours treated 1965–1982 with permanent Ir 192 implantation were presented by Mundinger and Weigel.

More and more exacting international norms of radioprotection limit however the use of permanent Iridium 192 implantations to specially authorized centers and require strict measures of protection of the patients entourage during several months. Temporary applications of Ir 192 with afterloading techniques associated or not to complementary external irradiation give very satisfactory long term results in small unresectable hemispheric or central gray nuclei gliomas, thus confirming the first results published 4 years ago at the Paris meeting (Rougier, Szikla).

Intracystic injection of colloidal beta emittors leads to rewarding long term results in cystic craniopharyngiomas and recurrent glioma cysts, with a minimal complication rate (Szikla, Netzeband).

5. *Permanent I 125 implantation* has been introduced in neurosurgical curietherapy in 1979.

Experience reported at this meeting shows that this technique does only partially fulfill the initial expectations based on the assumption that both the rapid attenuation of soft gamma rays and the protracted very low dose-rate irradiation delivered by permanently implanted I 125 seeds will limit radiation damage of neighbourhood structures, especially in the most critical locations such as brain stem and hypothalamus. Follow-up data after permanent Iodine 125 and Ir 192 implantations in 62 suprasellar tumours were analyzed by F. Mundinger. Endocrine and visual follow-up data are not yet available, but the presented survival figures clearly constitute a warning against indiscriminate radioisotope applications particularly in the hypothalamic area and suggest to reconsider the dosimetric concepts and indications especially of I 125 implantations. In agreement with physical dosimetry, the above mentioned experimental data suggest that interstitial Iodine 125 induces quite sharply limited necrosis of the adjacent tissues—brain as well as tumour—generates often widespread edema in the white matter but does not interfere significantly with tumour growth at only 1–2 millimeters beyond the border of the perifocal necrosis. These histological data resemble closely those observed after implantation of Y 90 seeds. Other types of stereotactic irradiation generating more homogeneous focal radiation fields (without necrotizing dose levels in the vicinity of radioactive sources) might be the most adequate treatment for slowly evolutive hypothalamic and brainstem tumours, where late radionecrotic changes imply not only increased functional but also vital risks.

The present discussion added valuable and new data to our knowledge and has shown that several aspects of tumour stereotaxis acquired a sort of maturity in the past few years. Stereotactic diagnostic and (—probably to a lesser degree—) therapeutic procedures will no doubt become more and more popular. It seems clear that they should be more and more closely associated to surgical and radiotherapeutic treatment schemas, matching by precise and low risk procedures the needs of critical cases. Much fascinating work remains to be done in this field of challenging problems, some of which were discussed today. Tomorrow's progress is well on the way and will lead to other symposia in the coming years.

Section III

Pain

Acta Neurochirurgica, Suppl. 33, 397—406 (1984)

Introductory Lecture

The Suggested Mechanisms of Chronic Pain and the Rationale of Neurosurgical Treatment

J. Gybels[1]

Summary

Knowledge about the pathogenesis of certain human diseases and how to treat them, has in general been advanced by the availability of a reasonably similar disease counterpart somewhere else in the animal kingdom. Unfortunately, a model of chronic pain is difficult to come by because of the inherent problem of defining animal pain, and it is only in recent years that such models have been proposed, and a study of them has started. The purpose of the present short review has been therefore to summarize some of the major developments in this field in such a way as to assist the reader in deciding just how exciting prospects in chronic pain research for the future might be.

Keywords: Chronic pain; animal models; neurosurgical treatment.

Introduction

Thc rationale for neurosurgical treatment of "intractable" chronic pain has historically first been derived from anatomo-clinical correlations in patients, and during the last decades from the rapid progress which has been made in the physiology of nociception.

There is now a growing concensus between many workers in the field of pain that there is a need for an animal model of chronic pain but that also from the ethical point of view a particular experiment

[1] Department of Neurology and Neurosurgery, A. Z. Sint Rafaël, Kapucijnenvoer 33, B-3000 Leuven, Belgium.

in which chronic pain is inflicted on an animal should have a benefit for mankind.

In this review, we will therefore mainly be concerned with principles derived from mostly recent experiments in which experimental animal models of chronic pain have been studied. We will describe some of these models, examine their most relevant behavioural, physiological and biochemical characteristics, scrutinize how well the proposed model fits the clinical facts and what indications the model might provide for the neurosurgical practice of chronic pain treatment. For comparison with clinical pain syndromes we have divided these animal experiments between a) models of somatic pain, where the noxious stimulus is detected by nociceptors, and b) models of dysesthetic pain, where sensation is conditioned by a so-called perturbation in the nervous system, caused by deafferentation.

Dysesthetic Pain Models

Several dysesthetic pain models have been proposed with manipulations at different levels—peripheral, radicular, spinal—of the nervous system, but most data now available deal with the properties of experimental neuromas and the consequences of dorsal root sections.

1. The Neuroma Model

In 1974 Wall and Gutnick[31] examined the physiological properties of experimentally produced neuromas. They found that spontaneous ungoing activity was present in A β-fibres and not in A δ-fibres, although according to Scadding[27], many fast afferent fibres also become active; moreover, in 76% of all fibres with ongoing activity mechanosensitivity was present[27].

Several additional results of importance emerged from the investigations on experimental neuromata (for references see[4]):

a) Afferent fibres from the neuroma can be activated via the neuroma by stimulation of other fibres and several types of "ephaptic transmission" have been observed: myelinated to myelinated fibres, myelinated to unmyelinated fibres, unmyelinated to unmyelinated fibres, unmyelinated to myelinated fibres.

b) The ongoing activity is enhanced by intravenous injection of nor-adrenaline, this effect being blocked by the α-blocker phentolamine and not by the β-blocker propranolol; this response to adrenergic stimulation is not solely due to a local change of blood flow, but damaged sensory axons develop α-adrenergic receptors that render them sensitive to sympathetic activity. Myelinated afferent endings in a neuroma can indeed be activated by stimulation of the sympathetic supply but up till now there is no clear evidence that nonmyelinated afferent endings in a neuroma can be activated by stimulation of the sympathetic supply; only in a few pilot experiments on rats activation of unmyelinated afferent fibres has been observed, even with low frequency stimulation of the sympathetic supply to the neuroma[4].

c) A short period (*e.g.* 10 sec) of repetitive electrical stimulation of the nerve in which a neuroma has been produced, at a strenght above threshold for the single fibre under study, completely stops the ongoing discharge for several minutes. The reason for this turn-off following antidromic invasion is not known, but there is a possibility that the tetanic stimulation hyperpolarizes the terminals and raises the threshold thereby decreasing their tendency to generate impulses spontaneously.

d) During the course of experiments on rats and mice designed to follow physiological and anatomical consequences of nerve injury, it was noticed that many animals attacked the area made anesthesic by the lesions. This phenomenon has been called "autotomy" and it has been argued that autotomy cannot simply be attributed to anesthesia since guanethidine treated animals have equally anesthesia yet do not display autotomy behaviour[32].

Let us now turn to man and examine where research and clinical data do agree and where not. Some of the properties of the sprouts in the neuroma, such as the spontaneous activity and mechanosensitivity can indeed well account for the painful paresthesias and the Tinel sign. However, it is a common neurosurgical experience that after resection of a damaged nerve, pain recurs in the same area as experienced before the operation. This might be due to neuroma formation, but as has been pointed out[24] careful analysis of failure of nerve resection and nerve grafts to cure chronic pain produced by nerve lesions leads to interesting suggestions. Indeed, these patients suffer two sequential lesions of the same nerve, the first of which the nature varies widely at the moment of the injury, the second at the moment of surgery. This second type of lesion is normally produced in nerve repair and only rarely gives rise to chronic pain. These clinical observations, and one can add many other arguments of a clinical nature, do suggest that these patients transfer the source of their abnormal processing of nerve impulses from the periphery to more central structures.

As far as the chemosensitivity for noradrenaline of the sprouts in the neuroma is concerned, this fits well with clinical observations where blocking the sympathetic outflow, either by surgery or injections of the sympathetic chain with local anesthesics or by the injection of guanethidine during occlusion of the circulation, results in pain relief in patients with peripheral nerve lesions which give rise to chronic painful states, such as causalgia, where hyperpathia is present[18], but patients with neuromata and with amputations are usually not helped by sympathetic blocks.

The results of tetanic stimulation on the ongoing activity in the experimental neuroma model and their interpretation as a prolonged turnoff of the abnormal pulse generator, cannot only explain the prolonged effect but also the extreme localisation of the therapeutic effect. However, problems remain. In the clinical situation it is a common experience that the intensity of the stimulating current for pain relief is below the threshold for activation of small fibres, and the poststimulation effects may be very long lasting. A patient of mine, operated upon for a painful neuroma, stimulated only every three days during a twenty minutes period to be pain free.

In order to understand the pathophysiology of certain pain syndromes following tissue or nerve injury, recording at the neural activity from the site of the lesion and the correlation of the activity with the patient's report of pain would be a powerful investigative tool. The microneurographic technique seems promising for this purpose, but although there are many data on nociceptor activation and evoked sensation in normal subjects[1], almost no data are available in pathological conditions.

2. *The "Dorsal Root Section" Model*

Many authors have studied in animals the neuronal activity at different levels of the nervous system after rhizotomy and described abnormal spiking. As early as 1968 Loeser *et al.*[17] recorded highfrequency paroxysmal discharges from chronically denervated cells in the conus medullaris of a paraplegic patient. In one study Lombard and Larabi[19] showed that abnormal spiking appears at the level of a group of cells in the dorsal horn, which in normal animals, receive convergent tactile and nociceptive inputs. This spiking activity appeared within the first months following the rhizotomy, the time during which the animal develops an abnormal behaviour, consisting of self-mutilation and scratching. It is believed that these abnormal behaviours are due to abnormal sensation felt in totally and partially deafferented areas and therefore this behaviour has been proposed by a number of authors as a model of chronic neurogenic pain[9,32,34] the most convincing evidence being that after traumatic avulsion of the brachial plexus in man, pain in the anesthetic limb often occurs. Sweet[28] however, in a critical study, concluded that from the available data in man, autotomy in an animal is not evidence that it has pain or paresthesias in the denervated part. In more central structures, such as thalamic nuclei and somatosensory cortex, abnormal bursting activity of neurons has been observed as well[2]. From these experiments, there is some neurophysiological indication that after rhizotomy there is a progressive development of epileptic activity in more central structures through a kind of kindling process. In this respect it is of interest that scratching behaviour develops in parallel with the spinal neuronal abnormal activity; however, the spinal neuronal abnormalities disappear, whereas the animals continue to present scratching behaviour, suggesting that somewhere at an unknown place in the nervous system abnormal central spiking activity persists. In this respect, the work of Tasker *et al.*[29] is of great interest, since these workers in a careful quantitative analysis of an important patient material pointed out that in patients with "deafferentation pain" there is a pecular sensitivity to electrical stimulation of the medial mesencephalic tegmentum and medial thalamus, where stimulation induces contralateral perception of ill-localized burning or pain that frequently resembles the pain from which the patient suffers, but not natural sensations. How after rhizotomy epileptic activity develops is not clear. From the anatomical point of view, histological changes are described after rhizotomy as are seen in epileptic foci, such as gliosis in the dorsal horn[14] and the correlation between gliosis and abnormal firing appears to be a tight one[26]. New ways of destroying nervous elements, without inducing gliosis, such as percutaneously iontophoretically applied microtubule inhibitors which inducc transganglionic degenerative atrophy of primary central nociceptive terminals[15] may therefore be of interest.

From the biochemical point of view, supersensitivity is thought to be an important mechanism in the genesis of epileptic foci. Following rhizotomy, supersensitivity to substance P has been demonstrated[22]. Substance P is postulated to be a neuro-transmitter in primary nociceptive afferent neurons, and therefore, one can hypothesize that perhaps local administration in the subarachnoidal space of substance P antagonists might be useful in certain chronic pain syndromes.

Desinhibition is another mechanism which is proposed to explain dysesthetic pain, and recently some neurophysiological evidence of desinhibition and its possible mechanism after nerve section has been presented. After section of the peripheral nerve, there is a marked expansion of the receptive fields of the neurons normally excited by the sectioned nerve[8], and there is some evidence that this desinhibition is due to a loss of presynaptic inhibition, in which the C afferents play a special role[10]. Together with these neurophysiological changes there are profound biochemical changes in dorsal horn cells: there is a loss of substance P and CCK, but not of neurotensin[3]. It could be that this reduction of afferent-mediated inhibition following peripheral nerve section contributes to the generation of chronic pain by increasing the excitability of dorsal horn neurones, and is tempting to hypothesize that the abnormal neuronal behaviour observed in the above mentioned experiments and pain states, which are termed as central pain, are due to such phenomena as denervation supersensitivity, sprouting of aberrant nerve connections, and unmasking of ineffective synapses.

One can speculate that perhaps activation of the deafferented neurons, *e.g.* by electrical stimulation of the remaining afferents or the neurons directly, may interfere with the development of these plastic changes. It has been shown recently that transcutaneous stimulation can delay and reduce autotomy in rats[2]. Once the plastic changes have developed there is still some indirect clinical evidence that electrical stimulation might interfere with this abnormal nervous process (for review, see[21]). It is not without interest to realize that in the last decade in clinical practice for the treatment of deafferentiation pain, destructive neurosurgical procedures have almost been replaced by various forms of stimulation of the nervous system, with the exception of dorsal root entry zone lesions in plexus avulsion pain[23].

Somatic Pain Models

The only model of somatic pain which from the neurophysiological point of view has been studied in some detail is the adjuvant-induced polyarthritis in rats (for references see[20]). In rats, Freund's adjuvant, *i.e.* a suspension in mineral oil of heat killed Mycobacterium butyricum is injected in the base of the tail, following which after a few days the animal develops a generalized immunological response with arthritis, vasculitis and skin lesions ressembling by its pathology joint and periarticular tissue human rheumatoid arthritis. Several reasons have been presented to hypothesize that arthritis induced by Mycobacterium butyricum in rats is associated with a condition of chronic pain, one important argument being that these arthritic rats develop an increased preference for suprofen, an inhibitor of prostaglandin biosynthesis, in their drinking water[6].

From the biochemical point of view, in arthritic rats there are increased levels of Met-enkephalin in both dorsal and ventral halfs of the spinal cord[5] but a normal enkephalinase activity[30], and increased levels of serotonin in the forebrain, brainstem and spinal cord, suggesting an active role of serotonergic structures in chronic pain[33]. Moreover the analgesic effect of morphine is much more pronounced in these animals than in normal rats[25], and low doses of naloxone (f.i. 10 μg/Kg I.V.) have a hypo-algesic, high doses (f.i. 1 mg · Kg I.V.) an hyperalgesic action[13].

From the neurophysiological point of view, it has been shown that chronic pathological conditions of the polyarthritic rats strongly modifie the responses of dorsal neurons[20] and ventrobasal thalamic neurons[11]; as compared to normal rats, in polyarthritic rats one observes a relatively high level of background activity, frequently with bursting patterns, and a high degree of responsiveness to light mechanical stimuli. It is probable that these high abnormal responses are the consequence of sensitization of thin peripheral fibres.

We have used this arthritis model to investigate stimulation produced analgesia (SPA) in chronic pain. Indeed, one is confronted with seemingly contradictory findings obtained in acute animal experiments and clinical findings in that as a rule in patients chronic pain relief is reported with PV-PAG stimulation even when the threshold for acute pain is not influenced by the stimulation. It was found that among behavioural elements analysed in adjuvant-induced arthritic rats only scratching behaviour was significantly and chronically increased in the arthritic rats, reversed by morphine, this effect being blocked by naloxone[7]; it was therefore reasonable to propose scratching as a painrelated behaviour in arthritic rats. This proposal is reenforced by the observation that the administration of acetyl salicylic acid decreases scratching behaviour while it is not influenced by peripherally acting antihistaminics; furthermore, there is an increase of substance P in primary afferent nerves of arthritic rats[10] and intrathecal substance P but not neurotensin or V.I.P., elicit a caudally-directly biting and scratching behaviour[12].

We then examined in quantitative terms the influence of central stimulation on "animal chronic pain" as measured by the amount of scratching, and on "acute pain" as measured by the tail-flick test. The results showed that: 1. suppression of scratching is rather specific, it is to say, without a significant modification of other behaviour parameters; 2. SPA for chronic pain is independent of SPA for acute pain, suggesting one is dealing with two independent antinociceptive mechanisms; 3. SPA can be obtained from PAG, n. Dors. Raphé and n. Raphé magnus, but also from many other localisations, from which it is not possible to predict wether SPA will be obtained for acute pain or for chronic pain.

Concluding Remarks

A measure of caution is necessary about any analogy which may be proposed between experimental animal models and human chronic pain. This review deals with this controversial subject. It will have been clear to the interested reader that not many really significant practical results have as yet resulted as far as patient treatment is concerned from the study of animals chronic pain models. We also know how inadequate we are in treating successfully chronic pain. The proper scientific conclusion is then that further research is needed to fill the deficient gaps in our present knowledge.

Acknowledgements

The author is indebted to Mrs. Feytons-Heeren for expert technical assistance. This work was supported by the F.G.W.O. (grant 3.0045.79) of Belgium and the Onderzoeksfond K. U. Leuven (grant OT/VII/34).

References

1. Adriaensen, H., Gybels, J., Handwerker, H. O., Van Hees, J., Response properties of thin myelinated (A δ) fibres in human skin nerves. J. Neurophysiol. *49* (1983), 111—122.
2. Albe-Fessard, D., Lombard, M. C., Use of an animal model to evaluate the origin of and protection against deafferentation pain. In: Advances in Pain Research and Therapy, Vol. 5 (Bonica, J. J., *et al.*, eds.), pp. 691—700. New York: Raven Press. 1983.
3. Barbut, D., Polak, J. M., Wall, P. D., Substance P in spinal cord dorsal horn decreases following peripheral nerve injury. Brain Res. *205* (1081), 289—298.
4. Blumberg, H., Jänig, W., Neurophysiological analysis of efferent sympathetic and afferent fibers in skin nerves with experimentally produced neuromata.

In: Phantom and Stump Pain (Siegfried, J., Zimmermann, M., eds.), pp. 15—31. Berlin-Heidelberg-New York: Springer. 1981.

5. Cesselin, F., Montrastruc, J. L., Gros, C., Bourgoin, S., Hamon, M., Met-enkephalin levels and opiate receptors in the spinal cord of chronic suffering rats. Brain Res. *191* (1980), 289—293.
6. Colpaert, F. C., De Witte, P., Maroli, A. N., Awouters, F., Niemegeers, C. J. E., Janssen, P. A. J., Self-administration of the analgesic suprofen in arthritic rats: evidence of Mycobacterium butyricum-induced arthritis as an experimental model of chronic pain. Life Sci. *27* (1980), 921—928.
7. De Castro Costa, M., De Sutter, P., Gybels, J., Van Hees, J., Adjuvant-induced arthritis in rats: a possible animal model of chronic pain. Pain *10* (1981), 173—185.
8. Devor, M., Wall, P. D., Plasticity in the spinal cord sensory map following peripheral nerve injury in rats. J. Neurosci. *1* (1981), 679—684.
9. Duckrow, R. B., Taub, A., The effect of diphenylhydantoin on self-mutilation in rats produced by unilateral multiple dorsal rhizotomy. Exp. Neurol. *54* (1977), 33—41.
10. Fitzgerald, M., Alterations in the ipsi- and contralateral afferent inputs of dorsal horn cells produced by capsaicin treatment of one sciatic nerve in the rat. Brain Res. *236* (1982), 275—287.
11. Guilbaud, G., Gautron, M., Benoist, J. M., Kayser, V., Characteristics of some ventrobasal thalamic neurons in polyarthritic rats. Effects of acute injection of Aspirin on neuronal responses to joint stimulation. In: Advances in Pain Research and Therapy, Vol. 5 (Bonica, J. J., *et al.*, eds.), pp. 393—400. New York: Raven Press. 1983.
12. Hylden, T. K. L., Wilcox, G. L., Intrathecal substance P elicits a caudally-directed biting and scratching behaviour in mice. Brain Res. *217* (1981), 212—215.
13. Kayser, V., Guilbaud, G., Dose-dependent analgesic and hyperalgesic effects of systemic naloxone in arthritic rats. Brain Res. *226* (1981), 344—348.
14. Kerr, F. W. L., Central nervous system changes and deafferentation pain: the role of reorganization and gliosis. In: Advances in Pain Research and Therapy, Vol. 5 (Bonica, J. J., *et al.*, eds.), pp. 663—675. New York: Raven Press. 1983.
15. Knyihár-Csillik, E., Szücs, A., Csillik, B., Iontophoretically applied microtubule inhibitors induce transganglionic degenerative atrophy of primary central nociceptive terminals and abolish chronic autochtonous pain. Acta neurol. scand. *66* (1982), 401—412.
16. Lembeck, F., Donnerer, J., Colpaert, F. C., Increase of substance P in primary afferent nerves during chronic pain. Neuropeptides *1* (1981), 175—180.
17. Loeser, J. D., Ward, A. A., White, L. F., Chronic deafferentiation of human spinal cord neurons. J. Neurosurg. *29* (1968), 48—50.
18. Loh, L., Nathan, P. W., Painful peripheral states and sympathetic blocks. J. Neurol. Neurosurg. Psychiat. *41* (1978), 664—671.
19. Lombard, M. C., Larabi, Y., Electrophysiological study of cervical dorsal horn cells in partially deafferented rats. In: Advances in Pain Research and Therapy, Vol. 5 (Bonica, J. J., *et al.*, eds.), pp. 147—154. New York: Raven Press. 1983.

20. Menétrey, D., Besson, J. M., Electrophysiological characteristics of dorsal horn cells in rats with cutaneous inflammation resulting from chronic arthritis. Pain *13* (1982), 343—364.
21. Meyerson, B. A., Electrostimulation procedures: effects, presumed rationale, and possible mechanisms. In: Advances in Pain Research and Therapy, Vol. 5 (Bonica, J. J., *et al.*, eds.), pp. 495—534. New York: Raven Press. 1983.
22. Nakata, Y., Kusakan, Y., Segawa, T., Supersensitivity to substance P after dorsal root section. Life Sci. *24* (1979), 1651—1654.
23. Nashold, B. S., Ostdahl, R. H., Dorsal root entry zone lesions for pain relief. J. Neurosurg. *51* (1979), 59—69.
24. Noordenbos, W., Wall, P. D., Implications of the failure of nerve resection and graft to cure chronic pain produced by nerve lesions. J. Neurol. Neurosurg. Psychiat. *44* (1981), 1068—1073.
25. Pircio, A. W., Fedele, C. T., Bierwagen, M. E., A new method for the evaluation of analgesic activity using adjuvant-induced arthritis in the rat. Eur. J. Pharmacol. *31* (1975), 207—215.
26. Prince, D. A., Neurophysiology of epilepsy. Ann. Rev. Neurosci. *1* (1978), 395—415.
27. Scadding, J. W., Development of ongoing activity, mechanosensitivity, and adrenaline sensitivity in severed peripheral nerve axons. Exp. Neurol. *73* (1981), 345—364.
28. Sweet, W. H., Animal models of chronic pain: their possible validation from human experience with posterior rhizotomy and congenital analgesia. Pain *10* (1981), 275—295.
29. Tasker, R. R., Tsuda, T., Hawrylyshyn, P., Clinical neurophysiological investigation of deafferentation pain. In: Advances in Pain Research and Therapy, Vol. 5 (Bonica, J. J., *et al.*, eds.), pp. 713—738. New York: Raven Press. 1983.
30. Van Veldhoven, P., Carton, H., Enkephalinase A activity in different regions of brain and spinal cord of normal and chronic arthritic rats. FEBS Letters *138* (1982), 76—78.
31. Wall, P. D., Gutnick, M., Properties of afferent nerve impulses originating from a neuroma. Nature (Lond.) *248* (1974), 740—743.
32. Wall, P. D., Scadding, J. W., Tomkiewicz, M. M., The production and prevention of experimental anesthesia dolorosa. Pain *6* (1979), 175—182.
33. Weil-Fugazza, J., Godefroy, F., Besson, J. M., Changes in brain and spinal tryptophan and 5-hydroxyindoleacetic acid levels following acute morphine administration in normal and arthritic rats. Brain Res. *175* (1979), 291—301.
34. Wiesenfeld, Z., Lindblom, U., Behavioral and electrophysiological effects of various types of peripheral nerve lesions in the rat: a comparison of possible models for chronic pain. Pain *8* (1980), 285—298.

Acta Neurochirurgica, Suppl. 33, 407—419 (1984)

I. Pelvic Cancer Pain (Somatogenic Pain)

Pros and Cons of Different Approaches to the Management of Pelvic Cancer Pain

B. A. Meyerson[1], S. Arnér[2], and B. Linderoth[1]

Introduction

Pain due to malignancy in the pelvic region is common and notoriously difficult to relieve. One important reason why this condition often fails to respond both to pharmacological and surgical treatment is that the genesis of the pain may be very complex as the pathological process may involve different types of tissue and organs. Thus, the pain may originate from the viscera, connective tissue, bone, and, of particular significance, from nervous tissue. Pelvic pain often radiates in the hip region or in the leg as a result of injury to the lumbo-sacral plexus, and it is wellknown that neurogenic pain, especially when there is a component of deafferentation, is extremely difficult to alleviate. As will be further discussed in this paper the pain analysis is therefore of utmost importance for the selection of a proper method of treatment. A further characteristic of pelvic cancer pain, which sometimes accounts for therapy failure is that such pain is often poorly localized and has a tendency to be felt in the midline or with bilateral spreading. Some of the destructive procedures available for malignant pain appear to be most suitable for pain confined to one side (cordotomy, neurolytic blocks) and when applied with the aim of producing bilateral effects the risk of serious side-effects and complications is considerably increased.

This paper is an attempt to evaluate and discuss the pros and cons of some neurosurgical and anesthesiological methods which

[1] Department of Neurosurgery, [2] Department of Anaesthesiology, Karolinska Sjukhuset, S-10401 Stockholm 60, Sweden.

are often applied for relieving pelvic cancer pain. The aim is not to review all possible means of dealing with such pain, and due to the lack of personal experience some methods are not delt with although their efficacy in these conditions has been stressed (*e.g.* myelotomy, which is discussed in detail in another paper in this volume).

Cordotomy

In the numerous studies published on the results of cordotomy applied for malignant pain the usefulness of the procedure is emphasized on the basis of the high rate of success, about 90%, whether the operation is performed with an open or percutaneous technique[6]. However, there are relatively few reports in which the results have been analyzed with regard to location and type of pain. That these factors are of importance for the outcome has been shown by for example Mansuy *et al.*[8], who discussed pain location and distribution, and by Tasker[13] who emphazises the important fact that deafferentation pain is less likely to respond to cordotomy than pain of a nociceptive type.

Evaluation of the clinical usefulness of a surgical destructive procedure for cancer pain is particularly difficult. One major reason is that a definite surgical lesion is produced in order to counteract a pain which is likely to change in location and character.

Thus, a surgical treatment can not be adapted to this changing pain pattern and long-lasting effects are therefore less probable than for example what can be achieved with pharmacological therapy.

In general, the marked tendency of the pain to reappear after destructive procedures is well recognized when pain is due to a non-malignant and non-progressive disease with normal life expectancy. However, this appears to be a major problem also when such methods are applied for cancer pain as evidenced by a few, but well documented, studies on the late results obtainable with cordotomy.

The percutaneous cordotomy technique has been used in our clinic since 1973 and the great majority of the patients (about 90%) have been effectively relieved of pain at discharge from the hospital. As almost all of these patients are referred to secondary hospitals for longterm care they have generally been lost for follow-ups. Therefore, we found it necessary to find out whether the initially favourable results lasted and whether the treatment led to a useful abolishment or reduction of the pain.

During the last two years 41 patients have been operated and 18 of them had pain in the pelvic region, either due to a primary pelvic malignancy or to metastases. In all these patients the pain has also involved the hip or/and radiated in the leg(s). The operation was performed with the conventional technique using fluoroscopic control and electric stimulation. Twelve patients had one, and five had two unilateral operations. In one patient a bilateral procedure was made. One patient had an open, high thoracic operation. The outcome of the treatment was assessed at discharge, 2–5 days postoperatively, and at 3–5 weeks, at 7–9 weeks and later on every second month. Based on the patient's own evaluation the amount of pain relief was classified at 100%, 50% or less. The patients were also asked about new pains, consumption of analgesics etc.

All patients were on opiates but had insufficient relief or intolerable side-effects. It is obvious that the patients had been referred at a comparatively late phase of their disease as the survival time in no less than 9 of the 18 patients did not exceed two months, and not more than five patients lived for more than five months (max. 12 months). In 8 of the patients the pain was experienced as strictly unilateral (*e.g.* hip and leg), in 5 there was some pain occasionally felt also in the other side and in another 5 patients the pain had a bilateral distribution but with a marked dominance in one side. Sixteen of the patients reported complete pain relief at the time of discharge from the hospital and in the other two the effect was not possible to evaluate as they were in a terminal stage (Table 1). At a control 3–5 weeks postoperatively all the surviving 13 patients retained this favourable effect but seven complained of pain in the contralateral side of the body. Thus, already at this short term follow-up only 5 patients were still pain free but 2 of these reported unpleasant paresthesiae. For later check-ups only 6 patients were in a condition which allowed reliable assessment of the pain. One had had a recurrence of the original pain, after two months, and 3 were judged to have only slight or moderate pain although they had resumed the use of opiates in moderate doses. The situation for the patients surviving for 5–10 months appears from Table 1.

It is of interest to note that of the 8 patients who had claimed that they had unilateral pain only, 3 experienced contralateral pain 3–5 weeks postoperatively, one survived only for two weeks and 4 were pain free but with dysesthesia.

Table 1. *Results of Cordotomy for Pelvic Cancer Pain*

At discharge		Surviving 3–5 weeks		Surviving 5–10 months
	16 pain free		5 pain free	2 pain free—dysest.
18		13		5→2 new pain
	2 doubtful		8 new pain	1 recurr. pain

Comments

It is evident that in this small group of patients with pelvic malignant pain cordotomy turned out to be ineffective in the large majority of cases. The effect on the original pain remained in all but two patients who had a recurrence after two and six months respectively. If the outcome of cordotomy is assessed with regard to permanent suppression of pain confined to one side of the trunk or to one extremity the results from the present series compared well with other studies in which it is concluded that cordotomy is effective for malignant pain. However, it is quite obvious that the overall results in the current report substantiate the impression that the clinical usefulness of cordotomy for pelvic malignant pain was practically nil. The obvious reason for this negative conclusion was the fact that already after 3–5 weeks more than half of the surviving patients (8 of 13) had a new pain which generally necessitated narcotic analgesics. These results may partly be due to the fact that most of the patients were in an advanced state of their progressive disease as shown by the relatively short survival times. A few other studies have reported comparatively negative results. Thus, Tasker[13] found 41% of the patients to have contralateral pain at follow-up, and Cowie and Hitchcock[2] reported a comparatively high rate of recurrencies although after a longer period of time than in the present material. The divergent results may be due to the selection of patients who in the former study had considerably longer survival. However, Cowie and Hitchcock[2] explicitly state that the results in pelvic pain are particularly unfavourable (cf.[8]). Our results confer well with those of Meglio and Cioni[9] who reported that already after three weeks the proportion of patients who were pain free had decreased from 80 to 33%. On the other hand, in that study it was stated that lumbo-sacral pain benefitted more often than cervico-thoracic pain.

In conclusion: For pelvic malignant pain cordotomy should only be considered in patients who present with strictly unilateral symptoms and when the underlying disease does not appear to be in a phase of aggressive progress and the survival time can be anticipated to exceed 4–6 months.

Thalamotomy

In the late sixties stereotactic thalamotomy, generally directed towards the intralaminar-medial nuclear complex (CM-Pf) and later on towards the pulvinar, attracted much interest in the treatment of chronic pain, in particular pain in malignancy. The attractive feature of these procedures is the possibility to alleviate severe pain without any demonstrable changes of sensibility (analgesia) or other neurological deficits. The mechanisms of pain relief obtainable with lesions in the non-specific thalamic nuclei are still poorly understood and have attracted little interest in modern pain research, in spite of the perplexing paradox of pain relief combined with normal pain sensitivity.

Although a number of reports on thalamotomy for pain have been published it is difficult to assess its clinical usefulness, the main reason being that the overall results have been inconsistant and few attempts have been made to analyze the outcome with regard to different types, etiology and location of pain. During later years thalamotomy is less commonly used, conceivably a consequence not only of the fact that the effect of the operation is often shortlasting and unpredictable but also because the interest in dealing with chronic pain is focused onto non-destructive methods.

The present report is a retrospective analysis of a series of 52 patients with cancer pain treated with CM-Pf lesions produced by stereotactic radiosurgery (gamma irradiation)[12]. In this group of patients 21 had pain originating from malignancy in the pelvic region and in nearly half of the patients it radiated into the leg(s) or low back. In general, the patients were treated in a rather late state of their disease as indicated by the relatively short survival times, 9 out of 21 being alive for three months or less.

Because of the varying and relatively short survival times it has been difficult to assess the clinical usefulness of the treatment taking into account the amount of pain reduction and the duration of the effect.

Five of the patients were judged to have a useful effect corresponding to good or moderate pain relief (Table 2). The

Table 2. *Clinical Usefulness of Thalamotomy (CM-Pf)*

Effect	Survival (months) < 1	1–3	4–6	7–12	> 12	Total
Useful effect (good-moderate)	0	1	3	0	1	5
Not useful effect (slight-none)	2	6	5	3	0	16
Total	2	7	8	3	1	21

remaining 16 patients reported only slight or no effect. The survival time does not seem to differ significantly between the two groups. Eleven cases had bilateral procedures, 8 of these in the same session. The remaining three patients were operated on the side contralateral to the pain in the first session, followed by an operation on the ipsilateral side when the effect of the first failed. Only one of the cases with bilateral lesions experienced a lasting useful effect. It may be of some significance that on 2 of the 5 patients with a useful effect the unilateral lesion was enlarged by combining two lesions at the side of each other in the medio-lateral dimension.

Comments

The results obtained in the present small series of patients certainly do not indicate that thalamotomy is a clinically useful method to treat pelvic cancer pain. Contrary to the results reported by *e.g.* Hitchcock and Teixeira[4], bilateral lesions in our material did not prove to be superior to unilateral. This finding is in accordance with the results obtained in the larger material from which the present group of patients was derived. Moreover, the poor outcome in this study may be partly due to the selection of target which in several cases was placed so that it presumably did not embraze the Pf nucleus. On the other side, the doubtful clinical value of thalamotomy for pelvic pain is in accord with the finding that in general this operation is more effective for pain located in the face, shoulder, and arm than in the lower part of the body[12]. Nevertheless, there are some few reports which convincingly show that destructive surgery in the thalamus, CM-Pf and the pulvinar, may be a valuable therapy of cancer pain which motivates further exploration of the method[3–5]. It might be that a thorough analysis of the pain, its character and genesis, may help to sharpen the indications and to select the appropriate target and lesion size. In comparison with stimulation procedures and the use of high doses of narcotic analgesics, a surgical intervention producing instantaneous and complete lasting relief without the risk of serious complications still represents an ideal treatment.

Epidural Morphine

In a series of 215 consecutive patients referred to one of us (S.A.) for symptomatic treatment of cancer pain 21 had pain in the pelvic region and were subjected to epidural morphine. Most of the patients presented with more than one pain component and an attempt was made to analyse the results with regard to the efficacy of epidural morphine for different types of pain.

In general the results of the treatment were very satisfactory as only three patients failed to obtain efficient relief. By subcutaneous tunnelling of the catheter to the flank the treatment could be continued for relatively long periods of time. Thirteen patients obtained good relief until death, which occurred at 4–170 days, mean 48 days, after implantation of the catheter (Table 3). One case

Table 3. *Epidural Morphine for Pelvic Cancer Pain 21 Patients*

13	Treated until death. 4–170 days (m = 48 days); (one patient treated 232 days)
2	Still on treatment
1	Lost for follow-up (good effect 40 days)
3	Insufficient relief
2	Off treatment (addiction, micturition disturbance)

was treated during 232 days without problems. There were no serious side effects or complications apart from disturbance of micturition which occurred in one patient in whom the treatment was discontinued.

On the basis of the patient's description of the character and time pattern of the pain, knowledge about the underlying pathology (site of tumour and metastases) and observations of the patients while in bed or ambulant, the pain were tentatively classified as: 1. continuous somatic, 2. intermittent somatic (being aggravated by movement in bed or by walking and standing), 3. continuous visceral, 4. intermittent visceral, 5. neurogenic, continuous or intermittent. A few cases also had aching pain from superficial cancerous ulcers. In the large majority of patients at least two of these different types were present in various combinations. It was found that these types of pain responded differently to epidural morphine. Thus, of 19 patients who were judged to have a continuous somatic pain, 14 experienced good relief, 3 were moderately helped and only 2 had a slight effect. In contrast, pain classified as being neurogenic, continuous or intermittent, which was present in 9 patients, appeared to be less responsive. The effect on this pain was deemed to be slight in 4 and none in 4 whereas one had a moderate relief. Based on these observations it is possible to present a tentative ranking list of different types of pain with regard to the likelihood of relief with epidural morphine:

1. somatic continuous pain,
2. visceral continuous (with the possible exception of pancreatitis),
3. somatic intermittent,
4. neurogenic, intermittent and continuous,
5. visceral intermittent (*e.g.* attacks of subileus),
6. cutaneous (cancerous ulcer or fistula).

The possible development of tolerance to epidural morphine is of course as crucial as with systemic administration of opiates. Although the material in this study is far too small to permit any conclusions on this issue it may be of significance that some of the patients who required increasing doses (up to 30–60 mg/24 hours) apparently sufferred from pain which did not respond to the treatment. In these cases the doses were increased not in order to retain a pain relief but instead to attempt to reach an effective dose level, as substantiated by the finding that 4 of these patients had a component of neurogenic pain, which was ineffectively suppressed. One patient, who prior to treatment had a high consumption of systemic opiates, tended to require increasing doses also with epidural morphine. This may have been an example of cross-tolerance. It should be noted also that in one patient the failing effect of large doses (up to 300 mg/24 hours) could be explained by the fact that the transport of the drug across the dura into the CSF seemed to be deficient as it was instead readily absorbed in the epidural vascular bed (Arnér, to be published).

Comments

It is obvious that in this series of patients epidural morphine proved to be a highly effective method of dealing with pelvic cancer pain (cf.[15]). Most of the patients had used systemic opiate analgesics in high doses but had failed to respond or had experienced intolerable side-effects. Nevertheless, the epidural route of morphine administration produced satisfactory relief in a large majority of the patients. The lack of serious side effects as compared to systemic opiates is illustrated by the fact that in several cases who were primarily considered to be in a terminal state the general condition improved markedly as the pain was abolished and nausea, dizziness and somnolence disappeared.

As with other forms of symptomatic pain treatment the indications for institution of epidural morphine should be based also on an analysis of the type of pain and the possible pain etiology. As emphazised above malignant processes in the pelvic region often give rise to pain of different types, and the probability of obtaining a satisfactory result with epidural morphine is dependent on the type that predominates. On the basis of this study it seems that neurogenic pain is less susceptible to the treatment than pain of a deep nociceptive type, and in this regard the epidural administration of an opiate does not offer any advantages as compared to systemic administration. The effect on pain from superficial ulcers and intermittent visceral pain appeared to be variable.

Epidural morphine has the advantage of being a reversible non-destructive procedure, simple to institute and associated with a low incidence of side-effects and complications. Subcutaneous tunnelling of the catheter makes longterm treatment possible and hospital facilities are not always required (cf.[7,11]).

The risk of developing tolerance to epidural morphine can not yet be evaluated but it is a general impression that this phenomenon is less likely to occur with epidural than with systemic administration. In view of experimental data there is perhaps a possibility of reducing the tendency to tolerance by the use of continuous drug infusion instead of bolus injections into the epidural space[14].

Neurolytic Blocks

Prior to the introduction of epidural morphine various forms of neurolytic blocks were often used for pelvic cancer pain[1]. In the series of 215 patients referred to above 27 patients received this type of treatment: in 8 sacral epidural phenol (6% in water), in 9 sacral epidural ethanol (50%), and in 10 intrathecal phenol (5% in glycerol). In general, the results obtained with blocks were favourable but in most cases the duration of pain relief was comparatively short, intrathecal phenol tending to produce somewhat longer effects than the epidural blocks (mean = 17 and 14 days respectively). In this material the continuous somatic type of pain dominated and pain of neurogenic origin was present in a few patients only. Therefore, no conclusions can be made with regard to the differential effect on pain of various types. However, it is noteworthy that one patient with pain interpreted as anus phantom pain was unrelieved, and also that superficial pain due to fistulas and ulcers appeared to be relatively resistent. Complications in the form of a transitory disturbance of micturition and slight paresis of a leg were comparatively common. The risk of complications and the relatively short duration as well as the limited area that can be made analgetic make neurolytic blocking procedures a much less useful approach than epidural morphine to the management of pelvic cancer pain.

Periventricular Stimulation

Although in use for almost a decade intracerebral stimulation still remains a rather exclusive method for dealing with chronic pain and the method is practised in a few centres only. Most of the clinical reports are concerned with periventricular stimulation (PVG) for pain of non-malignant origin such as "low-back syndrome" or "failed back-surgery" (review, see [10]). In view of the enourmous amount of experimental data demonstrating the selective blocking effect of stimulation in the diencephalic-mesencephalic junction region on nociceptive transmission in the spinal cord one would expect that such stimulation would be particularly effective for cancer pain. There are however comparatively few reports on the use of PVG-stimulation on this indication. A cooperative European study from 1979 contained 40 patients with cancer pain subjected to this type of stimulation and about half of them were reported to have obtained useful pain relief.

As previously reported we have chosen to try PVG-stimulation in cancer patients with pain of midline or bilateral distribution that did not respond to neurolytic blocks or other stimulation

Table 4. *Results of PVG Stimulation for Pelvic Cancer Pain*

		Initial and late results (duration of effects in months)	Survival (months)	Poststim effect (hours)
1	perineal sacral	good (60)	60 (alive)	3–5
2	groin gluteal	good (14) moderate (2) none (4)	20	8–10
3	sacral gluteal	good (12) moderate (3) none (2)	17	6–8
4	perineal groin leg	good (3) none (8)	11	½
5	perineal gluteal	good (3) moderate (2) none (1)	6	2–3
6	hip leg	moderate (1)	1	?
7	perineal groin	moderate (1) slight (1) none (1)	3	2–3
8	perineal	moderate (2) slight (1) none (1)	4	3
9	penis scrotal	moderate (2) slight (2)	4	2
10	perineal	none	3	—
11	bladder	none	3	—
12	hip. legs	none	2	—

procedures[10]. As a matter of fact a majority of these patients had pain due to malignancy in the pelvic region and the results are therefore of relevance in this context. As appears from Table 4 the initial results were as a rule satisfactory, 9 patients out of 12 having a beneficial effect (5 had good and 4 moderate pain relief). However, it is obvious that the efficacy of the treatment decreased with the time so that the results could be judged to be clinically useful only in 3 or 4 of the patients. Apparently the outcome was related to the survival time. The diminishing effect was due to development of tolerance only in a few of the patients, and instead it seemed to be the result of the occurrence of new pains or spreading of the original pain. The deterioration of the general condition of the patients when approaching the terminal state made them less motivated to continue a stimulation which rarely produced a total suppression of all pain and they tended to resume systemic opiates instead. It is of interest in this material to note that pain irradiating in the leg, conceivably due to the involvement of the lumbo-sacral plexus and thus of neurogenic origin, did not respond to the stimulation (case 4 and 6).

Comments

From the present material it can be concluded that PVG-stimulation is indicated in pelvic cancer pain only in exceptional cases. One reason for considering this type of treatment may be that systemic opiates are badly tolerated or not accepted by the patient for emotional reasons. However, an expected survival time of at least six months appears to be a prerequisite for obtaining a clinically useful result and in such a case intracerebral stimulation interferes less with an active life outside the hospital than epidural morphine.

References

1. Arnér, S., The role of nerve blocks in the treatment of cancer pain. Acta Anaesthesiol. Scand. *26*, Suppl. 74 (1982), 104—108.
2. Cowie, R. A., Hitchcock, E. R., The late results of antero-lateral cordotomy for pain relief. Acta Neurochir. (Wien) *64* (1982), 39—50.
3. Hitchcock, E. R., A comparison of analgesic ablative and stimulation techniques. Zentralbl. Neurochir. *42:* 4 (1981), 189—199.
4. Hitchcock, E. R., Teixeira, M. J., A comparison of results from center median and basal thalamotomies for pain. Surg. Neurol. *15:* 5 (1982), 341—351.
5. Laitinen, L. V., Anterior cingolotomy in the treatment of intractable pain. In: Neurosurgical Treatment in Psychiatry, Pain and Epilepsy (Sweet, W. H., *et al.*, eds.). Baltimore: University Park Press. 1977.
6. Lipton, S., Percutaneous cervical cordotomy. In: Advances in Pain Research and Therapy, Vol. 2 (Bonica, J. J., Ventrafridda, V., eds.), pp. 425—437. New York: Raven Press. 1979.
7. Mandaus, L., Blomberg, R., Hammar, E., Long-term epidural morphine analgesia. Acta Anaesthesiol. Scand. *26*, Suppl. 74 (1982), 149—150.
8. Mansuy, L., Sindou, M., Fischer, G., Brunon, J., La cordotomie spinothalamique dans les douleurs cancéreuses. Neurochir. *22:* 5 (1976), 437—444.
9. Meglio, M., Cioni, B., The role of percutaneous cordotomy in the treatment of chronic cancer pain. Acta Neurochir. (Wien) *59* (1981), 111—121.
10. Meyerson, B. A., Electrostimulation procedures: effects, presumed rationale, and possible mechanisms. In: Advances in Pain Research and Therapy, Vol. 5 (Bonica, J. J., *et al.*, eds.), pp. 495—534. New York: Raven Press. 1983.
11. Poletti, C. E., Cohen, A. M., Todd, D. P., Ojemann, R. G., Sweet, W. H., Zervas, N. T., Cancer pain relieved by long-term epidural morphine with permanent indwelling systems for self-administration. J. Neurosurg. *55* (1982), 581—584.

12. Steiner, L., Forster, D., Leksell, L., Meyerson, B. A., Boëthius, J., Gammathalamotomy in intractable pain. Acta Neurochir. (Wien) *52* (1980), 173—184.
13. Tasker, R. R., Percutaneous cordotomy—the lateral high cervical technique. In: Operative Neurosurgical Techniques, Vol. 2 (Schmidek, H. H., Sweet, W. H., eds.), pp. 1137—1153. New York: Grune and Stratton. 1982.
14. Yaksh, T. L., Spinal opiates analgesia: Characteristics and principles of action. Pain *11* (1981), 293—346.
15. Zenz, M., Piepenbrock, S., Schappler-Scheele, B., Hüsch, M., Peridurale Morphineanalgesie: III. Karcinomschmerz. Anesthesist *30* (1982), 508—513.

Acta Neurochirurgica, Suppl. 33, 421—425 (1984)

Personal Experience with Intrathecal Morphine in the Management of Pain from Pelvic Cancer

V. D'Annunzio[1], **F. Denaro,** and **M. Meglio**

With 2 Figures

Summary

The analgesic effect of intrathecal isotonic and hypertonic morphine has been studied in 20 patients suffering from chronic pain due to pelvic cancer.

Remarkable long lasting pain relief without motor or sensory loss was achieved in all the patients, 60% of them reported side effects.

The duration of analgesia appeared to be dose related but by increasing the dose the risk of side effects increased as well.

The conclusion is drawn that the best mode of utilizing intrathecal morphine is with fractioned doses.

Keywords: Intrathecal morphine pain pelvic cancer.

Introduction

Morphine directly injected into the CSF exerts a powerful analgesic effect both in animals[3] and in humans[1-3]. Side effects are reported to be limited[2] particularly when the drug is delivered in an hyperbaric solution[1].

We report here our personal experience in patients with chronic pain due to pelvic cancer. The effects of normo- and hyperbaric solutions of the drug have been compared.

---

[1] Istituto di Neurochirurgia, Università Cattolica del Sacro Cuore, Largo A. Gemelli, 8, I-00168 Roma, Italy.

Material and Method

Morphine-HCl in 5 cc of normal or hyperbaric solution (33% glucose) was injected via a subarachnoid catheter percutaneously inserted at the lumbar level and connected to a subcutaneous reservoir (Cordis system).

The analgesic effect of morphine was evaluated on the basis of the patient's report on a visual analogue scale and on his request for medication. By this means we deduced the % of pain reduction, the time interval between the injections and the onset of the analgesia (induction time) and, finally, the duration of analgesia.

Twenty patients (Fig. 1) affected by pelvic cancer and complaining of lumbosacral bilateral (17 cases) or diffuse (3 cases) pain were selected for this treatment. Eight had injections of morphine in normal saline solution, 9 hyperbaric morphine and the remaining 3 received both normal and hyperbaric morphine on different occasions.

Results

1. *Analgesic effect.* All the patients reported analgesia after morphine injection (Fig. 1). The degree of such analgesia varied from 50 to 100% and was at least 75% in the majority of the patients. Induction time of analgesia (ITA), evaluated as the interval between the time of injection and the onset of the effect according to the patient's report, ranged from 1 to 20 minutes.

No clear differences were observed in the degree of analgesia or ITA for different morphine doses nor for different morphine solutions. The pain distribution was the only factor affecting ITA. In patients with diffuse pain there was a clear caudal to rostral progression of analgesia.

The mean duration of pain relief following a single injection varied from 1 to 3.5 days. In three patients pain relief lasted for one week or more. The duration of analgesia did not seem related to the type of morphine solution used. At least at doses of 0.5 and 1 mg the mean time interval between two successive injections was nearly the same for patients receiving hypertonic and for those receiving isotonic solutions of the drug. Fig. 2 A compares the mean duration of analgesia achieved in our patients following different doses of morphine. A dose related effect seems to be quite clear.

In some patients the analgesic effect was not always reproducible in successive injections suggesting a tolerance phenomena. Fig. 2 B shows the mean duration of analgesia following the first five injections in our patients. It is noticeable that the first dose is usually the most effective.

2. *Side effects.* Side effects occurred in many cases (60%) (Fig. 1). Radicular pain during or immediately after the injection was

Case	Dosis (mg)	Induc. time (mn)	% Analg.	Interval (days)	Side effects
1	2–3	2	100	7	–
2	1–2	3	100	3	vomiting
3	3	2	100	15	–
4	0.5–3	3	75	2	radicular pain, vomiting, excitation
5	1	3	100	3.5	radicular pain
6	1–3	1	75	3.5	nausea
7	0.5–1	2	100	1	itching
	3	2	100	2	somnolence
8	1–2	2	75	2	somnolence
9	1	4	75	1	radicular pain
10	0.5–1	3	100	1	–

Fig. 1 A

Fig. 1 A. Results obtained in 10 patients receiving morphine in hypertonic solution

Case	Dosis (mg)	Induc. time (mn)	% Analg.	Interval (days)	Side effects
11	0.5–1	12	75	1	–
12	0.5–1	15	75	2	–
13	0.5–1	2	100	2	–
14	0.5–1	11	100	2	aseptic meningitis
15	0.5–1	1	100	1	–
16	0.5–1	1	75	3	reservoir rejection
17	1	20	100	2	–
18	0.5–1	3 150	100	1	headache, bladder paresis, rachialgia
19	0.5	15 30	100	7	itching, nausea, pain at the reservoir site
20	0.5–1	4 60	50	2	vomiting, bladder paresis, constipation

Fig. 1 B

Fig. 1 B. Results obtained in 10 patients receiving morphine in isotonic solution

reported by three patients, all receiving hyperbaric morphine. Five patients complained of nausea and/or vomiting for many hours after the injection. Diffuse itching was a frequent complaint, and in two cases was very intense. Transient bladder paresis was observed in two cases. Aseptic meningitis which cleared spontaneously in a few days was present in two patients. Somnolence for many hours

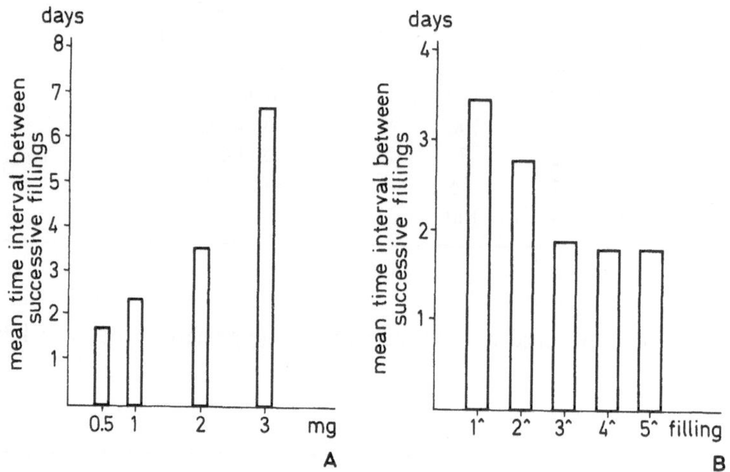

Fig. 2 A. Mean duration of analgesia after injections of different dosis of morphine (0.5–1–2 and 3 mg)

Fig. 2 B. Mean duration of analgesia following the first five dosis. Note that after an early reduction the effect seems to stabilize

occurred in three cases, two of whom receiving the hyperbaric solution. In two patients the catheter and the reservoir were removed, in one because of rejection and in the other because of CSF leakage from the reservoir.

Although side effects did not occur with all the injections in the same patient they were often quite disturbing, and limited the utilization of this route. In many cases they could be diminished by decreasing the dose of morphine, but the duration of analgesia decreased as well.

Our experience leads to the conclusion that the best mode of application of intrathecal morphine will be achieved with fractionated doses.

References

1. Lazorthes, Y., Gouarderes, Ch., Verdie, J. C., Monsarrat, B., Bastide, R., Canpan, L., Alwan, A., Cros, J., Analgésie par injection intrathécale de morphine. Neurochirurgie *26* (1980), 159—164.
2. Wang, J. K., Nauss, L. A., Thomas, J. E., Pain relief by intrathecally applied morphine in man. Anesthesiology *50* (1979), 149—151.
3. Yaksh, T. L., Spinal opiate analgesia: characteristics and principles of action. Pain *11* (1981) 3, 293—346.

Acta Neurochirurgica, Suppl. 33, 427—430 (1984)

The Role of Cervical Percutaneous Antero-lateral Cordotomy in Malignant Low-back Pain

G. Broggi[1], **A. Franzini, C. Giorgi,** and **D. Servello**

With 2 Figures

Summary

Consecutive series including 76 patients which underwent percutaneous cervical antero-lateral cordotomy for malignant cancer pain of the lower body are reported. The follow-up was continued till death in the whole series. Results and indications to percutaneous cervical antero-lateral cordotomy are reported and discussed.

Keywords: Percutaneous cervical antero-lateral cordotomy. Malignant low-back pain.

Introduction

Out of 200 percutaneous cervical antero-lateral cordotomies performed in cancer patients between 1975 and 1981, 76 patients were suffering from intractable malignant pain localized to the lower part of the body. The peculiar features of malignant low-back pain syndromes, the problem of bilateral pain and the value of percutaneous cordotomy in these patients are discussed according to our series in which the follow-up was continued till the exitus.

Material and Methods

Percutaneous antero-lateral cordotomy has been performed according to the technique described by Rosomoff *et al.*[5] through lateral cervical approach and radiofrequency lesion of the spino-thalamic tract at C 1–C 2 level. The procedure has been carried out with local anaesthesia. The target was choosen where

[1] Department of Neurosurgery, Istituto Neurologico "C. Besta", Via Celoria N. 11, I-20133 Milano, Italy.

electrical stimulation of the cord evoked paraesthesias in the painful areas below the umbelical region thus sparing the thoracic and superior limb sensory systems whose fibers run medially and much more closer to the descending respiratory pathways[3,4].

Patients for surgery have been selected according to the following main criteria: a) pain resistence to medical treatment including narcotic drugs; b) lateralization of the painful symptomatology or presence of radiologic signs suggesting the major involvement of one side, particularly when pain was localized in perineal and sacral regions; c) presence of verified malignant tumours

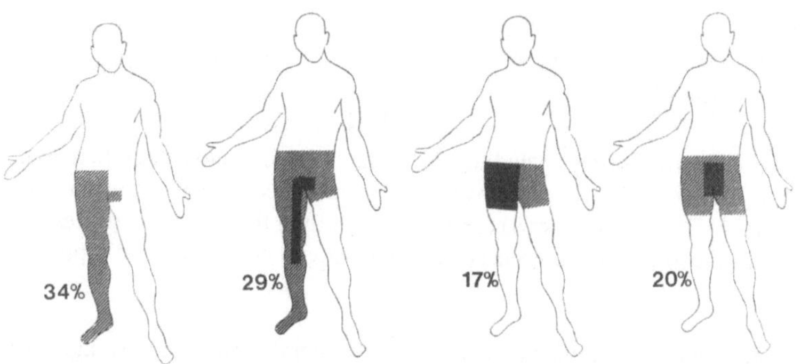

Fig. 1. Schematic representation of the localization of pain in the whole series of treated patients; painful areas are shaded and in bilateral pain patients the prevailing painful zones are marked by darker shading

or metastasis localized to the lower part of the body with short life expectancy, no longer than one year, in order to avoid the risk of intractable pain recurrence or the development of deafferentation pain syndromes[1-6].

Our series consists of 76 patients, 37 males and 39 females, age between 14 and 78 years: 22 patients had primary tumours of the urogenital system, 16 patients had primary tumours of the bowel and anorectal region and 38 patients had metastatic tumours localized to the pelvic bones and soft tissues. Unilateral pain with involvement of the inferior limb was present in 34% of patients; bilateral pain with prevalence on one side and corresponding leg was present in 29% of patients; 17% of patients had perineal pain, without leg involvement but predominately unilateral, 20% of patients had bilateral perineal and/or sacral pain and lateralization of treatment was suggested only by radiologic and radioisotopic studies CT scan of the pelvic and sacral region. The localization of painful symptomatology is represented in Fig. 1.

Results and Discussion

Complete pain relief was obtained immediately after the procedure in patients with lateralized symptomatology only and in this group narcotic drugs could be withdrawn. In patients with bilateral pain, immediate pain relief was obtained on the treated side. Contralateral pain could be controlled by medical therapy in all but 16 patients who required delayed open thoracic cordotomy about one month later; in this group of patients 5 cases had equal pain bilaterally and midline even before the percutaneous cordotomy, 11 cases had enhancement of contralateral pain after the percutaneous procedure.

In spite of the accuracy of preoperative subjective responses to neurophysiological tests, only 38% of the whole series obtained anaesthesia in the painful areas below the umbilical line and 62% had complete hemianaesthesia including the cervico-brachial region. All patients underwent serial neurological examination from the pain-free postoperative period. At three months follow-up 85% of patients had pain relief without major analgesic drugs. At six months this favourable rate was significatively lowered to 54% but only 16 patients were still alive. At nine months only 16% of patients were free from pain and there were only 8 survivors.

There was no postoperative mortality or respiratory disturbances; in the whole series permanent bladder disfunction was present in 10% of operated cases and slight permanent gait impairement (hemiparesis and ataxia) in 9%. Transitory motor and sphincter disturbances developed in many more patients but recovered completely few days after the operation.

In conclusion percutaneous antero-lateral cordotomy allowed complete pain relief untill death in 80% of the whole series including patients requiring medical treatment for controlateral pain and a group of 16 patients who had controlateral open thoracic cordotomy.

Our experience emphasizes:

1. the value of preoperative selection particularly regarding the length of life-expectancy. High rates of pain recurrences may be expected after the ninth month from surgery as reported elsewhere for painful syndromes of the upper body treated by percutaneous antero-lateral cordotomy[1];

2. the value of radiologic examinations to choose the side for treatment in patients with bilateral pain, which is not a contraindication to percutaneous cordotomy;

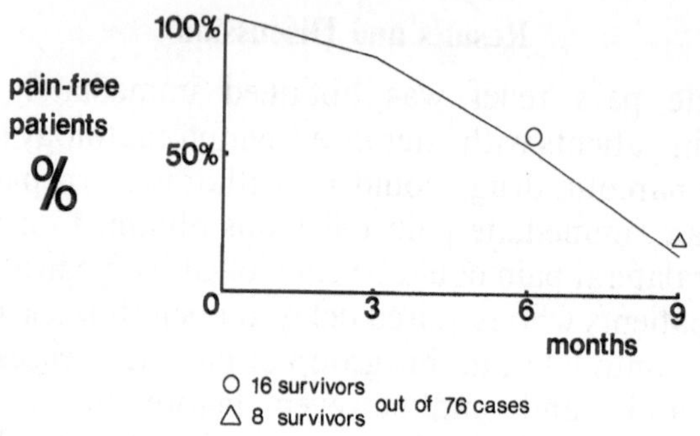

Fig. 2. Diagram representing the progressive decay of pain relief at different periods from percutaneous antero-lateral cordotomy. Patients which had medical treatment and/or open thoracic cordotomy for contralateral pain are included in the series. Note that most patients die between the third and sixth months

3. the possibility of delayed open antero-lateral thoracic cordotomy when contralateral pain is unchanged or enhanced and resistent to narcotic drugs. Bilateral cervical percutaneous cordotomy was avoided in this series because the of risk of respiratory disturbances[2].

Long term results from the whole series are represented in Fig. 2.

References

1. Broggi, G., Franzini, A., Lasio, G., Servello, D., Cordotomie antérolatérale percutanée dans le traitment de la douleur d'origine cancéreuse. Med. Hyg. *40* (1982), 1962—1968.
2. Krieger, A. J., Rosomoff, H. L., Sleep-induced apnea I. A respiratory and autonomic dysfunction syndrome following bilateral cervical percutaneous cordotomy. J. Neurosurg. *39* (1974), 168—180.
3. Krieger, A. J., Rosomoff, H. L., Sleep induced apnea II. Respiratory failure after anterior surgery. J. Neurosurg. *39* (1974), 181—185.
4. Lorenz, R., Methods of percutaneous spino-thalamic tract section. In: Advances and Technical Standards in Neurosurgery, Vol. 3 (Krayenbühl, H., *et al.*, eds.), pp. 123—145. Wien-New York: Springer. 1976.
5. Rosomoff, H. L., Carrol, F. J., Brown, J., Sheptak, P., Percutaneous radiofrequency cervical cordotomy: technique. J. Neurosurg. *23* (1965), 639—644.
6. White, J. C., Sweet, W. H., Pain and the neurosurgeon, pp. 699. Springfield, Ill.: Ch. C Thomas. 1969.

Acta Neurochirurgica, Suppl. 33, 431—435 (1984)

Stereotactic High Cervical Extralemniscal Myelotomy for Pelvic Cancer Pain

J. R. Schvarcz[1]

With 1 Figure

Summary

Midline and/or bilateral pelvic pain of neoplastic origin is difficult to deal with. However, stereotactic extralemniscal mylelotomy seems to be a rational approach, devoid of untoward side effects.

The author has already suggested that this is not a segmental commisural procedure but rather the interruption of an ascending nonspecific multisynaptic pathway.

Seventy-nine cases with midline and/or bilateral pelvic pain related to cancer, out of a series of 116 consecutive myelotomies, are reported. Satisfactory results were achieved in 78% of the cases overall. Physiological data germane to accurate lesion placement are discussed.

Keywords: Myelotomy; stereotaxis; pain; spinal cord.

Introduction

Midline and/or bilateral pelvic pain of neoplastic origin is notoriously difficult to deal with. In such cases, conventional methods are usually not only ineffective but also hazardous. With stereotactic extralemniscal myelotomy, however, the deterrent side effects of bilateral lesions are avoided.

This is not a segmental commissural procedure, but rather the interruption of an ascending non-specific multisynaptic pathway at the high cervical spinal cord.

Seventy-nine cases with intractable pelvic pain of neoplastic origin who underwent this procedure, out of a series of 116 consecutive stereotactic extralemniscal myelotomies, are reported.

[1] School of Medicine, University of Buenos Aires, Beruti 2926, Buenos Aires 1425, Argentina.

Material and Methods

Seventy-nine patients with midline and/or bilateral intractable pelvic pain related to neoplasms are reported.

Their pain histories ranged from 4 to 12 months. They all had pain refractory to medical treatment. Some of them have also had epidural block(s) which have either failed or recurred. Four have had unilateral cordotomies performed elsewhere, which have failed to relieve their pain.

The technique has already been described[10,12]. All patients were operated on under local anaesthesia, in the sitting position, with the head fully flexed within a modified Hitchcock's stereotactic apparatus, which was rigidly fixed to the operating table.

The midline of the odontoid process was assumed to superimpose on the midline of the spinal cord, provided that there was no rotation. The spinal cord was outlined by water soluble positive contrast cisternography, and then approached by a posterior route through the atlanto-occipital interspace with an external cannula advanced until cerebrospinal fluid was aspirated. A 0.6 mm steel electrode with a thermistor was then advanced to the target (Fig. 1).

The target is the central cord region, viz., at the midsagittal plane 5 mm in front of the dorsal border of the spinal cord, as determined radiographically and corroborated by impedance measurement. Its definite placement, however, was always based on the results of electrical stimulation.

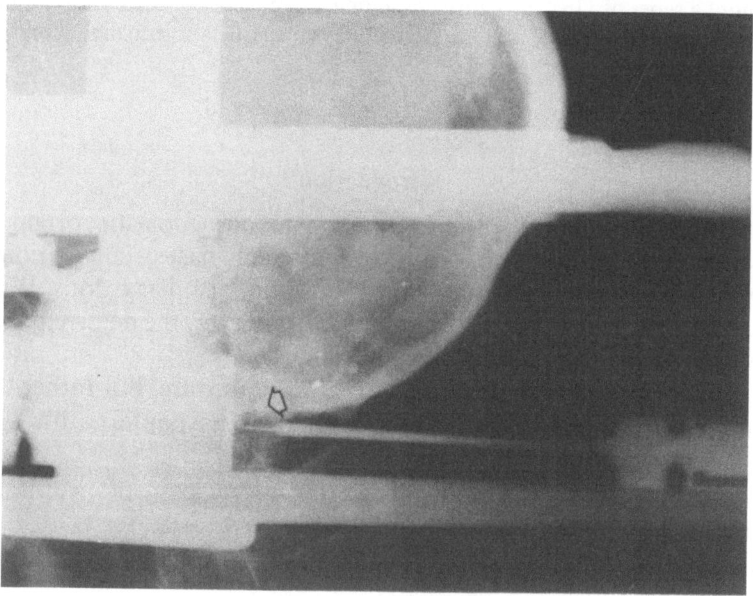

Fig. 1. Lateral radiograph with the electrode in place, demonstrating the atlanto-occipital posterior approach (arrows: dorsal border of the spinal cord)

The dorsal column has a definite homuncular arrangement, which enabled an accurate recognition of the electrode position[11].

A basic pattern of responses was consistently produced from the central canal region, which was related to stimulation of the base of the dorsal funiculi. This consisted of paraesthesiae starting at the soles of both feet and propagated to the dorsal aspect of the legs as the intensity of stimulation was increased. This constant basic pattern of responses was obtained either in isolation or in combination with additional, superimposed responses, namely trigeminal paraesthesiae, or crossed limb involvement, or less frequently, of both upper limbs, or even any or all of them in combination[11–13]. Sometimes distinctive bilateral burning truncal sensations occurred.

Radiofrequency thermocontrolled lesions were placed just in front as well as where distal lower limb threshold responses were obtained.

Results

Satisfactory pain relief, *i.e.*, no pain or infrequent pain relieved by non-narcotic analgesics, was obtained in 76% of the cases overall.

Only clinical subjective analgesia was usually induced, without demonstrable sensory changes. Indeed, no relationship was demonstrated between pain relief and the presence or absence of objective sensory losses if any occurred.

The follow-up time ranged between 0.5 and 30 months, but 82% of the patients died within the first 6 months. Although transient post-operative gait unsteadiness was a common observation there were no lasting motor or autonomic side effects.

Discussion

The decussating spinal fibres to the spinothalamic tracts were first severed by Armour[1]. Leriche[2] and Putnam[8] independently reported a similar technique, which finally became an accepted but infrequently used pain relieving method.

Hitchcock[4] developed a stereotactic procedure enabling the placement of radiofrequency lesions in the commissural region at the first cervical segment. These lesions produced a widespread alleviation of pain which, curiously enough, included the lower half of the body. I have used a similar technique since 1971[9].

There is no evidence whatsoever to suggest that the spinothalamic fibres from the lower parts of the body are still decussating or lying near the central canal in the cervical region, and this stereotactic lesion should not then be expected to produce analgesia beyond the related segmental dermatomes. Other anatomical structures are presumably involved in commissural myelotomy, suggesting a different pathophysiology as well.

The existence of alternate pathways by which nociceptive information may be rostrally transmitted is a logical assumption from the demonstration of both the recovery of sensation after bilateral cordotomy and the nociceptive changes produced by myelotomy[14].

I have therefore stated that this stereotactic central cord destruction is not a segmental commissural procedure but rather the interruption of an alternate non-specific multisynaptic pathway, naming the procedure extralemniscal myelotomy[9–11].

These single high cervical central cord lesions produced striking effects. A widespread alleviation of pain occurs, both upper and lower body pain being easily dealt with[4–6,9–11]. However, only subjective analgesia is induced, usually without demonstrable sensory changes, and both sharp and blunt discrimination and the ability to localize stimuli were preserved.

Satisfactory results were obtained in 76% of the cases herein reported, without untoward side effects.

Hitchcock[6] reported on 30 stereotactic myelotomies, with satisfactory results in 64% of the cases overall.

Eiras *et al.*[2] reported 12 stereotactic myelotomies, with good results in 75% of the cases, followed up between 2 and 22 months.

Sourek[13] performed suprasegmental surgical central cord radiofrequency lesions in 20 patients, achieving good results in 85% of the cases, without neurological deficits, followed up between 12 and 36 months.

Gildenberg and Hirshberg[3] described limited suprasegmental myelotomies in 18 patients, with good results in 86% of the cases, without complications, and without loss of nociception.

Stereotactic extralemniscal myelotomy appears to be especially suitable for pelvic pain of neoplastic origin, whereby both pain related to midline structures or with bilateral distribution are conveniently managed by a single lesion, without encroachment on the autonomic pathways.

References

1. Armour, D., Surgery of the spinal cord and its membranes. Lancet *ii* (1927), 691—697.
2. Eiras, J., Garcia, J., Gomez, J., Carcavilla, L., Ucar, S., First results of extralemniscal myelotomy. Acta Neurochir. (Wien), Suppl. *30* (1980), 377—382.

3. Gildenberg, P. L., Hirshberg, R. M., Limited myelotomy for the treatment of intractable pain. Neurochirurgia (Stuttgart), Suppl. Neurological Surgery 66, 1981.
4. Hitchcock, E. R., Stereotactic cervical myelotomy. J. Neurol. Neurosurg. Psychiat. *33* (1970), 224—230.
5. Hitchcock, E. R., Stereotactic myelotomy. Proc. R. Soc. Med. *67* (1974), 771—772.
6. Hitchcock, E. R., Stereotactical spinal surgery. In: Neurological Surgery, with Emphasis on Non-invasive Methods of Diagnosis and Treatment (Carrea, R., ed.), pp. 271—280. Amsterdam: Excerpta Medica. 1978.
7. Leriche, R., Du traitement de la douleur dans les cancers abdominaux et pelviens inopérables et récidives. Gaz. Hôp. *109* (1936), 917—922.
8. Putnam, T. J., Myelotomy of the commissure. A new method of treatment for pain in the upper extremities. Arch. Neurol. Psychiat. *32* (1934), 1189—1193.
9. Schvarcz, J. R., Spinal cord stereotactic surgery. In: Recent Progress in Neurological Surgery (Sano, K., Ishii, S., eds.), pp. 234—241. Amsterdam: Excerpta Medica. 1974.
10. Schvarcz, J. R., Stereotactic extralemniscal myelotomy. J. Neurol. Neurosurg. Psychiat. *39* (1976), 53—57.
11. Schvarcz, J. R., Functional exploration of the spinomedullary junction. Acta Neurochir. (Wien), Suppl. *24* (1977), 179—185.
12. Schvarcz, J. R., Spinal cord stereotactic techniques re trigeminal nucleotomy and extralemniscal myelotomy. Appl. Neurophysiol. *41* (1978), 99—112.
13. Sourek, K., Central thermocoagulation of the cord for relief of intractable pain. Neurochirurgica (Stuttgart), Suppl. Neurological Surgery, 66, 1981.
14. Yaksh, T. L., Hammond, D. L., Peripheral and central substrates involved in the rostrad transmission of nociceptive information. Pain *13* (1982), 1—86.

Acta Neurochirurgica, Suppl. 33, 437—443 (1984)

Rostral Stereotactic Mesencephalotomy in Treatment of Cancer Pain; a Survey of 40 Treated Patients

F. Frank[1], G. Frank, G. Gaist, C. Sturiale, and **A. Fabrizi**

With 1 Figure

Summary

The authors report their experiences in the treatment of cancer pain with rostral stereotactic mesencephalotomy. Forty-five operations, of which 5 were bilateral, were performed in 40 patients. In addition to brief technical notes, a six month to two year follow-up is presented. The analgesic results were initially good in all the patients. In the follow-up, the results remained good in 85% of the patients, while 15% complained of disturbances which could be attributed to anesthesia dolorosa. All the immediate post-operative side-effects were associated with oculomotor disturbances (20% with Parinaud's syndrome and/or Foville's syndrome). These side-effects were only transitory in the majority of the cases, and spontaneously regressed in two to three weeks. In only three patients were these side-effects permanent. The authors emphasize the absence of any mortality, the rapidity of execution of the operation, and the possibility of avoiding major risks even with a bilateral procedure. The chief indications are facio-thoraco-brachial pain syndromes; but there was difficulty in obtaining adequate analgesia in the legs. The authors suggest that this may depend on a dispersion of fibers representing the legs in the spinothalamic tract at the mesencephalic level.

Keywords: Rostral stereotactic mesencephalotomy; upper body cancer pain; analgesic effects; oculomotor disturbances; dysesthesias.

Introduction

We started performing rostral stereotactic mesencephalotomy 4 years ago for the treatment of upper body cancer pain. Our first results have previously been published[3]. A larger series with larger follow-up is presented and confirms the validity of the procedure.

[1] Division of Neurosurgery, Bellaria Hospital, Bologna, Italy.

Method

The Mundinger-Riechert stereotactic frame was used with a frontal paramedian approach in front of the coronal suture. After intra-operative ventriculography (Iopamidol, 3 cc.), the spinothalamic tract was reached 4 mm below the posterior commissure, 1 mm in front of the aqueduct, and between 7.5–10 mm lateral to the midline. Before making the lesion, using the same electrode[1], neurophysiological stimulation was given. Four coagulations, 30" each at 70–75 °C were usually sufficient to achieve good hemi-analgesia.

Material and Results

Table 1 shows our present series (40 patients treated, 5 bilaterally), etiology and site of pain, immediate post-operative results and operative complications.

Table 1. *Personal Experiences in the Treatment of Cancer Pain with Rostral Stereotactic Mesencephalotomy from 1980–1982*

		INTERVENTIONS		
SIDE OF CANCER	PATIENTS	UNILATERAL	BILATERAL	ANALGESIC RESULTS
LUNG	23	18	5	GOOD IN ALL PATIENTS (100%)
CERVICO-FACIAL	15	15	-	MORTALITY 0
BREAST	2	2	-	MORBIDITY
TOT.	40	35	5	OCULO-MOTOR DISTURBANCES 8 (20%); DYSESTHESIA 2 (5%)

The majority of the patients suffered of lung cancer and a few of facio-cervical cancer. There was no operative mortality. From the antalgic viewpoint, they all showed excellent immediate post-operative results. In 3 patients, pain recurred after a very short time (24–48 hours), due to insufficient coagulation; they were all successfully reoperated. After the operation, contralateral hypo-analgesia appeared in all the patients, with a greater sensitivity loss in the upper body. Table 2 presents a follow-up of all 40 patients, either seen directly or indirectly (referred to us by relatives). Our follow-up ranged from 6 months to 2 years. The analgesia remained good in 85% of the patients, while the other 15% (6 patients) showed algo-dysesthesias of variable intensity. Of these 6 patients, only 2 (5%) manifested

---

[1] Radio-frequency generator (RFG-5) and temperature monitoring (TM) electrode manufactured by Radionics Inc., 76 Cambridge Street, Burlington, Massachusetts, U.S.A.

Table 2. *Follow-up with respect to Analgesia and Side-effects (6 months to 2 years)*

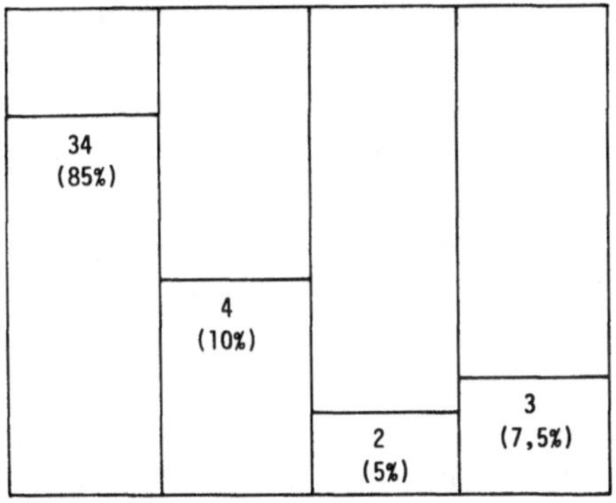

Table 3. *Immediate Morbidity Following Rostral Stereotactic Mesencephalotomy*

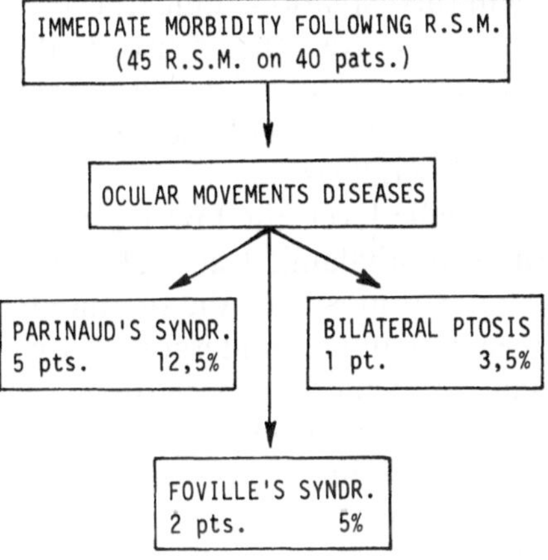

anesthesia dolorosa. Undesired side-effects, in most cases, were oculomotor disturbances. Immediate painful dysesthesias appear in two patients (both cases were of the hand). Gaze palsies remained permanent in 3 patients; while in the others, the loss was temporary, regressing completely in 1 to 2 weeks.

Discussion

Our first rostral stereotactic mesencephalotomies were performed as an alternative to percutaneous cervical cordotomy for upper body cancer pain, pain syndromes associated with respiratory disorders, and as the second procedure in cases of bilateral pain. However, there are difficulties in obtaining long term analgesia with percutaneous cervical cordotomy above C8-D1 dermatomes. Furthermore, respiratory complications due to lesions of the reticular descending pathways, running medial to the spinothalamic tract, are possible at the cervical level[7,8]. As for bilateral percutaneous cervical cordotomies, all the authors agree that there is a high percentage of postoperative mortality[7,9]. With rostral stereotactic mesencephalotomy, one achieves facio-thoraco-brachial analgesia, without respiratory disturbances, because the lesion is localized above the respiratory centers. Bilateral rostral stereotactic mesencephalotomies performed at a 7 day interval from the first intervention, presents no jeopardy to the patient's life.

Rostral stereotactic mesencephalotomy is recommended for upper body pain, because at the level of the upper midbrain tegmentum, thermo-algesic sensitivity is well represented in its cephalic component (quintothalamic tract), and in its brachio-thoraxic component (neo-spinothalamic tract)[9,10]. These bundles, that run together towards the sensory thalamus, have a somatotopic distribution identical to the thalamic relay nuclei (VPL-VPM complex), with the cephalic region arranged medially, and the lower body laterally[11].

At the mesencephalic level, the lower extremities are sparsely represented in the spinothalamic tract. The thinning of the tract towards the thalamus, is mostly of the thermoalgesic fibers of the pelvis and the lower extremities, undergoing a dispersion along the multisynaptic paleo-reticulothalamic tract. The homunculus appears disproportioned, with only a few fibers representing the lower body (Fig. 1). According to Mazars[4], the fibers in this tract run latero-ventral. Our experience with neurophysiological stimulation and lesions places these fibers latero-dorsal.

The spatial location of the spinothalamic tract presents some discordance among various authors: some place it more medial[5], and some more lateral[10]. On section of the midbrain tegmentum perpendicular to the Sylvian aqueduct, 4 mm below the inferior border of the posterior commissure, we find the spinothalamic tract between 7.5–10 mm from the midline and 1 mm ventral to the anterior aspect of the aqueduct (as described by Mazars)[4].

Neurophysiological stimulation of the spinothalamic tract is characteristic, because it provokes thermic sensations (hot and cold), mixed, at times, with tingling sensations[10]. It is strange that

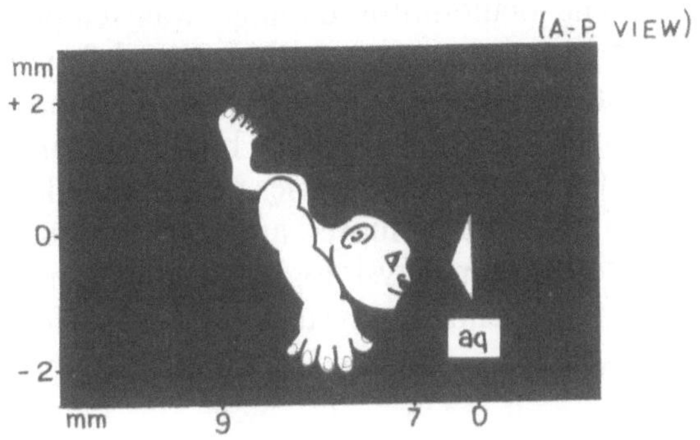

Fig. 1. Somatotopic representation of the spinothalamic tract in man. From 7 to 9 mm: Extension of the spino-thalamic tract at the superior collicular level. This homuncular representation is called by the aa. as "plongeur"

stimulation of a tract carrying pain sensation, never evokes feelings of pain. Albe-Fessard[1], and Tasker[10] were able to provoke pain by stimulating the spinothalamic tract only in cases of lesions of the medial lemniscus. It is important to make a distinction between the thermo-tingling sensation and an electric shock sensation. While the first is an expression of the spinothalamic tract activation, the second is of the medial lemniscus[10]. A lesion involving the medial lemniscus, which runs ventral to the spinothalamic tract, is responsible for paresthesias that, if important, reduce the success of the operation[3]. The medial lemniscus represents an inhibitory system for the spinothalamic and more ancient tracts (paleo- and archi-spinothalamic tracts)[2,10].

Painful paresthesias due to accidental lesions of the medial lemniscus may be a phenomenon of liberation of these primitive systems. Usually, these paresthetic sensations are immediate, but in rare cases, they may appear at a later stage (even after months), and may spread to a whole hemisoma. These late appearing paresthesias might be explained by the theory proposed by Noordenbos, on the poli-modal function of the central nervous system tracts[6]. The algogenic impulses, finding the main pain pathway interrrupted by a lesion, after a period of latency, may reappear along other tracts (not necessarily sensitive), explaining the temporary effectiveness of all pain surgery of the central nervous system.

In the past, rostral stereotactic mesencephalotomy was abandoned due to the high percentage of oculomotor disturbances[5]. The oculomotor damage was temporary in the majority of our cases (regressing within 2 weeks); while the few permanent damages represent the results of lesions spreading medially involving the intercollicular bundles. Carrying out a correct stereotactic lesion, these injuries may be avoided, even with bilateral operations. Furthermore, an exact evaluation of the sensations evoked by neurophysiological stimulation is important to avoid damage to the lemniscal system, responsible for the painful paresthesias.

Conclusions

Our present experience with rostral stereotactic mesencephalotomy in the treatment of upper body cancer pain is positive with 85% good results at follow-up. The undesirable side-effects associated with the operation (oculomotor deficits and painful dysesthesias) can be avoided by performing lesions of smaller size (2–3 mm in diameter), exactly on target. They must not be less than 7.5 mm from the midline, and performed only after correct responses to neurophysiological stimulation.

References

1. Albe-Fessard, D., Dondey, M., Nicolaidis, S., LeBeau, J., Remarks concerning the effect of the diencephalic lesions on pain and sensitivity with special reference to lemniscally mediated control of noxious afferences. Confin. Neurol. *32* (1970), 174—184.
2. Foerster, O., Die Leitungsbahnen des Schmerzgefühls und die chirurgische Behandlung der Schmerzzustände, pp. 77–80. Berlin-Wien: Urban and Schwarzenberg. 1927.
3. Frank, F., Tognetti, F., Gaist, G., Frank, G., Galassi, E., Sturiale, C., Stereotaxic rostral mesencephalotomy in treatment of malignant faciothoracobrachial pain syndromes: A survey of 14 treated patients. J. Neurosurg. *56* (1982), 807—811.
4. Mazars, G., Merienne, L., Cioloca, C., Etat actuel de la chirurgie de la douleur. Neurochirurgie *22*, suppl. 1 (1976), 53—61.
5. Nashold, B. S., jr., Extensive cephalic and oral pain relieved by midbrain tractotomy. Confin. Neurol. *34* (1972), 382—388.
6. Noordenbos, W., Remarks on afferent system in the anterolateral quadrant. In: Pain Basic Principles. Pharmacology. Therapy. (Jansen, R., Kerdel, W. D., Herz, A., Steichele, G., eds.), pp. 112–115. Stuttgart: G. Thieme. London: Churchill Livingstone. 1972.
7. Rosomoff, H. L., Bilateral percutaneous cervical radiofrequency cordotomy. J. Neurosurg. *31* (1969), 41—46.

8. Rosomoff, H. L., Krieger, A. J., Kuperman, A. S., Effects of percutaneous cervical cordotomy on pulmonary function. J. Neurosurg. *31* (1969), 620—627.
9. Tasker, R. R., Somatotopographic representation in the human thalamus, midbrain and spinal cord. In: Current Controversies in Neurosurgery, pp. 485—495. Philadelphia-London-Toronto: W. B. Saunders. 1976.
10. Tasker, R. R., Organ, L., Hawrylyshyn, P., The spinothalamic pathway. In: The Thalamus and Midbrain of Man. A Physiological Atlas Using Electrical Stimulation, pp. 109—199. Springfield, Ill.: Ch. C Thomas. 1982.

Acta Neurochirurgica, Suppl. 33, 445—450 (1984)

II. Plexus Avulsion Pain (Neurogenic Pain)

High Frequency Coagulation of Dorsal Root Entry Zone in Patients with Deafferentation Pain

G. Dieckmann[1] **and G. Veras**

With 1 Figure

Summary

In 18 patients suffering from chronic unbearable pain Nashold's technique of dorsal root entry zone lesioning was performed. In 11 patients with deafferentation pain a good or an excellent result was obtained. No improvement was seen in 3 patients of this group because of drug related reasons. 4 patients with somatogenic pain showed no improvement. Postoperative side effects consisted of partially reduced sensory capacities but in only 2 patients was this of practical consequences because of motor weakness. One patient died because of an angiospastic event followed by a painful paraplegia 4 days postoperatively. High frequency coagulations were performed by an usual cordotomy electrode attached to a special electrode holder allowing a safe and easy handling under the microscope.

Keywords: Deafferentation pain; high frequency coagulation; dorsal root entry zone.

Introduction

In 1974 Sindou *et al.* published a new method to ameliorate somatogenic pain by selective undercutting of nociceptive fibers entering the spinal cord in the dorsal root-cord junction[9]. Two

[1] Dvision of Functional Neurosurgery, Georg-August-University Medical Centre, Robert-Koch-Strasse 40, D-3400 Göttingen, Federal Republic of Germany.

years later, Nashold *et al.*[7] reported good results in the treatment of neurogenic pain by high frequency coagulation of the substantia gelatinosa Rolandi within the dorsal laminae of grey matter of the spinal cord. The Duke University group later on achieved[3-6] good results by this method in both neurogenic as well as somatogenic pain. In Europe first confirmations of these results came from Samii 1980[8] and from Wiegand *et al.* 1982[11]. Our own experience since December 1981 with dorsal root entry zone lesioning concerns 18 patients who form the basis for this report.

Material

From December 1981 to December 1982 using Nashold's technique of dorsal root entry zone lesioning we operated on 18 patients who suffered from chronic unbearable pain. Nine of these patients suffered from pain after avulsion of two or more roots of the brachial plexus; five of phantom limb and/or stump pain. Two other patients suffered from pain following a complete thoraco-lumbar paraplegia. One patient had zoster neuralgia of the intercostal nerves, a another patient had intractable sciatic pain after lumbar disc surgery. Previous treatment had included transcutaneous electrical stimulation, dorsal column stimulation, rhizotomies and sympathectomies. In half of the patients narcotics had played an important role in the therapy.

Method

Lesioning of the dorsal root entry zone was performed according to Nashold and Ostdahl[4]. However, for the coagulation we used the usual cordotomy electrode (OWL Instruments Ltd.). For the purpose of safe and easy handling under the microscope we attached the electrode to a special holder as shown in Fig. 1. A strip of radiofrequency coagulations was produced from the uppermost to the lowermost extent of the desired region. The current flow ranged from 30–40 mA, the coagulation time was 15 sec. The voltage depended on the extrusion of the free tip of the electrode, mostly it ranged from 25–30 V. Because of the size of the electrode holder sometimes it was difficult to achieve the appropriate approach of the electrode regarding the angle of entrance proposed by Nashold, and the laminectomy had to be enlarged.

Results

The 18 patients operated were followed up for 2–16 months. In this period, the patients with deafferentation pain had the best results regarding pain relief. Eleven of these had an excellent or good result as indicated in Table 1 and 2. "Excellent" indicates a total pain relief; "good" a pain relief of at least 50% without the

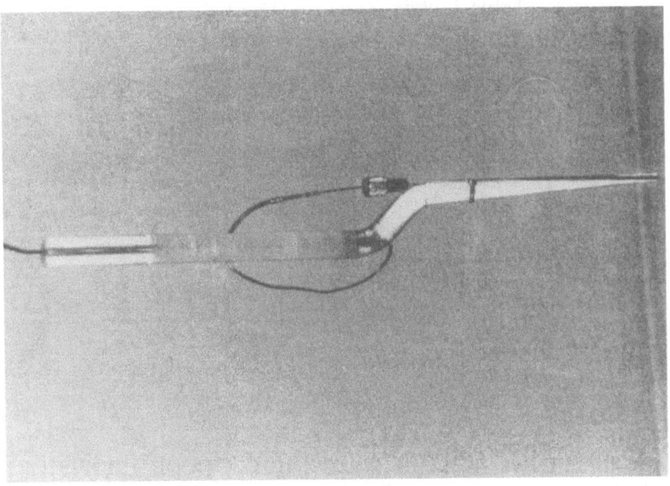

Fig. 1. Electrode holder with an usual cordotomy electrode attached

Table 1. *Clinical Results of DREZ Coagulations for Pain Relief with a Follow-up of 2–16 Months*

Case no.	Diagnosis	Result	Follow-up Period (months)
1	phantom	poor	16
2	root avulsion	good	15
3	phantom	good	15
4	root avulsion	poor	5 (suicide)
5	phantom	excellent	13
6	paraplegia	poor	13
7	root avulsion	excellent	12
8	root avulsion	excellent	10
9	phantom	excellent	9
10	root avulsion	good	9
11	root avulsion	poor	9
12	phantom	excellent	4 days
13	zoster neural.	none	8
14	arach. spin	none	8
15	root avulsion	excellent	6
16	paraplegia	none	3
17	root avulsion	excellent	3
18	root avulsion	excellent	2

Table 2. *Pain Relief by DREZ Lesions*

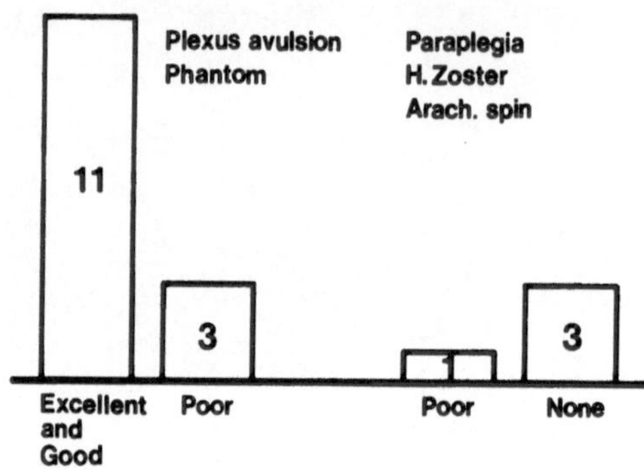

necessity of further narcotic medication; "poor" indicates initial pain relief, but recurrence after weeks; "none" indicates no pain relief, not even for a few weeks.

Postamputation pain and deafferentation pain following root avulsion were relieved (good or very good respectively). Poor results occured in three patients with deafferentation pain. In these an addiction to the narcotics previously given appeared postoperatively. One patient committed suicide 5 months postoperatively. The one patient with postherpetic pain and the other patient with somatogenic pain obtained no pain relief.

Complications

Transitory side effects were frequent during the first postoperative days. As noted previously by Nashold and Ostdahl[4], several disturbances of epicritic and proprioceptive sensibility occured. Most of these disappeared within the subsequent postoperative weeks.

Table 3 shows the remaining complications. Three of our patients had a permanent sensory deficit. Two of these had a defect of proprioceptive sensibility, together with motor weakness of the ipsilateral leg. The third patient had a sensory deficit of the postcordotomy dysaesthesia type. Bladder dysfunction occured in two patients in whom function was already disturbed preoperatively by the disease or the preceding operative treatment, respectively. The sensation and motor side effects can be explained by the anatomical proximity of the pyramidal tract adjacent to the coagulation site within the substantia gelatinosa Rolandi as well as the fact that coagulation medial to the entrance of the dorsal root

Table 3. *Remaining Complications After DREZ Lesions*

Sensory change	3
Motor weakness	2
Bladder dysfunction (bilat. interv.)	2
Postop. death	1

destroys the A-beta fibers responsible for the myostatic reflex as well as for epicritic sensibility.

One patient died 4 days postoperatively. He developed a painful paraplegia on the second postoperative day and died 2 days later because of stress induced coronary insufficiency. Histological examination revealed total necrosis of the spinal cord at the thoracic-lumbal level with intact vessels thus indicating an angiospastic event.

Discussion

As stated by Stavraky[10] the so-called deafferentation pain is caused by a supersensitivity of neuronal pools following peripheral lesions within the nervous system. Lesions such as cervical root avulsion may produce a denervation hypersensitivity of neurones within the substantia gelatinosa Rolandi thus disinhibiting the T-cells which are the origin of the spinothalamic tract. Although the development of central pain is assumed to be related to central structures[1], a disturbance of the sensory gate mechanism within the spinal cord[2] seems to be the prefered explanation for deafferentation pain at present. The dorsal root entry zone lesion destroys the hyperexcited neuronal pools within the gate control system and/or rebalances the modulating influence of the Lissauer tract.

The results of Nashold were confirmed by Samii[8] in regard to deafferentation pain and by Wiegand *et al.*[11] for central pain in paraplegics. Our findings are in accordance with the results of these authors, except for our poor results in somatogenic pain.

The intervention of Sindou *et al.*[9] seems more to abolish a hypersensitivity of nociceptive afferences, for instance by scarring in cancer patients; therefore this operation is more valid for somatogenic pain. In these circumstances it might be useful to coagulate more superficially and laterally within the dorsal surface of the spinal cord than that done for coagulations against deafferentation pain.

References

1. Livingston, W. K., Pain Mechanisms: A physiologic interpretation of causalgia and its related states. New York-London: Plenum Press. 1976.
2. Melzak, R., Wall, P. D., Pain Mechanism: A new theory. Science *150* (1965), 971—979.
3. Nashold, B. S., jr., Bullitt, E., Dorsal root entry zone lesions to control central pain in paraplegics. J. Neurosurg. *55* (1981), 414—419.
4. Nashold, B. S., jr., Ostdahl, R. H., Dorsal root entry zone lesions for pain relief. J. Neurosurg. *51* (1979), 59—69.
5. Nashold, B. S., jr., Ostdahl, R. H., Pain relief after dorsal root entry zone lesions. Acta Neurochir. (Wien), Suppl. *30* (1980), 383—389.
6. Nashold, B. S., jr., Bullitt, E., Ostdahl, R., The role of dorsal root entry zone lesions in relief of central pain. In: Neurological Surgery (Dietz, J., *et al.*, eds), p. 67. Stuttgart-New York: Thieme. 1981.
7. Nashold, B. S., jr., Urban, B., Zorub, D. S., Phantom relief by focal destruction of substantia gelatinosa of Rolando. In: Advances in Pain Research and Therapy, Vol. 1 (Bonica, J. J., Albe-Fessard, D. G., eds.), pp. 959—963. New York: Raven Press. 1976.
8. Samii, M., Thermocoagulation of the substantia gelatinosa for pain relief—(Preliminary report). In: Phantom and Stump Pain (Siegfried, J., Zimmermann, M., eds.), pp. 156—159. Berlin-Heidelberg-New York: Springer. 1981.
9. Sindou, M., Fischer, G., Goutelle, A., Mansuy, L., La radicellotomie postérieure sélective. Premiers résultats dans la chirurgie de la douleur. Neurochirurgie (Paris) *20* (1974), 391—408.
10. Stavraky, G. W., Supersensitivity following lesions of the nervous system: An aspect of the relativity of nervous integration. Toronto: University of Toronto Press. 1961.
11. Wiegand, H., Winkelmüller, W., Dietz, H., Results of dorsal root entry zone lesions for pain relief in paraplegics. Acta Neurochir. (Wien) *62* (1982), 147—148.

Acta Neurochirurgica, Suppl. 33, 451—457 (1984)

Epidural versus Thalamic Stimulation for the Management of Brachial Plexus Lesion Pain

T. W. Hood and J. Siegfried[1]

Summary

Epidural stimulation was used to treat 16 patients with brachial plexus lesion pain, 13 secondary to trauma, 2 with metastatic disease, and 1 with radiation plexopathy. Only 2 patients obtained good pain relief, 1 fair, and the remainder poor. Permanent implantation was performed in 8 patients with an average follow-up of 56 months. Of this group 11 patients had cervical nerve root avulsion 1 of whom had good pain relief, but the remainder all had poor results. A second group of 8 patients with cervical nerve root avulsion was treated with thalamic sensory nucleus stimulation. By this therapy 2 had excellent results, 2 good, 1 fair, and 3 poor; 7 patients received definitive implantation with an average follow-up of 21 months. Based on this experience trials of epidural stimulation in patients with brachial plexus avulsion are unwarranted. Thalamic sensory nucleus stimulation is a potential, non-ablative, and low-risk therapy for intractable brachial plexus avulsion pain.

Keywords: Brachial plexus avulsion; deafferentation pain; thalamic sensory nucleus stimulation; dorsal cord stimulation.

Introduction

The management of brachial plexus lesion pain has included many therapies which in time have failed. Previous treatments as amputation, neuroma excision, and peripheral neurectomies have been ineffective for long term relief[17]. Anterolateral cordotomy provides temporary relief at best, *i.e.* 6 months in 50% of patients and 3 years in only 20%; its use currently is usually reserved for pain of malignant origin[13,14]. Stereotactic mesencephalotomy has likewise been unsuccessful for the long term management of brachial plexus pain[12]. Stereotactic thalamotomy has been applied to

[1] Department of Neurosurgery, University of Zürich, CH-8091 Zürich, Switzerland.

patients with various pain of the deafferentiated type, but the results have been discouraging. Centre median lesions[16] or centre median, nucleus intralamellaris medialis, and pulvinar lesions[15] have demonstrated poor results and although centre median—parafascicularis lesions produced better relief, the failure rate was still approximately 50%[8]. More recently, dorsal root entry zone lesions have been introduced for the therapy of brachial plexus lesion pain[10]. In one series of 18 brachial plexus avulsion patients 56% had good relief, 22% fair relief, and 22% poor relief[9]. Additional time is needed to see if a dysesthetic pain syndrome will result from this procedure as has occurred with other ablative techniques involving primary sensory pathways.

Since 1973 neurostimulation techniques have been utilized for the treatment of chronic pain at the University of Zürich. For patients with brachial plexus lesion pain who had failed to respond to conservative management, trials of epidural stimulation were indicated. If adequate pain relief was not obtained by epidural stimulation, the patients were considered candidates for thalamic sensory nucleus stimulation. This report reviews the results of these two therapies.

Material and Methods

Epidural stimulation was first used on patients whose pain failed to respond to conservative therapy. This group contained 16 patients, 11 male and 5 female and their average age was 48 years. Pain was secondary to trauma in 13 patients of whom 11 patients had cervical nerve root avulsion documented by myelography in 10 and by clinical examination in 1; there were 2 patients with metastatic disease and 1 patient with radiation plexopathy. Except for the first patient who had an endodural electrode placed with general anesthesia, all patients had a percutaneous placement of an Avery monopolar electrode during intermittant methohexital anesthesia as well as 2% procaine local anesthesia. Except for the first case all patients had a trial of stimulation lasting several days before a decision concerning permanent implantation was made. For 8 patients who received definitive implantation, follow-up occurred every 6 months. Patients who had not been interviewed within the past 6 months were contacted by letter to obtain their current results with stimulation.

In a second group of 8 patients with cervical nerve root avulsion, all of whom had unsuccessful trials of epidural stimulation at the University Hospital of Zürich or other centers, deep brain stimulation of the contralateral thalamic sensory nucleus was performed. All patients had myelographic evidence of avulsion except one case in which the diagnosis was determined by clinical examination. This group contained 5 males and 3 females; their average age was 31 years. The surgery was performed using 2% procaine local anesthesia as well as methohexital in the occasional patient. After air ventriculography the Foramen of Monro—Posterior Commissure baseline was determined. The target point was 3 mm anterior to the Posterior Commissure, 2 mm below the baseline, and 13 mm laterally from the midline. An Avery monopolar electrode was positioned so that stimulation elicited paresthesias in the pain distribution of the affected arm. The electrode was secured to the skull with a self-tightening screw and a connecting lead is tunnelled beneath the scalp for several centimers before externalized. A trial period of several days was used to ascertain the effectiveness of stimulation before a final decision on definitive implantation is made. For the 7 patients who received definitive implantation, follow-up has occurred on a 6 month basis. Patients who had not been examined within the past 6 months were contacted by letter to obtain the most current results with stimulation.

The level of pain relief was determined by the estimation of the patient with both epidural and thalamic stimulation. A 75 to 100% reduction of pain without narcotics was considered an excellent result. A 50 to 74% reduction was a good result and a 25 to 49% reduction a fair result. Pain relief of 0 to 24% or continued use of narcotics was judged a poor result.

Results

Of the group of 16 patients who received trials of epidural stimulation, long term follow-up of an average of 56 months has revealed that no patient obtained excellent relief; 2 had good relief 1 fair, and 13 poor (Table 1). Only 8 patients obtained sufficient initial pain relief to warrant definitive implantation. In this group were 11 patients with cervical nerve root avulsion of whom only 1 patient received good pain relief by epidural stimulation. The remainder all had poor results (Table 2). There were no complications or mortality in this group.

Table 1. *Results of Epidural Stimulation in Patients with Brachial Plexus Lesion Pain*

	Trauma	Malignancy	Radiation
Excellent (100–75)			
Good (74–50)		2	
Fair (49–25)	1		
Poor (24–0)	12	1	
	13	2	1

8 Permanent implantations
56 Months average follow-up

Table 2. *Effect of Epidural Stimulation in Patients with Brachial Plexus Avulsion*

Excellent (100–75)	
Good (74–50)	
Fair (49–25)	1
Poor (24–0)	10

Table 3. *Results of Thalamic Sensory Nucleus Stimulation in Brachial Plexus Avulsion Patients*

Excellent (100–75)	2
Good (74–50)	2
Fair (49–25)	1
Poor (24–0)	3

7 Permanent implantations
21 Months average follow-up

Of the group of 8 patients with cervical nerve root avulsion who received a trial of contralateral thalamic sensory nucleus stimulation, 2 patients continue to have excellent pain relief; 2 have good results, 1 fair, and 3 poor (Table 3). Definitive implantation was performed in 7 patients and their average follow-up had been 21 months. There were no mortalities; there was one complication, a scalp necrosis overlying the screw which required wound revision.

Discussion

From our experience of generally poor results of epidural stimulation for the treatment of brachial plexus avulsion pain, we no longer consider these patients as candidates for a trial of stimulation. Zorub *et al.* reported similar results in a series of 7 patients with brachial plexus avulsion treated with epidural stimulation only 1 of whom obtained excellent pain relief and the remainder poor[18]. We have presented an insufficient number of cases with brachial plexus pain without avulsion to make a definite judgement of its efficacy in these patients; however, we have subsequently had 5 additional patients with brachial plexus pain secondary to malignancy or radiation plexopathy. In this larger group with an average follow-up of at least one year 2 patients have obtained good pain relief, 3 fair, and 3 poor. Presently, we would consider this latter group candidates for epidural stimulation due to the low morbidity and mortality of the procedure. One possible explanation for the poor results of epidural stimulation in avulsion cases is the lack of large myelinated afferent fibers from the affected painful region; thus the inability to stimulate them to effect the pain relief theorized by Melzack and Wall[7]. The loss of input would result in the hyperactivity of the dorsal horn at that level as shown by Loeser and Ward[4], Loeser *et al.*[5], and Lombard and Larabi[6].

Hyperactivity is not limited to the dorsal horn alone. At progressively higher CNS levels abnormal hyperactivity also has been reported. Kjerulf and Loeser[3] recorded neuronal hyperactivity in the lateral cuneate nucleus in 2 day postoperative rhizotomized rats. Nashold and Wilson[11] recorded spontaneous electrical activity in the medial mesencephalic tegmentum characterized by bursts concurrent with episodes of pain in patients with deafferentation pain. In C5—Th1 dorsal rhizotomized rats Albe-Fessard and Lombard[1] have demonstrated trains of rhythmic, 10 Hz slow waves accompanied by bursts of spikes in the thalamic ventralis posterior nucleus zone for forelimb representation in the normal animal, the centralis lateralis nucleus, and in the primary somethesic area of the cortex, again at the region representing the forelimb in the normal animal. The abnormal thalamic activity was seen starting six months following rhizotomy followed by the appearance of abnormal activity of the cortex.

Although the abnormal thalamic activity following deafferentation has been characterized in the chronic animal model only, its potential occurrence in patients with widespread deafferentation pain may serve as an hypothesis for the efficacy of thalamic sensory nucleus stimulation. Modulation or inhibition of this hyperactivity by thalamic stimulation could explain the pain relief provided these patients. We reserve the use of thalamic stimulation for brachial plexus avulsion patients with severe pain that has failed to respond to all conservative therapies. The use of neurostimulation techniques when appropriate is preferable to ablative techniques, especially of the central primary sensory pathways, the lesions of which may result in deafferentation pain[2]. In conclusion we recommend thalamic sensory nucleus stimulation for the treatment of intractable, severe brachial plexus avulsion pain since it avoids additional neurological deficit, does not require a general anesthetic, is completely reversible, and has a low surgical morbidity.

References

1. Albe-Fessard, D., Lombard, M. C., Use of animal model to evaluate the origin of and protection against deafferentation pain. In: Advances in Pain Research and Therapy, Vol. 5 (Bonica, J. J., Lindblom, U., Iggo, A., eds.), pp. 691—700. New York: Raven Press. 1983.
2. Cassinari, V., Pagni, C. A., Central Pain. Cambridge, Massachusetts: Harvard University Press. 1969.
3. Kjerulf, T. D., Loeser, J. D., Neuronal hyperactivity following deafferentation of the lateral cuneate nucleus. Exp. Neurol. *39* (1973), 70.
4. Loeser, J. D., Ward, A., jr., Some effects of deafferentation in neurons of the cat spinal cord. Arch. Neurol. *17* (1967), 629—636.
5. Loeser, J. D., Ward, A., jr., White, L. E., Chronic deafferentation of human spinal cord neurons. J. Neurosurg. *29* (1968), 48—50.
6. Lombard, M. C., Larabi, Y., Electrophysiological study of cervical dorsal horn cells in partially deafferented rats. In: Advances in Pain Research and Therapy. Vol. 5 (Bonica, J. J., Lindblom, U., Iggo, A., eds.), pp. 147—154. New York: Raven Press. 1983.
7. Melzack, R., Wall, P. D., Pain mechanisms: A new theory. Science *150* (1965), 971—979.
8. Mundinger, F., Becker, P., Long-term results of central stereotactic interventions for pain. In: Neurosurgical Treatment in Psychiatry, Pain, and Epilepsy (Sweet, W. H., Obrador, S., Martin-Rodriguez, J. G., eds.), pp. 685—691. Baltimore: University Park Press. 1975.
9. Nashold, B. S., Ostdahl, R., Dorsal root entry zone lesions for pain relief. J. Neurosurg. *51* (1979), 59—69.
10. Nashold, B. S., Urban, B., Zorub, D. S., Phantom pain relief by focal destruction of the substantia gelatinosa of Rolando. In: Advances in Pain Research and Therapy, Vol. 1 (Bonica, J. J., Albe-Fessard, D. G., eds.), pp. 959—963. New York: Raven Press. 1976.
11. Nashold, B. S., jr., Wilson, W. P., Central pain: Observations on man with chronic implanted electrodes in the midbrain tegmentum. Confin. Neurol. *27* (1966), 30—44.
12. Nashold, B. S., jr., Wilson, W. P., Slaughter, D. G., Stereotaxic midbrain lesions for central dysesthesia and phantom pain. J. Neurosurg. *30* (1969), 116—126.
13. Siegfried, J., Neurosurgical treatment for intractable pain of terminal cancer patients. In: The Continuing Care of Terminal Cancer Patients (Twycross, R. G., Ventafridda, V., eds.), pp. 369—376. Oxford: Pergamon. 1980.
14. Siegfried, J., Krayenbühl, H., Einige Erfahrungen über die chirurgische Behandlung medikamentös nicht beeinflußbarer Schmerzzustände. In: Schmerz (Janzen, R., Keidel, W. D., Herz, A., Steichele, C., eds.), p. 217. Stuttgart: Thieme. 1972.
15. Siegfried, J., Zumstein, H., La douleur fantôme et son traitement neurochirurgical. Med. Hyg. *31* (1973), 867—868.
16. Sugita, K., Results of stereotaxic thalamotomy for pain. Confin. Neurol. *34* (1972), 265—274.

17. White, J. C., Sweet, W. H., Pain and the Neurosurgeon. A Forty-year Experience. Springfield, Ill.: Ch. C Thomas. 1969.
18. Zorub, D. S., Nashold, B. S., jr., Cook, W. A., Avulsion of the brachial plexus: I. A review with implications on the therapy of intractable pain. Surg. Neurol. *2* (1974), 347—353.

Acta Neurochirurgica, Suppl. 33, 459—469 (1984)

III. Other Topics on Pain

One Possible Mechanism of Central Pain. Autokindling Phenomenon on the Phantom Limb or Sensory Loss Oriented Patients

S. Tóth[1], A. Sólyom, and Z. Tóth

With 6 Figures

Summary

The authors compares the electrical activity of the specific and non-specific thalamic nuclei in cases of central pain (phantom pain, thalamus pain and anesthesia dolorosa) and in cases of other disturbances. They found that in central pain from these structures chronic paroxysmal activity can be recorded. This process evolves by the patients own abnormal sensory stimuli and is probably an autokindling phenomenon. The authors findings satisfy the necessary conditions of central pain evolvement namely, that the pain appears gradually after the sensory lesion, the pain is progressive in nature and that the evolvement needs the patients personality. In the management of central pain chronic stimulation needs reconsidering because of these results.

Keywords: Central pain; thalamus; irritative mechanism; autokindling; chronic stimulation.

Introduction

The underlying mechanism of central pain (phantom pain, anesthesia dolorosa, thalamus pain) still remains enigmatic despite the considerable effort to solve it. Melzack[6] and later Melzack and Loeser[7] postulated that a lesion of the sensory system results in

[1] National Institute of Neurosurgery, Budapest, Hungary.

hyperactivity in cells lying central from the lesion. According to the gate control theory the pain results from the unbalanced stimuli between C and A fibers[8]. Others emphasize the absence of central inhibitory mechanisms[2,4,11]. Sano[9] postulates reverberating circuits between the specific and non-specific thalamic nuclei originating from the hyperirritability of the sensory nuclei.

The basic mechanism is still a puzzle and considerable pessimism has attended the therapy of central pain because it is very difficult to control either by conservative or by surgical means. One thing is certain; central pain takes time to appear after the lesion in the sensory system, appears gradually and is not consistent with the lesion, sometimes it appears, sometimes not, with the same lesion. It is also probable that the normally evolved body scheme which is in constant need of reinforcement because of the significantly altered sensory experience, undergoes certain changes which play a role in the originating pain[3].

The chronic multielectrode stereoxial method used by us[12,13] made it possible to observe the spontaneous and evoked activity of specific and non-specific sensory structures for a long time in central pain patients and in patients with other disorders. From an incidental observation it was supposed that in patients suffering from central pain the activity of the subcortical sensory structures differs strongly from that observed in other patients.

Materials and Method

The examinations were carried out on 14 patients. Four patients suffered from phantom pain, 3 from anesthesia dolorosa, 3 from thalamus pain and these results were compared with 2 patients suffering from parkinsonism, 1 from hyperkinetic motor disturbance and 1 from obsessive-compulsive symptoms. The activity of the same central structures were compared in these patients.

The following central structures were examined: the ventral posterolateral and posteromedial thalamic nuclei, the centrum medianum, pulvinar and the mesencephalic reticular formation. Chronic gold or platina-irridium electrode bundles were inserted in these structures by the aid of a stereotactic instrument[12,13]. The spontaneous electrical activity was registered, then during the stimulation of one structure we registered the evoked potentials and the evoked electrical activity in the other not stimulated structures.

Registration was carried out with a 16 channel ELEMA-Mingograph and with a MEDICOR MG-42 four channel amplifier. The stimulations were carried out with a DISA Multistim or with a MEDICOR ST-21 stimulator.

Stimulation parameters were 0.5–1 Hz; 0.05 ms; 10–30 V single square pulses and 100 Hz; 0.05 ms, 5–30 V, 500 ms trains.

Results

In the control group of patients with movement disorders or psychiatric symptoms the spontaneous electrical activity of the VPL and VPM, CM, pulvinar and mesencephalic reticular formation did not differ from the electrical activity of the fronto-parietal cortex. The subcortically recorded amplitudes were one third one fourth of the cortically recorded ones (Fig. 1 A and Fig. 2). During the stimulation of one structure the evoked responses occuring in the others were 100–200 ms in duration and were composed of 2–3 waves. The 500 ms trains did not alter the spontaneous activity after a temporary depression (Fig. 2). In contrast, in patients with central pain it was striking that the spontaneous activity in the VPL and VPM and in the CM was dysrhythmic, contained many sharp steep waves and the amplitude was pronounced, sometimes more pronounced than in the cortical activity (Fig. 3 and Fig. 4 A). The activity contained bursts composed of sudden spike like waves (Fig. 3 B and Fig. 5 A, B). If we stimulated one structure from the above mentioned ones with single stimuli, in the others 4–6 Hz waxing-waning steep potential series could be recorded (Fig. 4 B and Fig. 5 C). During 100 Hz, 500 ms train stimulation in the VPL, VPM and in the CM typical electroconvulsive paroxysmal activity occured which was strictly localized within these structures. Only slight traces appeared in the fronto-parietal cortical activity (Fig. 6). These changes were most pronounced in phantom pain but could be observed in anesthesia dolorosa and in thalamic pain as well (Fig. 1 B).

Discussion

From these studies we postulate that in central pain the spontaneous and evoked electrical activity in the specific and non-specific thalamic nuclei are characteristically paroxysmal and this activity can be strongly enhanced within these structures from each other. Because central pain evolves gradually (if our results can be related to central pain) these changes must evolve also gradually. In patients suffering from other disorders than central pain the electrical activity of the thalamic nuclei is of low amplitude resembling cortical activity as found by other authors as well[1,10,14].

Gücer *et al.*[5] in central pain—unlike us—described delta spindles parallel with delta spindles recorded over the cortex. Their patients had thalamic pain.

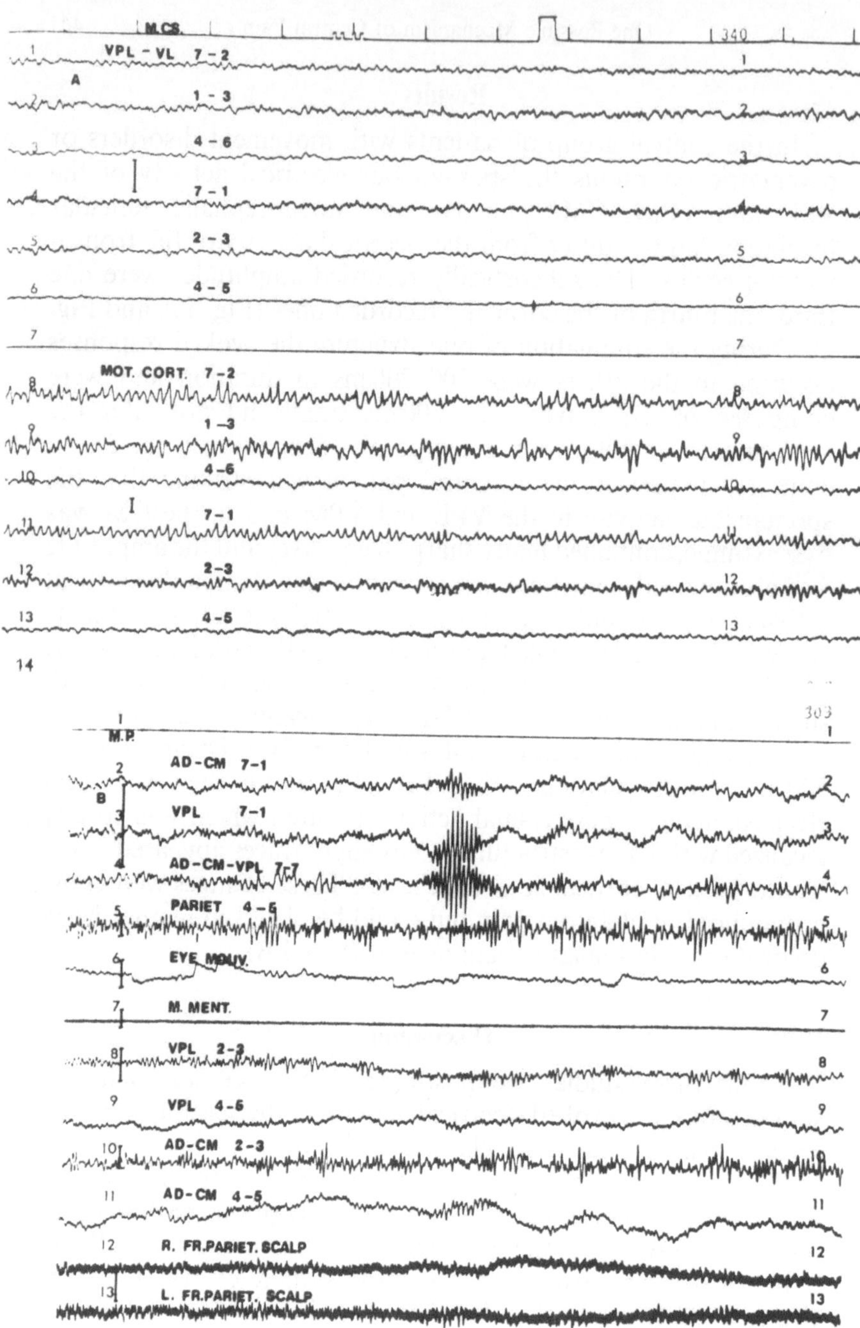

Fig. 1. A) Patient with movement disorder. Electrical activity of the thalamus and motor cortex. Calibration: 70 microV for the thalamus, 200 microV for the motor cortex. B) Electrical activity of the thalamus and the cortex of a patient with thalamic pain. Pronounced burst like spindles in the VPL (channel 3) and in the CM-VPL connection (channel 4). Calibration: 30 microV for channels 1–3.150 microV for channel 4,70 microV for channel 7–8,100 microV for channel 9–11 and 70 microV for channel 12–13

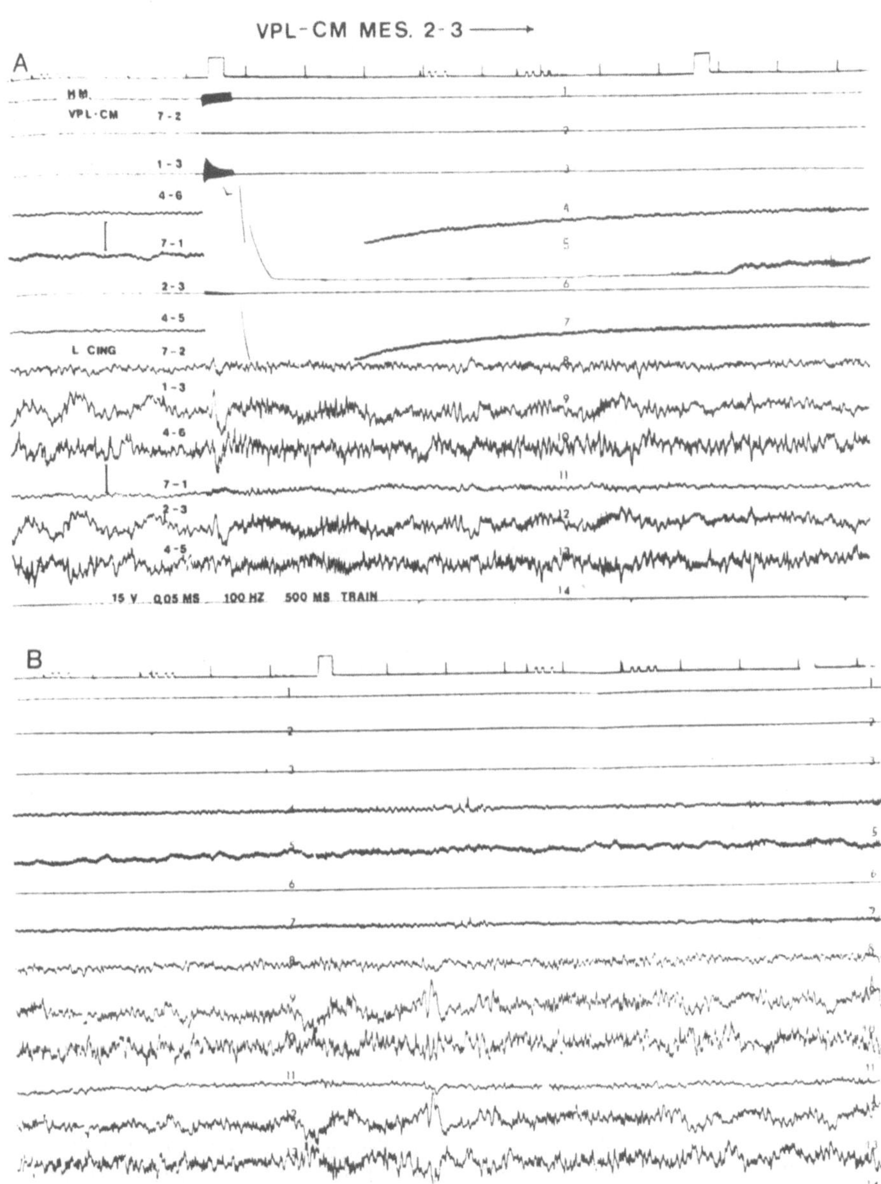

Fig. 2. Electrical activity of a patient with obsessive-compulsive symptoms. Thalamus and cingular cortex activity after the stimulation of the VPL. A continues in B

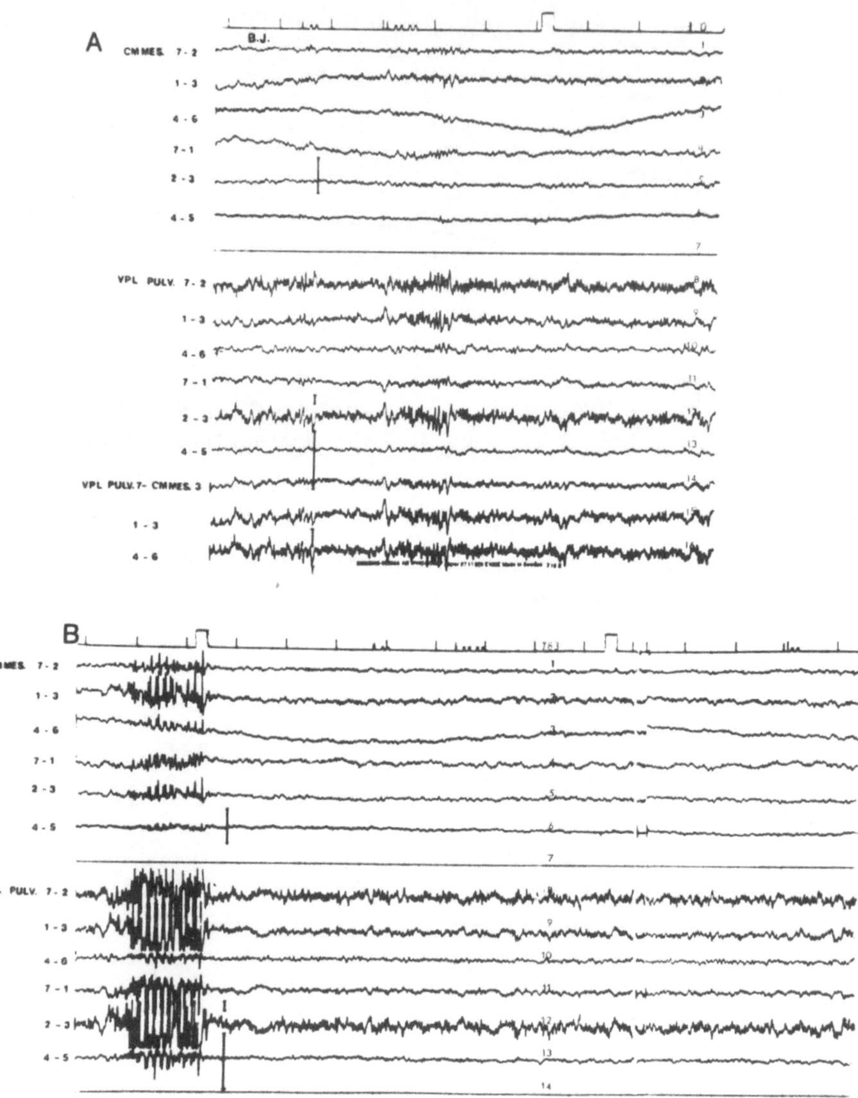

Fig. 3. A) Electrical activity of the CM, mesencephalic reticular formation VPL and pulvinar of a patient with phantom limb pain. Calibration: 50 microV for channels 1–6,200 microV for channel 8–12,30 microV for channel 13 and 100 microV for channel 14–16. B) Burst like activity of CM and VPL in the same patient. Calibration as in A

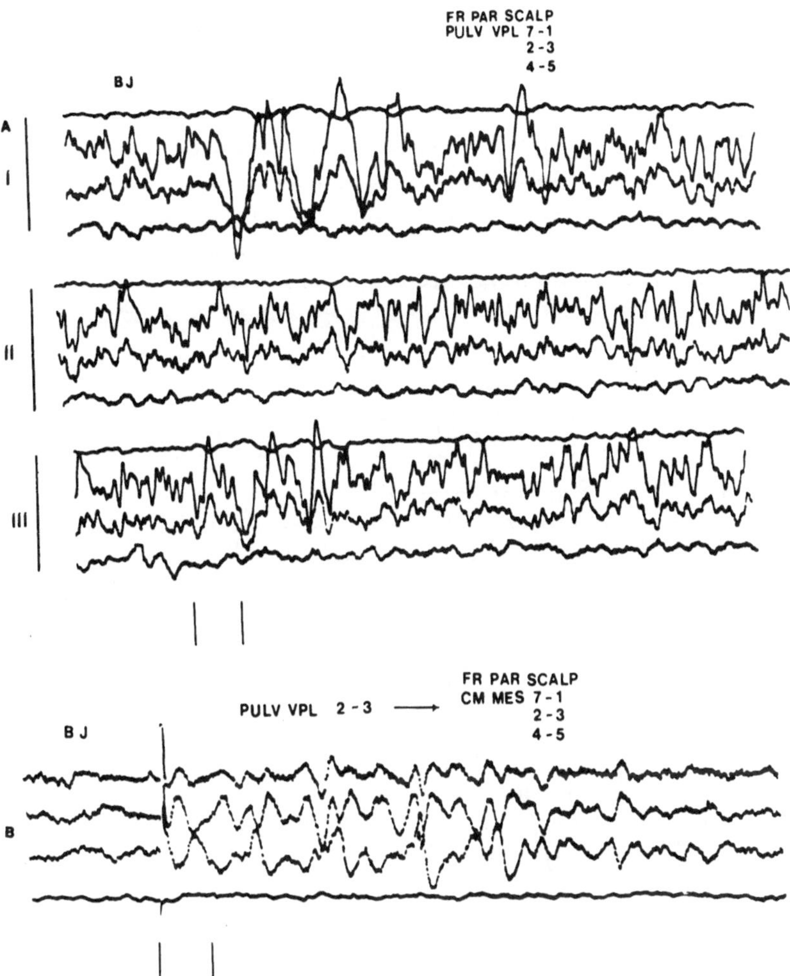

Fig. 4. A) Electrical activity of the VPL, pulvinar and fronto-parietal cortex of a patient with phantom limb pain. Dysrhythmic high amplitude activity in the VPL. Low amplitude activity in the cortex and pulvinar. I continues as II and III. Calibration: 50 microV for the cortex and 20 microV for the thalamus, 100 ms. B) Evoked potential in the CM and mesencephalic reticular formation in the same patient as in A, after the stimulation of the VPL (0.5 Hz, 10 V, 0.05 ms). Calibration: is the same as in A

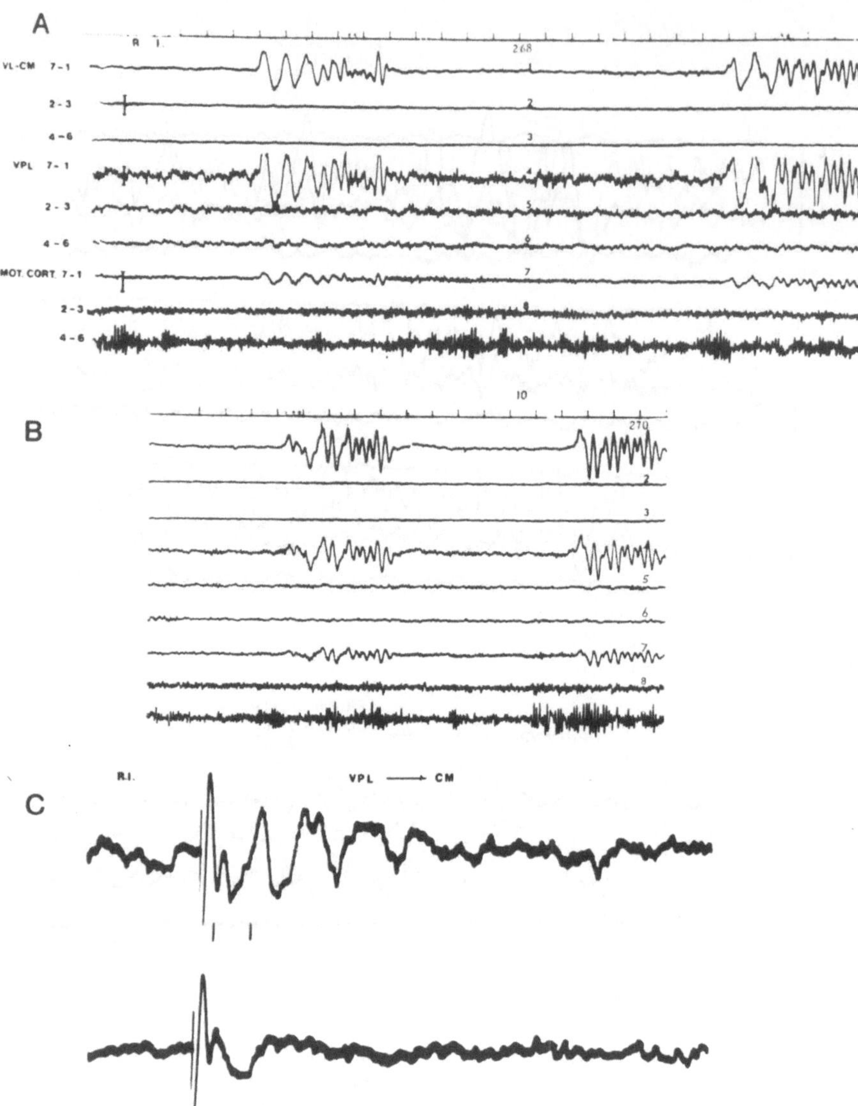

Fig. 5. A) Electrical activity of the thalamus and the motor cortex of a patient with phantom limb pain. Burst like activity in the CM and in the VPL only with traces of this activity in the neighbouring structures and in the motor cortex. Calibration: 100 microV. B) The same as in A. C) Evoked potential in the CM of the same patient as in A after the stimulation of the VPL

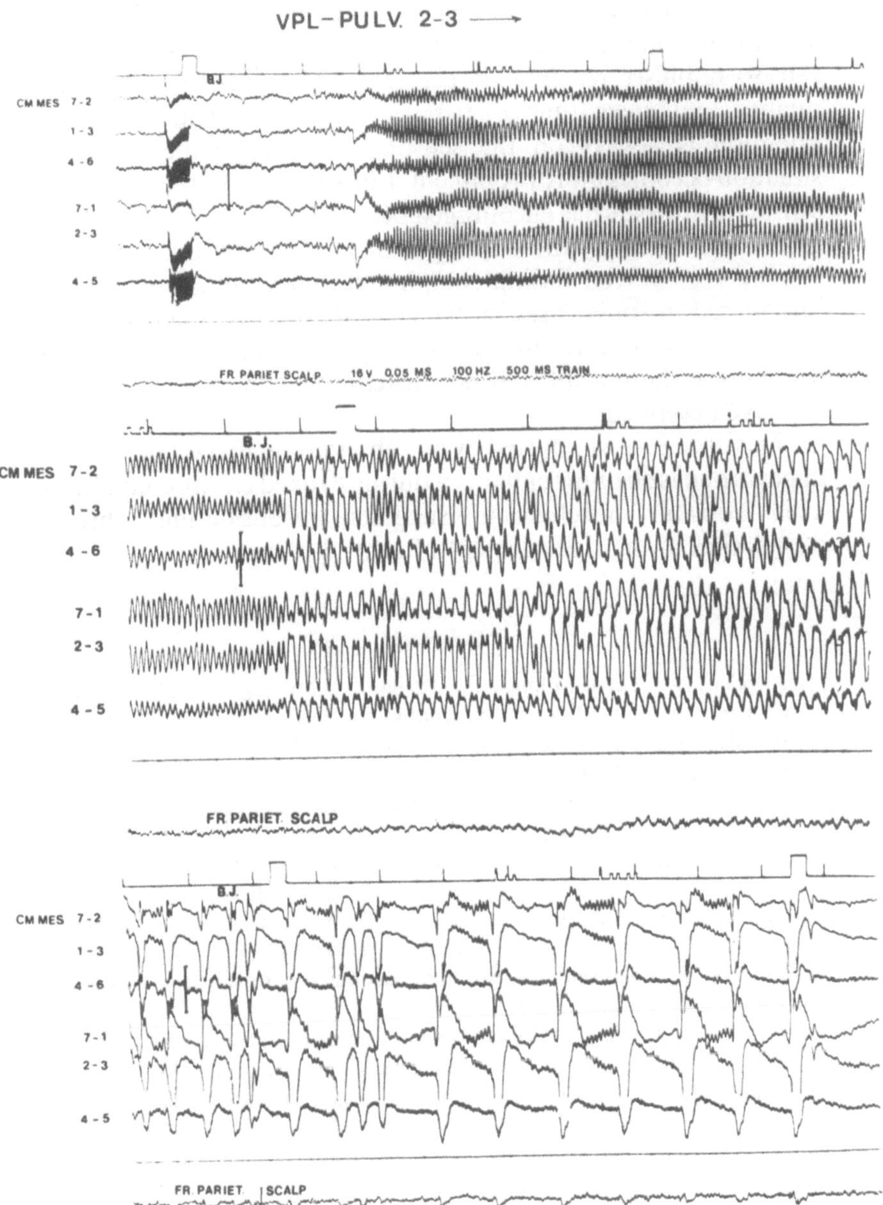

Fig. 6. Electrical activity of the CM and mesencephalic reticular formation after the train stimulation of the VPL. The ectroconvulsive paroxysmal activity is more pronounced in the CM and no trace of this activity can be seen on the fronto parietal cortex. Calibration: 50 microV. Patient with phantom limb pain

Central pain develops when following a lesion in the sensory system, the normal quality and normal space-time distributed sensory impulses, reaching the central systems, change to abnormal quality and space-time distributed impulses. If the patient's attention is always on the sensory disturbance the abnormal situation becomes more prominent. Enhancement of the area of the sensory disturbance is encouraged because the body scheme alters, as demonstrated by the development of the phantom sensation. Finally the evolved feeling-complex becomes unbearable and is interpreted in some cases by the central nervous system as pain. This process is reflected by the probably autokindling phenomenon localized in the specific and non-specific thalamic sensory system we have described.

This opinion is supported by our observation that phantom pain appears and is strongly enhanced during evoked electroconvulsion. This possible mechanism suggests reconsidering chronic stimulation in the management of central pain.

References

1. Angeleri, F., Ferro-Milone, F., Parigi, S., Prolonged implantation of electrodes in man. EEG clin. Neurophys. *16* (1964), 100—129.
2. Bowsher, D., The anatomy of thalamic pain. J. Neurology, Neurosurg. Psychiat. *22* (1959), 81—82.
3. Deák, Gy., Tóth, S., Die Behandlung des Phantomschmerzes durch postzentrale Topectomie. Arch. Psychiat. Nervenkr. *208* (1966), 482.
4. Fields, H., Adams, J. E., Pain following cerebral injury relieved by electrical stimulation of the internal capsule. Brain *97* (1974), 169—178.
5. Gücer, G., Niedermayer, E., Lowy, D. M., Thalamic EEG recordings in patients with chronic pain. J. Neurol. *219* (1978), 47—61.
6. Melczak, R., Phantom limb pain: implications for treatment of pathologic pain. Anestesiology *35* (1971), 409—419.
7. Melczak, R., Loeser, D. J., Phantom body pain in paraplegics: evidence for a central "pattern generating mechanism" for pain. Pain *4* (1978), 195—210.
8. Melczak, R., Wall, P. D., Pain mechanism: A new theory. Science *150* (1965), 971—979.
9. Sano, K., The role of internal medullary lamina in pain. Anales del XII Congreso Latinamericano del Neurochirurgia, pp. 937—952. Lima: Peru. 1967.
10. Okuma, T., Shimazono, Y., Fukuda, T., Narabayashi, H., Cortical and subcortical recordings in non-anesthetized periods in man. EEG clin. Neurophys. *6* (1954), 269—286.
11. Shimazu, H., Yanashigawa, N., Garoute, B., Corticopyramidal influences on thalamic somatosensory transmission in the cat. Jap. J. Neurophys. *15* (1965), 101—124.

12. Tóth, S., Effect of electrical stimulation of subcortical sites on speech and consciousness. In: Neurophysiology Studied on Man (Soemjen, G., ed.), pp. 40—46. Amsterdam: Excerpta Medica. 1972.
13. Tóth, S., Vajda, J., Multitarget technique in Parkinson surgery. Appl. Neurophys. *43* (1980), 109—113.
14. Walker, A. E., Marshall, C., The contribution of depth recording to clinical medicine. EEG clin. Neurophys. *16* (1964), 88—89.

Acta Neurochirurgica, Suppl. 33, 471—472 (1984)

Tic Douloureux Treated by the Injection of Glycerol into the Retrogasserian Subarachnoid Space Longterm Results

S. Håkanson[1]

During the period 1976–1983 about 250 patients suffering from genuine trigeminal neuralgia have been treated by the injection of pure sterile glycerol into the trigeminal cistern.

The subarachnoid space (the trigeminal cistern) behind the trigeminal ganglion was punctured by a needle (22 G OD 0.7) introduced through the foramen ovale by the anterior percutaneous route. Following spontaneous CSF drainage a contrast medium, metrizamide (Amipaque®), was injected to assure an intracisternal position of the tip of the needle. A small amount of glycerol (0.20–0.30 ml) was injected after removal of the contrast medium. The procedure is only slightly painful for the patient and can be performed under light premedication and local anesthesia only. Electric stimulation or intraoperative sensory testing is not required.

Following a latent period of up to five days about 95% of the patients are pain free. In a group of patients (100) observed during a mean follow-up of close to 4 years (range 3–8 years) 78% of the patients are still completely pain free following the first injection (58%) or one or two reinjcctions (20%).

The treatment causes only slight sensory disturbances as measured by clinical examinations or quantitative measurements of tactile or thermal thresholds. About 60% of the patients noted a slight numbness, but no cases of dysesthesia, anesthesia dolorosa or involvement of other cranial nerves have been observed in these patients. It is proposed that glycerol injected into the trigeminal cistern acts mainly on the large fiber spectrum. Large fibers with

[1] Department of Neurosurgery, Karolinska Sjukhuset, Stockholm, Sweden.

segmental demyelination, supposedly involved in the pathophysiology of trigeminal neuralgia, may be particularly vulnerable to the slightly neurotoxic effect of glycerol.

Reference

Håkanson, S., Trigeminal neuralgia treated by injection of glycerol into the trigeminal cistern. Neurosurgery *9* (1981), 638—646.

Acta Neurochirurgica, Suppl. 33, 473—478 (1984)

Neurophysiological and Ultrastructural Study of the So-called Microcompression of the Gasserian Ganglion in the Treatment of Trigeminal Neuralgia

S. Esposito[1], A. Delitala[1], A. Canova[1], P. Bruni[1], M. Colangeli[1], and D. Sollazzo[2]

With 2 Figures

Summary

The present paper reports a comparative study about the immediate and short term results in a series of 15 patients treated with the new technique of microcompression, 15 with glycerol injection and 15 with thermorhizotomy. From a structural and ultrastructural study of the Gasserian ganglion after microcompression in rabbits and from the trigeminal somatosensory evoked potentials (TSEP) in 45 patients treated with the three different techniques, the authors put forward the assumption that it should be possible to make an estimation of the long-term results in the microcompression and glycerol procedures too.

Keywords: Trigeminal neuralgia; balloon percutaneous microcompression; evoked potentials; glycerol; ultrastructure.

Introduction

In addition to the many techniques already employed in the treatment of trigeminal neuralgia, the "percutaneous microcompression of the Gasserian ganglion" has been proposed by Mullan and realized by Bricolo[4]. This technique arises from some observations, mostly empiric, published in the past about the relief from trigeminal neuralgia in patients undergoing a compression of the ganglion of Gasser[14].

[1] Division of Neurosurgery "G. Lancisi", S. Camillo Hospital, Roma, Italy.
[2] Service of Neurophysiopathology, S. Camillo Hospital, Roma, Italy.

Material and Methods

Since the relation of Bricolo at the 31. Annual Meeting of the Italian Neurosurgical Society, held in Rome in November 1982[4], we began to treat patients suffering from trigeminal neuralgia with the original procedure of percutaneous microcompression of Gasserian ganglion, as well as with the classic technique of thermorhizotomy according to Sweet[17] and the method of intracisternal glycerol according to Håkanson[11]. Under brief general anesthesia with 10 ml of Propanidide (Epontol) in the patient already premedicated with 50 mg of chloride-prometazine (Fargan), a 14 gauge needle is placed into the trigeminal cistern via the foramen ovale, under intermittent fluoroscopic control, by the usual anterior percutaneous route.

The fluoroscopic control testifies the correct placement of the needle behind the Gasserian ganglion. The CSF leak confirms the introduction of the needle into the cistern, but is not absolutely necessary. A No. 4 Fogarty catheter is inserted into the cistern via the needle; it is then filled with 0.5–0.6 ml of an hydrosoluble contrast media (Metrizamide or Iopamiro 300) per 6 minutes. When the compression is finished, the balloon is deflated and removed (Fig. 1).

We prefer to perform this procedure under brief general anesthesia, as it does not require any collaboration from the patient, but it is also possible under local anesthesia. The relief from pain is generally immediate. No impairment of the tactile and deep sensitivities is observed. The corneal reflex is always saved. We have treated 15 patients with this technique of microcompression and 15 with the Håkanson's glycerol procedure. In all cases there has been an immediate relief from pain. At a short term follow-up (an average of 3 months) all but one patient treated with microcompression technique were free from pain. The case with recurrence 2 months after the procedure was again treated by the same method; he is now free from pain 3 months after the last operation. No complication has been observed.

As it is too early to take an opinion about the effectiveness of this procedure, like the Håkanson's one, for the lack of a long term follow-up, we have studied the possible structural and ultrastructural changes of the Gasserian ganglion after microcompression in rabbits.

Two rabbits, under general anesthesia, underwent open exposures of the Gasserian ganglion; a finger compression per 6 minutes was performed. The animals were killed 24 hours after the operation, and a light- and electron-microscope study of the ganglion made. No significant changes in the cells and the fibers of the ganglion has been observed.

Trigeminal somatosensory evoked potentials (TSEP) have been recorded in 15 patients treated with microcompression of the Gasserian ganglion, 15 with the Håkanson's procedure of glycerol injection and 15 with thermorhizotomy before and 1 month after the operation.

In all 45 cases, but one, the same changes of the responses after the operation have been observed; they were mostly a reduction in number of the earlier waves recorded (with latencies less than 18 msec), and a general reduction in amplitude of the responses (Fig. 2).

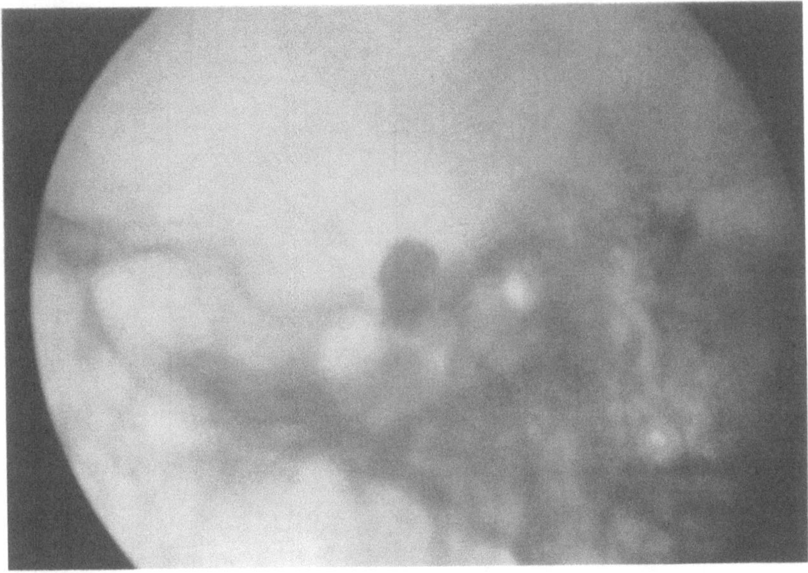

Fig. 1. The balloon of the Fogarty catheter, correctly placed behind the gasserian ganglion, is filled with 0.6 ml of contrast media for 6 minutes

Discussion

The decompressive method of Gasserian ganglion in the treatment of trigeminal neuralgia has been proposed many years ago[18]. However, compression rather than decompression was already mentioned as early as 1955 by Shelden and Pudenz[14]. Bricolo first applied this percutaneous compression[4] in a series of 51 patients with good results; he reports a relatively high percentage of recurrence of pain, but apparently due to an insufficient compression (less than 6 minutes). Our 15 cases with immediate and short-time results, confirm his opinions.

Beaver[1] and Kerr[12] described the light and electron microscope observations in biopsies of the trigeminal ganglion in patients suffering from neuralgia. They found a peculiar irregular vacuolization which gave to cytoplasm a fenestrated appearance[1]. We did not observed any changes in the Gasserian ganglion of the animals which underwent compression. This finding adds little to the possible mechanism of action of the microcompressive method, but it shows that the compression acts only on a ganglion already modified by the "lesions" underlying the trigeminal neuralgia. It is

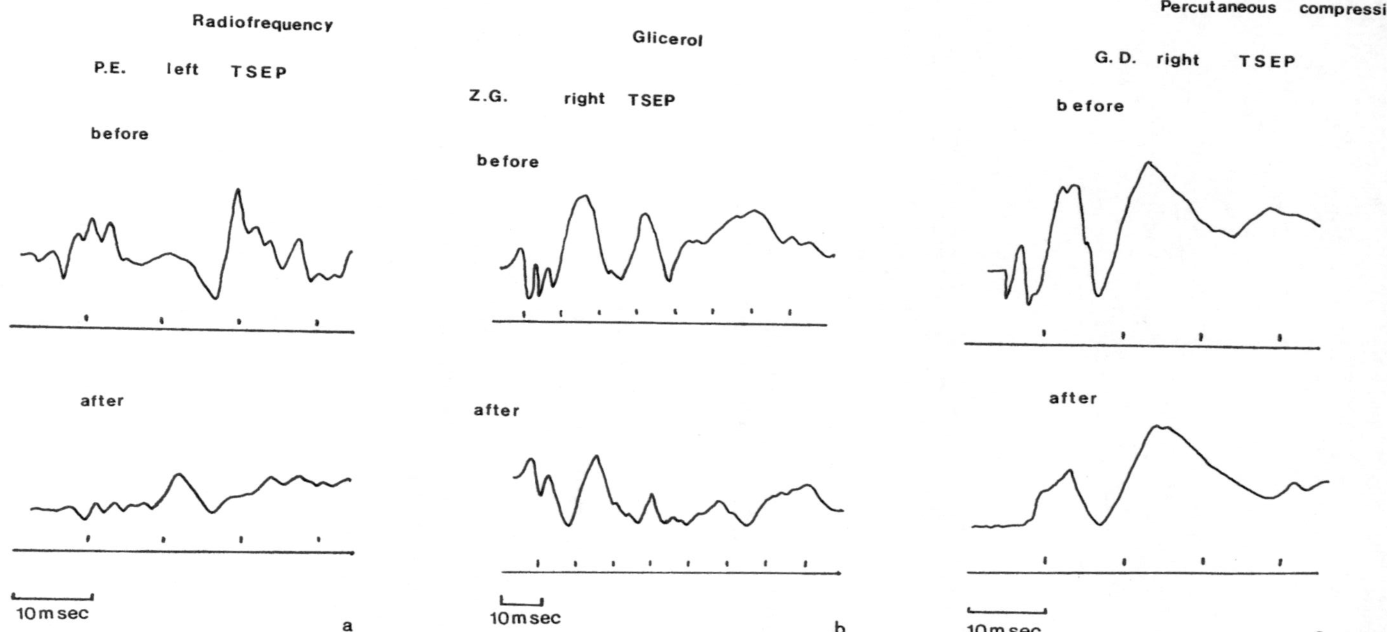

Fig. 2. The study of the trigeminal somatosensory evoked potentials (TSEP) shows the same changes, after the operation, in the three different procedures (Thermorhizotomy, left; glycerol, centre; microcompression, right)

in accord with the hypothesis about the possible mechanism of action of the thermorhizotomy[5,7,9,15,17] and glycerol[11] on the trigeminal neuralgia.

In other words, the compression did not change the trigeminal system of the rabbits because it was perfectly integral.

For the lack of long-term results in this new procedure and since many series have been published reporting the good results of the thermorhizotomy[10,15,17], we compared the neurophysiological findings (TSEP) of our series treated with the three different procedures. In literature there are few studies on the trigeminal evoked potentials[2,3,5–9,13,16]. Our findings reporting the same changes of the TSEP in every method let us put forward the opinion that the three different techniques produce the same neurophysiological changes.

A prevision about the long-term results in the microcompressive method should be likewise possible. The clinical long-term results will say the last word.

References

1. Beaver, D. L., Electron microscopy of the Gasserian ganglion in trigeminal neuralgia. J. Neurosurg. *26* (1967), 138—150.
2. Bennet, M. H., Jannetta, P. J., Evoked potentials in trigeminal neuralgia. Presented at the Annual Meeting of the American Association of Neurological Surgeons, New York, April, 1980.
3. Bennet, M. H., Jannetta, P. J., Trigeminal evoked potentials in humans. Electroenceph. clin. Neurophysiol. *48* (1980), 517—526.
4. Bricolo, A., Microcompressione percutanea del ganglio di Gasser nel trattamento della nevralgia del trigemino. Presented at the 31. Annual Meeting of the Italian Society of Neurosurgery, Rome, 1982. Acta Neurochir. (Wien) *69* (1983), 102.
5. Broggi, G., Siegfried, J., The effect of graded thermocoagulation on trigeminal evoked potentials in the cat. Acta Neurochir. (Wien) Suppl. *24* (1977), 175—178.
6. Drechsler, F., Short and long latency cortical potentials following trigeminal nerve stimulation in man. In: Evoked Potentials. Proceeding of an International Evoked Potentials Symposium held in Nottingham, England (Barber, C., ed.), pp. 515—522. Lancaster, England: MTP Press. 1980.
7. Drechsler, F., Wickboldt, G., Neuhauser, B., *et al.*, Somatosensory trigeminal evoked potentials in normal subjects and in patients with trigeminal neuralgia before and after thermocoagulation of the ganglion Gasseri. Electroenceph. clin. Neurophysiol. *43* (1977), 496 (abstract).
8. Findler, G., Feinsod, M., Sensory evoked response to electrical stimulation of the trigeminal nerve in humans. J. Neurosurg. *56* (1982), 545—549.

9. Frigyesi, T. L., Broggi, G., Siegfried, J., Evoked potentials in the trigeminal dorsal root: their selective vulnerability to graded thermocoagulation. Exp. Neurol. *49* (1975), 11—21.
10. Guidetti, B., Fraioli, B., Sul trattamento chirurgico della nevralgia del trigemino. Il dolore *1* (1979), 33—40.
11. Håkanson, S., Trigeminal neuralgia treated by the injection of glycerol into the trigeminal cistern. Neurosurgery *9* (1981), 638—646.
12. Kerr, F. W., Pathology of trigeminal neuralgia: light and electron microscopic observations. J. Neurosurg. *26* (1967), 151—156.
13. Salar, G., Job, I., Mingrino, S., Cortical evoked responses before and after percutaneous thermocoagulation of the Gasserian ganglion. Preliminary report. Appl. Neurophysiol. *44* (1981), 355—362.
14. Shelden, C. H., Pudenz, R. H., Freshwater, D. B., Compression rather than decompression for trigeminal neuralgia. J. Neurosurg. *12* (1955), 123—126.
15. Siegfried, J., 500 percutaneous thermocoagulations of the Gasserian ganglion for trigeminal pain. Surg. Neurol. *8* (1977), 126—131.
16. Stohr, M., Petruch, F., Somatosensory evoked potentials following stimulation of the trigeminal nerve in man. J. Neurol. *220* (1979), 95—98.
17. Sweet, W. H., Wepsic, J. G., Controlled thermocoagulation of trigeminal ganglion and rootlets for differential destruction pain fibers. Part 1: Trigeminal neuralgia. J. Neurosurg. *39* (1974), 143—156.
18. Taarnhoj, P., Decompression of the trigeminal root and the posterior part of the ganglion as treatment in trigeminal neuralgia: preliminary communication. J. Neurosurg. *25* (1966), 370—373.

Acta Neurochirurgica, Suppl. 33, 479—480 (1984)

Longterm Results of Stimulation via an Implanted Gasserian Electrode for Atypical Trigeminal Pain

B. A. Meyerson[1] and **S. Håkanson**

It is well known that facial pain due to injury to the peripheral trigeminal neuron is extremely difficult to alleviate. Typically, such pain does not respond to carbamazepin and analgesics. There is often a history of surgery or trauma in the territory of the peripheral trigeminal nerve and often the pain can be interpreted as being of dental origin. These patients often present with complex changes of facial sensibility in the form of hyperpathia, dysesthesia and hyperalgesia. The pain is generally continuous and lacks the characteristic paroxysmal character of tic douloureux. Sometimes this pain condition responds favourably to transcutaneous nerve stimulation but a more effective pain relief can be obtained by direct stimulation of the trigeminal ganglion and rootlets via a bipolar electrode. This method was first reported in 1979.

Although the selection of patients for this type of treatment in most cases can be made on the basis of their response to TNS, direct stimulation via a percutaneously introduced lead electrode in the trigeminal cistern has proven to be a more reliable method. Such temporary test stimulation can be performed for several days and the stimulation-produced paresthesiae are felt very similar to those evoked by stimulation with an electrode implanted epidurally into the trigeminal cistern.

To date, 11 patients have been permanently implanted, and follow-up for 7 of them ranges between 3–5½ years. All these patients have retained a good or even excellent clinical effect. Two other patients who have been followed for 6–12 months respectively also experience excellent pain relief. In one patient treated for trigeminal pain following surgery of the maxillary sinus, the effect was good for almost one year but then it failed in spite of

[1] Department of Neurosurgery, Karolinska Sjukhuset, Stockholm, Sweden.

satisfactory functioning of the equipment and stimulation-produced paresthesiae covering the entire painful area. In addition to this patient there are two other who have had no benefit of the treatment. Thus, of 12 patients permanently implanted 9 have had a clinically useful result and 3 have failed.

Temporary percutaneous test stimulation was performed in 5 patients and 3 had good result (two have been permanently implanted and one is scheduled for implantation). The duration of the poststimulatory effect varies considerably, in a few patients being 12–48 hours and in others generally not more than 1–2 hours. One single patient has no poststimulatory effect at all and has to stimulate himself continuously. It can be concluded that for atypical trigeminal pain stimulation via an electrode implanted onto the Gasserian ganglion may provide an effective relief. In comparison with other forms of afferent stimulation the efficacy of this type of stimulation appears to persist. The possibility of performing temporary test stimulation has been found to be very useful in selecting patients for implantation. Work is in progress to develop a system for percutaneous permanent implantation.

Reference

Meyerson, B. A., Håkanson, S., Alleviation of atypical trigeminal pain by stimulation of the Gasserian ganglion via an implanted electrode. Acta Neurochir. (Wien) Suppl. *30* (1980), 303—309.

Acta Neurochirurgica, Suppl. 33, 481—486 (1984)

Radiofrequency Electrical Stimulation of the Gasserian Ganglion in Patients with Atypical Trigeminal Pain. Methods of Percutaneous Temporary Test-stimulation and Permanent Implantation of Stimulation Devices

U. Steude[1]

With 4 Figures

Summary

The problem of treating patients with atypical trigeminal neuralgia, particularly in the presence of sensory deficits (anesthesia dolorosa) has not been satisfactorily solved. While percutaneous thermocoagulation represents the method of choice for the treatment of idiopathic trigeminal neuralgia it is not effective in cases with atypical trigeminal neuralgia and may even result in a worsening of symptoms. In the present report, a method is described—similar to the technique of percutaneous spinal cord stimulation with the use of "Pisces"—permitting percutaneous test stimulation of the trigeminal ganglion. This method was used in 10 patients with atypical trigeminal neuralgia. In 3 patients responding satisfactorily to the test stimulation, permanent electrodes were implanted into the trigeminal ganglion and connected to a monopolar receiving unit. Postoperative observation periods ranged from 6 months to 3.5 years.

Introduction

The treatment of atypical trigeminal neuralgia and anesthesia dolorosa remains an unresolved problem. Whereas selective percutaneous thermocoagulation of the trigeminal ganglion represents the treatment of choice in cases of idiopathic trigeminal

---

[1] Neurochirurgische Klinik, Klinikum Grosshadern, Marchioninistrasse 15, D-8000 München 70, Federal Republic of Germany.

neuralgia (supported by our own experience with 750 procedures) thermocoagulation used in atypical trigeminal neuralgia may even result in a worsening of the clinical condition[2,3]. The need for destructive procedures in atypical trigeminal neuralgia has therefore been questioned. Characteristically, in atypical trigeminal neuralgia there is a long lasting, burning pain sensation without any typical attacks. The patient's history frequently reveals multiple interventions involving the maxillary sinus for the treatment of chronic infections, dental extractions or orthodontic interventions. As a rule, we find a more or less marked sensory loss as a result of previous interventions in the vicinity of the trigeminal nerve. Following our experience that satisfactory results could be obtained in cases of anesthesia dolorosa by stereotactic electrostimulation with electrodes implanted in the periventricular grey matter, some years ago we tried electrostimulation of the brain stem and of the trigeminal nuclei[4]. Electrodes were inserted between C_1 and C_2 according to the procedure used for percutaneous chordotomy and then guided cranially through the foramen occipitale magnum and finally placed within the area of the cerebello-pontine angle. Subsequently, Meyerson[1] reported on electrostimulation of the trigeminal ganglion using a craniotomy and surgically implanted electrodes. Selection of patients for this procedure was done according to transcutaneous nerve stimulation. In patients with atypical facial pain, particularly those presenting with a sensory deficit, it was thought to be of advantage to use a percutaneously placed electrode guided into the trigeminal ganglion for test stimulation or permanent implantation. Straumann & Avery made an electrode modified in accordance with our suggestions, which can be introduced into the ganglion under X-ray control for stimulation purposes (Fig. 1).

Clinical Material

Patients were divided into two groups.

Group 1. Six patients with atypical trigeminal neuralgia secondary to chronic maxillary sinusitis or multiple dental procedures. All patients in this group had had previous procedures for trigeminal pain such as electrocoagulation, thermocoagulation or extradural sensory root section. Neurologic examination in all six patients revealed analgesia and marked hypaesthesia.

Group 2. Four patients with postherpetic neuralgia mainly involving the first and less often also the second devision of the trigeminal nerve. In all patients pain had persisted for years and a sensory deficit was noted with corresponding alterations of the skin.

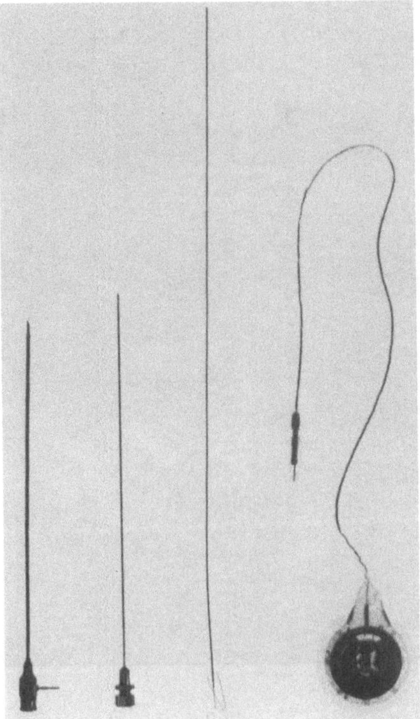

Fig. 1. Set for implantation of the electrode and the receiver system

Technique

The procedure was done under local anaesthesia combined with shortlasting barbiturates. As in selective percutaneous thermocoagulation, the foramen ovale was penetrated and the needle is further advanced intracranially under X-ray control until it's tip come close to the clivus. A brief stimulation test was done and thereafter the electrode introduced, again under X-ray control, until it's tip lay at least at the same height as the clivus. Test stimulation was then repeated and the cannula withdrawn. The electrode was secured to the skin using a single suture. Thereafter test stimulation was continued for the next 3 to 4 days with the patient able to adjust the intensity of the current as well as the frequency (Figs. 2–4).

Results

Amelioration or relief of pain could not be achieved in patients with anesthesia dolorosa secondary to postherpetic neuralgia inspite of adequate stimulation paresthesia which was obtained in

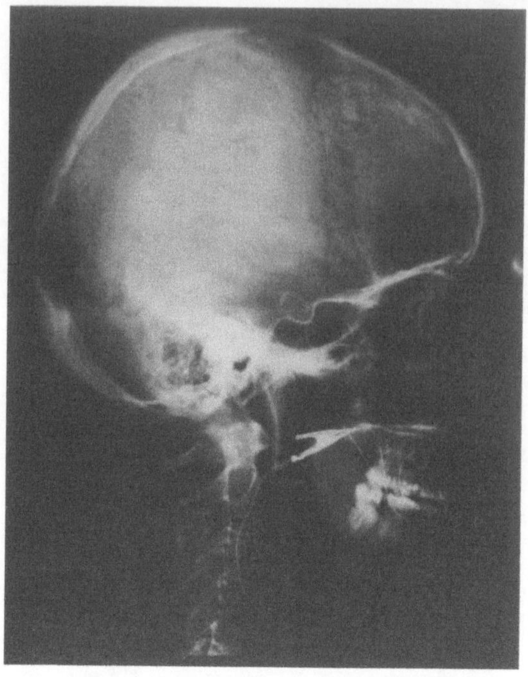

Fig. 2. Lateral X-ray view of the skull within the electrode in the Gasserian ganglion

the non-involved divisions of the trigeminal nerve. Three patients of group 1 with anesthesia dolorosa secondary to atypical trigeminal neuralgia and multiple previous pain procedures reported a marked improvement or even complete relief of pain. All of these patients had anesthesia dolorosa within the second and third division of the trigeminal nerve. In the other patients who did not show any satisfactory response to stimulation, the first division of the nerve was also involved. It is suggested that in the non-responding patients the lesion was retroganglionic and more pronounced. In view of the good results that were obtained in three patients, permanent implantation of electrodes was performed. Following test stimulation, under X-ray control an electrode was advanced into the trigeminal ganglion. The receiving unit for the monopolar stimulation was implanted into the infraclavicular groove and both parts were then connected subcutaneously. All three patients subsequently reported a marked improvement of their symptoms with the postoperative follow-up period varying

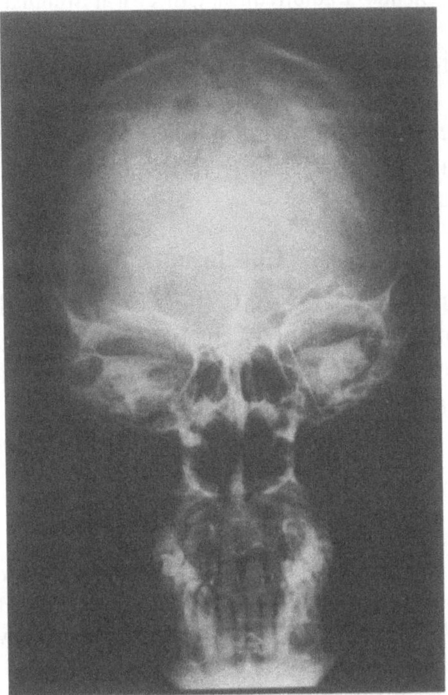

Fig. 3. a.p. X-ray view of the skull with the electrode within the Gasserian ganglion

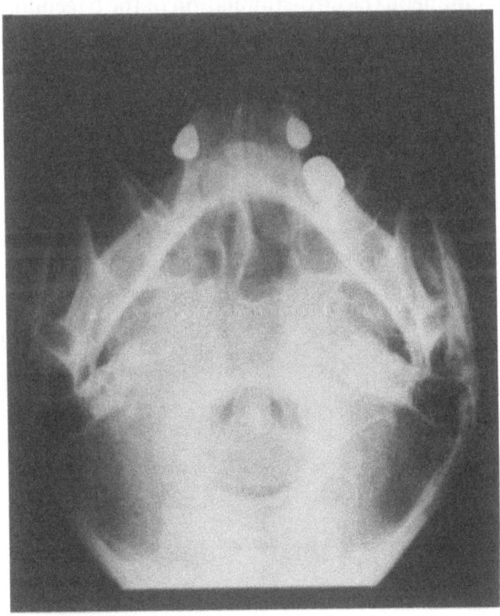

Fig. 4. X-ray view of the base of the skull within the electrode in the Gasserian ganglion penetrating the foramen ovale

from 6 months to 3½ years. No change of the position of the electrode was noted. In one patient, the receiving unit had to be temporarily removed following a local infection. After complete healing the unit was successfully re-implanted.

Conclusion

These results indicate that the present method facilitates percutaneous test stimulation of the trigeminal ganglion in patients undergoing pain treatment by electrostimulation. In addition, this method also allows permanent implantation of electrodes for stimulation of the ganglion in a similar way to lumbar stimulation.

References

1. Meyerson, B. A., Håkanson, S., Alleviation of atypical trigeminal pain by stimulation of the Gasserian ganglion via an implanted electrode. Acta Neurochir. (Wien) Suppl. *30* (1980), 303—309. Wien-New York: Springer. 1980.
2. Siegfried, J., Neurochirurgische Behandlung der symptomatischen und atypischen Gesichtsschmerzen. Münch. med. Wschr. *120* (1978), 675—678.
3. Sweet, W. H., Controlled thermocoagulation of trigeminal ganglion and rootlets for differential destruction of pain fibers: Facial pain other than trigeminal neuralgia. Clin. Neurosurg. *237* (1976), 96—102.
4. Steude, U., Percutaneous electro-stimulation of the trigeminal nerve in patients with atypical trigeminal neuralgia. Neurochirurgia *21* (1978), 66—69.

Acta Neurochirurgica, Suppl. 33, 487—490 (1984)

Results to Explain the Mechanism of Certain Chronic Pain Syndrome with the Method of Evoked Sensory Potentials and Power Spectra Density Analysis

R. Kálmánchey[1], **S. Tóth, I. Kismarty-Lechner,** and **A. Sólyom**

With 4 Figures

Keywords: Thalamic and phantom limb pain; deep electrodes; acoustic and visual evoked potentials; power spectra density analysis.

We have attempted to study differences in the mechanism of generation of phantom pain and thalamic pain.

Methods

Two patients with thalamic pain and phantom pain were investigated by chronically implanted multielectrodes probes. Electrical activity was registered in sensory cortex, motor cortex, n. ret. thalami, centrum medianum, CGM, mesencephalon, n. ant. thalami, fornix, pulvinar thalami, scalp. Power spectra density of EEG, averaged visual and acoustic evoked potentials and power spectra density of evoked potentials and that of the periods before stimuli were analyzed.

Results

1. Lower power density of alpha activity was found in thalamic pain (in each structure) than in phantom pain (Fig. 1).

2. Peak latencies of the slow components of visual evoked potentials (VEP) were greater in thalamic pain than in phantom pain. Appearing VEP was more consequent and less variable in sensory cortex at thalamus pain, than in phantom pain (Fig. 2).

---

[1] National Institute of Neurosurgery and [2] Semmelweis University Medical School Data Center, Budapest, Hungary.

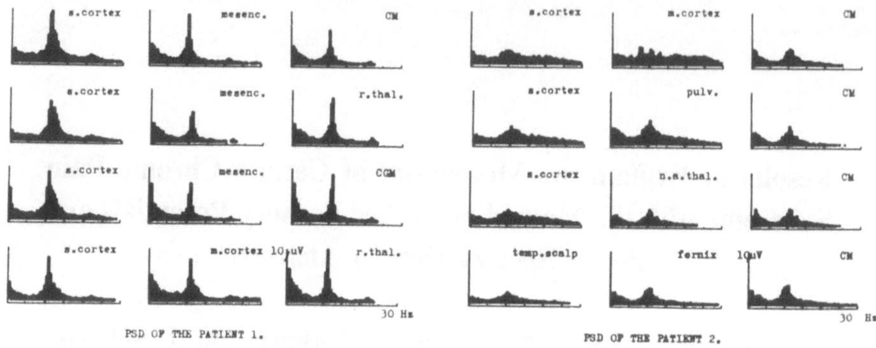

Fig. 1. Averaged power spectra densities by 1 minutes of 3–3 different structures registered simultaneously in phantom pain (Psd of patient 1) and thalamic pain (Psd of patient 2)

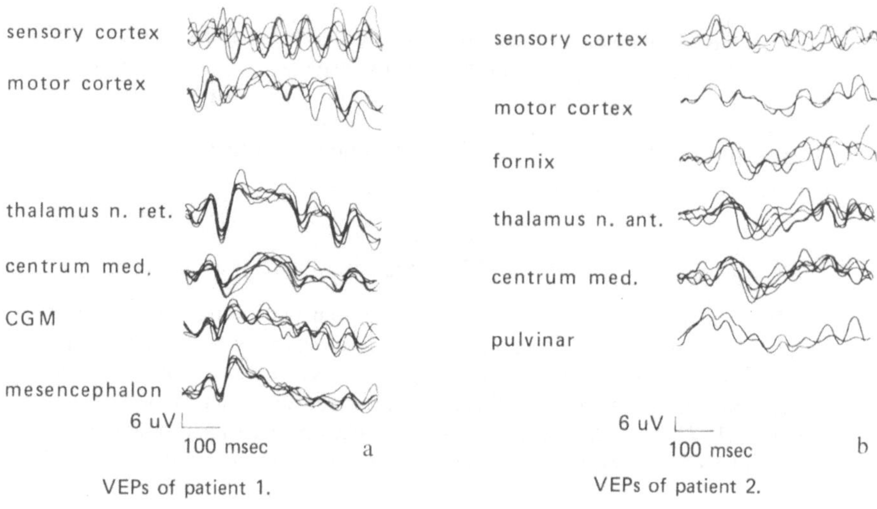

Fig. 2. Visual evoked potentials in phantom pain (a) and thalamic pain (b). Each trace is the average of 40 responses, negativity is up reffered to linked ears

3. Alpha density responding to acoustic stimulation decreased in sensory cortex at thalamic pain; decrease was more intensive in deep structures (Fig. 3). Alpha activity did not change in phantom pain.

4. 4 Hz burst activity was observed during the intermediate phase of sleep-awakeness in phantom pain. Tendency of the changes of N_1, N_2 components of acoustic evoked potentials (AEP)

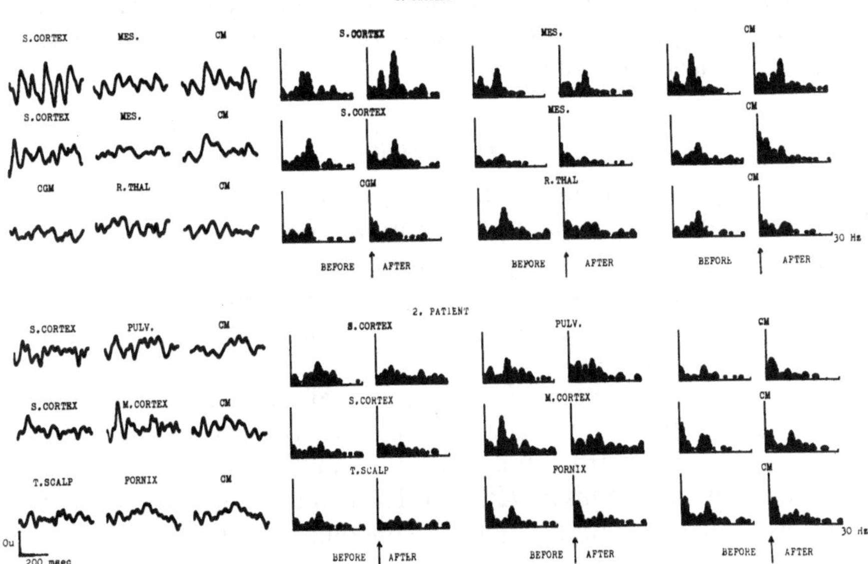

Fig. 3. Acoustic evoked potentials (average of 40 responses) and power spectra density of the averaged periods before and after stimulus in phantom pain (patient 1) and in thalamic pain (patient 2)

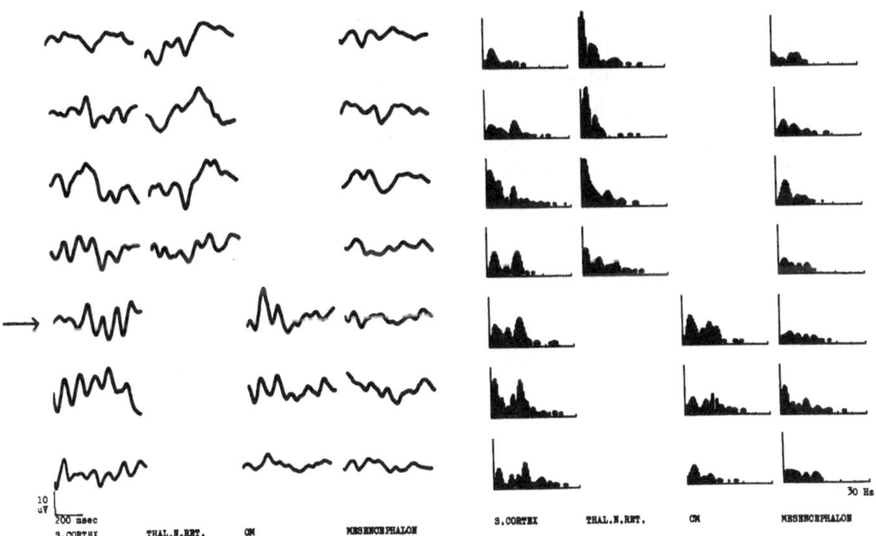

Fig. 4. Acoustic evoked potentials in sleep (upper 4 traces) in intermediate phase (arrow) and in awakeness (lower 2 traces) of different structures and their power spectra density in phantom pain

and power spectra density (Psd) of AEP was opposite in CM and in cortex; this phenomenon was most pronounced in intermediate phase of sleep-awakeness (Fig. 4).

Discussion

1. The cortical alpha rhythm generated by the thalamus[1] decrease after thalamotomy[5]. According to our data in thalamic pain the decrease of alpha power in cortex, decrease of latencies of VEP slow components[3] and more consequent appearance of VEP in the cortex[4] may be signs of disconnection of thalamocortical reverberating circuits.

2. CM was irritated in phantom pain mainly during the decreased cortical inhibition; pronounced form of thalamic spindle[1] can be regarded as a sign of the above irritation. Earlier we observed irritativ signs in VPL too. The irritative signs of CM may be caused by excitation of pain conducting system.

References

1. Andersen, P., Andersson, S. A. (Appleton-Century-Crofts) New York. 1977.
2. Andersson, S. A., Manson, J. R., Rhythmic activity in the thalamus of the unanaesthetized decorticate cat. Electroenceph. clin. Neurophysiol. *31* (1971), 21—34.
3. Ciganec, L., The evoked response to light stimulus in man. Electroenceph. clin. Neurophysiol. *13* (1964), 165—172.
4. Skinner, J. E., Lindsley, D. B., Enhancement of visual and auditory evoked potencials during blockade of the nonspecific thalamo-cortical system. Electroenceph. clin. Neurophysiol. *31* (1971), 1—6.
5. Ohmoto, T., Mimura, Y., Bala, Y., Miyamoto, T., Matsumoto, A., Nishimoto, A., Matsumoto, K., Thalamic control of spontaneous alpha-rhythm and evoked responses. Appl. Neurophysiol. *41* (1978), 180—192.

Acta Neurochirurgica, Suppl. 33, 491—495 (1984)

Deep Brain Stimulation in Chronic Pain Syndromes

F. Frank[1], **G. Frank, G. Gaist, A. Fabrizi,** and **C. Sturiale**

Summary

21 patients were treated with deep brain stimulation. Patients had chronic pain syndromes of which 14 were benign pain, and 7 were caused by slow growing neoplasms. In 3 cases, implantation was temporary due to poor analgesic results after an adequate test period. The remaining 18 patients had permanent implantation after a trial period of 7 to 15 days. In so-called benign pain syndromes, the sensory thalamus was stimulated twice, and in the remaining cases the posterior limb of the internal capsule was chosen. In cancer pain, the target of choice was always the ventro-rostral segment of the mesencephalic periaqueductal gray matter. A one to two year follow-up showed all periaqueductal stimulations remained effective. Stimulation of the somato-sensory system progressively deteriorated in two patients with thalamic electrodes, and in one patient with the electrode in the posterior limb of the internal capsule. Periaqueductal stimulations provoked oculomotor disturbances; thalamic stimulations evoked unpleasant electrical paresthesias. Stimulations of the posterior limb of the internal capsule in two patients provoked visual impairments such as scotomas, and one patient had muscular contractions.

Keywords: Deep brain stimulation; chronic pain syndromes; posterior limb of the internal capsule; periaqueductal gray; hypotheses of analgesia.

Introduction

For more than 10 years, chronic pain of every etiology has been treated with deep brain stimulation. Our experience, although limited, is encouraging.

Materials and Method

Twenty-one patients were treated with deep brain stimulation in 2 years. Table 1 shows our series with immediate post-operative results. The implantation was temporary in 3 cases due to a lack of pain relief. Table 2 shows a one to two year

[1] Division of Neurosurgery, Bellaria Hospital, Bologna, Italy.

Table 1. *Immediate Post-operative Results of 21 Patients*

Case n.	Sex	Age	Location of pain	Etiology	Target	Immediate results	Side effects
1	M	54	Left forearm (Radial nerve)	Herpes Zoster	Right VPL	Good	Unpleasant Paresthesias
2*	M	25	Left inferior limb.	Spinal Cord trauma	Right VPL	Poor	—
3	F	73	Right facio-cervical	Herpes Zoster	Left	Good	Scotomas
4	M	40	Right hemifacial	Anesthesia dolorosa	Left I. C.	Good	—
5	F	39	Right inferior limb.	Spinal arach-noiditis	Left I. C.	Good	—
6*	M	52	Right superior limb.	Anesthesia dolorosa	Left I. C.	Poor	—
7	M	69	Spinal cord	Vertebral metastases from prosta-tic carcinoma	P. A. G.	Good	Anxiety at stimulation
8	M	59	Left hemifacial	Cancer of left maxil-lary sinus	P. A. G.	Good	—
9	M	74	Right facio-cervical	Herpes Zoster	Left I. C.	Good	—
10	M	52	Left cervico-thoracic	Herpes Zoster	Right I. C.	Good	—

11	M	49	Left hemithorax	Anesthesia dolorosa	Left I. C.	Good	—
12	F	62	Right superior limb.	Post-irra-diation	Right I. C.	Good	—
13	F	55	Right superior l. and hemithorax	Anesthesia dolorosa	Left I. C.	Good	Muscular contractures
14	M	42	Left superior l. and hemithorax	Anesthesia dolorosa	Right I. C.	Good	—
15	M	61	Left inferior limb.	Bone cancer	P. A. G.	Good	Sleep-wake cycle disturb-ances
16	M	49	Right hemifacial	Cancer of Right maxil-lary sinus	P. A. G.	Good	—
17*	M	45	Left cervico brachial	Lymphoma	P. A. G.	Poor	—
18	M	75	Right hemithorax	Lung cancer	P. A. G.	Good	Parinaud Syndrome
19	F	74	Right hemithorax	Breast can-cer	P. A. G.	Good	—
20	M	56	Left cervico facial	Post-irra-diation	Right I. C.	Good	—
21	M	65	Right inferior limb.	Spinal Arachoidit.	Left I. C.	Good	—
Total patients: 21.			Good: 18 pa-tients (85.7%).				Side effects: 6 pa-tients (28.6%).

* These patients underwent only temporary implantation due to a lack of pain relief by D. B. S.

Table 2. *Follow-up of 18 Patients* (mean 1.5 years, range 1 to 2 years)

	Good	Fair	Poor
Benign pain (12 patients)	9	3	0
Cancer pain (6 patients)	5	1	
(Total 18 patients)	14 (77%)	4 (23%)	0

follow-up on 18 patients with definitive implantations. The electrode implantation is performed with a stereotactic procedure under local anesthesia. After a 7 to 15 day test period, if the stimulation is effective (the patient takes no analgesics), permanents implantation of the radio-frequency receiver, connected to the cerebral electrode, is performed under general anesthesia. The receiver is embedded in a subcutaneous pouch in the subclavicular region. A unipolar electrode was employed once (Avery Inc.), and a multipolar electrode (Medtronic Inc.) used on 20 occassions.

Discussion

From an analysis of our results, the pain syndrome best responding to deep brain stimulation is post-zosterian neuritis [5]. In post-mesencephalotomy anesthesia dolorosa and in spinal cord trauma, the results are poor. Pain due to slow growing neoplasms improved with stimulation of the so-called endorphinergic system [4]. Surprisingly, these patients felt well for a long time in spite of the global decrease of pain relief, which is the common picture with all types and targets of stimulation. One of these patients was good at follow-up at 15 months. With moderate use (5–6 stimulations daily) of deep brain stimulation, good levels of analgesia can be maintained; even if the target is subject to progressive functional decrease through time.

In chronic benign pain, the target of choice is the somatosensory system, which is referred to as an antagonist of the nociceptive multisynaptic pathway [2, 3]. Possible sites of stimulation are: the medial lemniscus, the sensory thalamus (VPL–VPM nuclei), and the posterior limb of the internal capsule. A preference for stimulation of the internal capsule is made for two resons: 1. Paresthesias evoked by stimulation are better tolerated by the patient than those evoked by medial lemniscal and sensory thalamic stimulation which are of an unpleasant electric character. 2. It is possible that more than one mechanism is responsible for the production of analgesia: a) a direct antidromic inhibition towards the thalamus and brainstem, b) an activation of a corticofugal inhibitory system towards deep seated centers [1], c) a dromic parietal suppression.

Conclusions

Deep brain stimulation seems to be a safe technique for the treatment of chronic pain. It presents the advantage of being completely reversible in case of failure, since it is a non-lesioning method. Finally, it represents the only present means of treatment for pain syndromes such as post-zosterian and deafferentation pain syndromes.

References

1. Adams, J. E., Hosobuchi, Y., Fields, H. L., Stimulation of the internal capsule for relief of chronic pain. J. Neurosurg. *41* (1974), 740—744.
2. Foerster, O., Die Leitungsbahnen des Schmerzgefühls und die chirurgische Behandlung der Schmerzzustände, pp. 77—80. Berlin-Wien: Urban and Schwarzenberg. 1927.
3. Melzack, R., Wall, P. D., Pain mechanisms: a new theory. Science *150* (1965), 971—979.
4. Richardson, D. E., Akil, H., Pain reduction by electric brain stimulation in man. 1. Acute administration in periaqueductal and periventricular sites. J. Neurosurg. *47* (1977), 178—183.
5. Siegfried, J., Monopolar electrical stimulation of nucleus ventroposteromedialis thalami for postherpetic facial pain. Appl. Neurophysiol. *45* (1982), 179—184.

Acta Neurochirurgica, Suppl. 33, 497—500 (1984)

Preliminary Results of Specific Thalamic Stimulation for Deafferentation Pain

G. Broggi[1], **A. Franzini, C. Giorgi, D. Servello,** and **R. Spreafico**

With 2 Figures

Summary

Ten patients suffering from central or deafferentation pain underwent stereotactic implant of VPM–VPL thalamic nuclei (9 cases) or PVG (1 case). After temporary stimulation trial, 7 patients had definitive implant of the system. Long term results, overall more than satisfactory, are discussed.

Keywords: Central pain; deafferentation pain; specific thalamus; periventricular gray; deep brain stimulation; neurostimulation.

Introduction

Central pain syndrome, following vascular, viral, traumatic and degenerative lesions of Nervous System, is characterized by pain often very intense, that occurs in paroxysms and that is usually present in regions with sensory loss. Frequently this pain has the character of hyperpathia and/or allocheria.

No universally accepted explanation of this pain has been given, but presumably it is due to alteration of the integration processes between lemniscal and extralemniscal neuronal systems carrying nociceptive and proprioceptive inputs.

Deafferentation pain has similar etiopathogenical and semeiological features. Both these types of pain usually do not respond to morphine.

[1] Department of Neurosurgery, Service Functional Neurosurgery, Istituto Neurologico "C. Besta", Via Celoria N. 11, I-20133 Milano, Italy.

Material and Methods

On the basis of other authors'[3–5] experience, since October 1981, 10 patients suffering from these type of pain underwent a trial of deep brain stimulation. Six were males and 4 females. The median age was 65.3 years (range: 48–75 years). Nine cases were operated on with stereotactic implant of a stimulating electrode in the VPM and/or VPL thalamic nuclei. In one patient, suffering from intractable pain due to carcinoma in the latero-cervical region, with a component of deafferentation pain due to brachial plexus compression and in which the morphine infusion test was positive, the PVG matter target was preferred to specific thalamic nuclei. All other cases were affected with post-herpetic neuralgia (5 cases), thalamic pain syndrome (2 cases), anesthesia dolorosa following trigeminal rhizotomy (1 case) and pain due to brachial plexus avulsion. The average duration of pain was 5.8 years (range: 1–9 years).

After the surgery test stimulation was performed via an external connecting cable for temporary stimulation. Two electrode systems have been used: a monopolar electrode system (Avery) for specific thalamic implants, and a multicontact electrode system (Medtronic) in a bipolar configuration for PVG implant.

The stereotactic operation were performed using the Riechert stereotactic frame, with local anesthesia. Target coordinates were calculated using stereotactic references structures after positive contrast (Metrizamide, Iopamidol) stereotactic ventriculography, adapted on a computerized version of the stereotactic atlas of Schaltenbrand and Wharen[2]. Patients collaboration allowed maping paresthesias elicited by intraoperative thalamic stimulation. Intraoperative thalamic S. E. P. has been used to confirm the accurate recognition of the target. Square-wave electrical pulse stimuli were applied transcutaneously to contralateral trigeminal nerve (infra-orbital nerve), median nerve at the wrist, and common peroneal nerve at the ankle. SEP's were recorded from thalamic electrode with the usual averaging technique[1].

Stimulation trials were performed with constant parameters: at 50–75 Hz, 250 msec and 1.5 mA, 5 minutes each time, 5 times/day. The average duration of the trial was 30 days (range: 15–90 days)' No neurological deficit followed the surgical procedures; the trial began on the first postoperative day.

Results

Pain reductions of various degrees occurred in all patients during the initial observation period (Fig. 1). Minimal moderation of pain (15–30%) occurred in two patients and the system was removed after one month. One patient died of cardio-pulmonary failure 10 days after operation. Excellent results were obtained in the remaining 7 patients (pain relief maintained between 80 and 90%) and they underwent definitive implant. Evaluation of pain relief was based upon a visual-analogue scale the follow-up period extended up to 18 months.

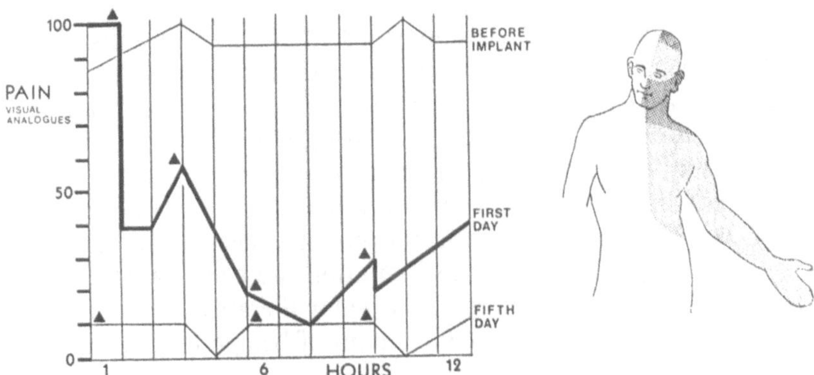

Fig. 1. Visual-analogue scale of a case of post-herpetic facial-cervical neuralgia (dark steppled area). Each stimulation trial is marked by a triangle. VPM stimulation induced paresthesias overlap the painful area (light steppled area). Note the immediate induced pain relief

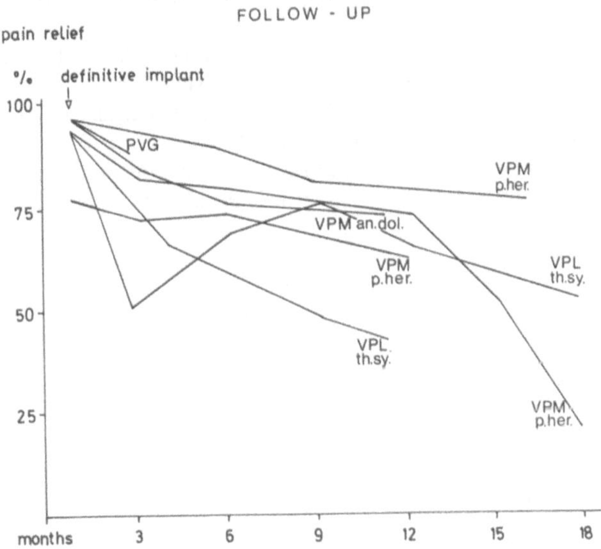

Fig. 2. Summary of all cases long term results. Note target and etiology for each patient. *p. her.* = post herpetic neuralgia; *th. sy.* = thalamic syndrome; *an. dol.* = anesthesia dolorosa

One patient died of an intracerebral haemorrhage after 11 months.

The initial pain relief diminished after some months: some patients experienced pain recurrence (tolerance development?) requiring a change of parameters of stimulation (*e.g.* rate) and associated therapy with L-Dopa (250 mg/die) which resulted in a recovery of the stimulation induced analgesia.

Most patients experienced pain relief of more than 50%, but long term follow-up suggests the possible decrease of induced analgesia (Fig. 2). Despite this limitation, we believe that chronic thalamic stimulation constitutes a valid therapeutic support for patients affected from intractable pain of benign origin.

References

1. Broggi, G., Franzini, A., Giorgi, C., Servello, D., Crenna, P., Carenini, L., S. E. P. utilization in chronic thalamic stimulation for deafferentation pain. A preliminary study. Acta Neurochir. (Wien) (in press).
2. Giorgi, C., Garibotto, G., Garozzo, S., Micca, G., Piretta, G., Three dimensional processing of a stereotactic atlas. Appl. Neurophysiol. *45* (1982), 419—425.
3. Hosobuchi, Y., Adams, J. E., Rutkin, B., Chronic thalamic stimulation for the control of facial anesthesia dolorosa. Arch. Neurol. *9* (1973), 158—161.
4. Mazars, G. J., Intermittent stimulation of nucleus ventralis posterolateralis for intractable pain. Surg. Neurol. *4* (1975), 93—95.
5. Siegfried, J., Monopolar electrical stimulation of nucleus ventro-posteromedialis thalami for post-herpetic facial pain. Appl. Neurophysiol. *45* (1982), 179—184.

Acta Neurochirurgica, Suppl. 33, 501—503 (1984)

Effect of Electrical Stimulation of Periaqueductal Gray and Septal Area on Beta-Endorphin Plasma Levels in a Model of Deafferentation Pain. Experimental Study in Rats

P. Roldán[1], J. Moreno, E. Vicent, M. Cerdá, S. Ramos, and J. L. Barcia-Salorio

With 1 Figure

Summary

The effect of electrical stimulation of the periadequeductal gray and septal area on plasma levels of immunoreactive beta-endorphin was measured on an experimental model of chronic deafferentation pain, induced by unilateral C5–Th1 dorsal rhizotomy in rats. An abnormal behaviour consisting of edema, scratching wounds and self-amputation of deafferented limbs was observed. A slight decrease in plasma levels of beta-endorphin was noted in deafferented animals. Groups in which electrical stimulation of the periadequeductal gray and septal area was performed showed an increase in plasma levels of beta-endorphin. The hypoactivity of the endorphinergic system observed in the animals with chronic pain could be reversed by stimulation of the periaqueductal gray.

Keywords: Deafferentation model; endorphin; deep brain stimulation.

Based on the anatomical distribution of immunoreactive beta-lipotropin in rat brain[3], therapeutic stimulation at different sites of the so called "beta-endorphin system" has been performed in the periaqueductal gray (PAG) and septal area (S) for the surgical management of chronic pain[2]. However the mechanism of action of these techniques remains obscure. Therefore, the effect of electrical stimulation of PAG and S on plasma levels of immunoreactive beta-endorphin (ir b–E) was measured in an

[1] Department of Neurosurgery, Hospital Clínico Universitario, Valencia, Spain.

experimental model of chronic deafferentation pain, induced by unilateral C_5–Th_1 dorsal rhizotomy in rats, as developed by Albe-Fessard *et al.*[1].

Material and Methods

Male Wistar rats, were distributed in four groups: pain (P), septal (SS) and PAG (PAGS) stimulation groups, and pain plus PAG stimulation (P + PAGS). The control groups were: normal (N), pain (P–SH), PAG (PAGS–SH) and septal stimulation (SS–SH) sham groups, and neutral globus pallidus stimulation (GS).

In groups P and P + PAGS a unilateral C_5–Th_1 dorsal rhizotomy was performed, and the animals' behaviour observed for a period of four months. In group P–SH hemilaminectomy but not rhizotomy was carried out. In groups PAGS, SS, PAGS–SH, SS–SH and GS a 0.5 mm epoxy insulated stainless steel bipolar electrode was implanted in the respective target area by stereotactic means. After the electrode was implanted, animals in groups PAGS, SS and GS were stimulated with square pulse trains of 0.5 s, 0.2 ms pulse duration, 100 Hz (SS) or 20 Hz (PAGS) frequency, and 3 V. For PAGS, voltage was fixed at a point just below the level suficient to produce oculomotor effects. The current was applied for 20 minutes every hour during a total stimulation period of 4 hours. Stimulation in group P + PAGS was delayed till the hyperalgesic syndrome developed.

Once the hyperalgesic syndrome had developed in group P, and after the stimulation period in the other groups, the animals were decapitated and their blood collected for biochemical determinations. Radioimmunoassay (RIA) was employed for ir b–E plasma determinations. Comparisons between two different groups were made with the same RIA kit.

Results

All deafferented animals gradually developed a complex behavioural disturbance called hyperalgesic syndrome, consisting of edema, scratching wounds and self-amputation of deafferented limbs. Pathological findings in the dorsal horn of the spinal cord included a long-term fibrotic lesion induced by radicular avulsion.

Fig. 1 shows a histogram of ir b–E plasma levels in all series ($p < 0.05$). In series 1 a slight decrease in ir b–E was noted in deafferented animals, thus showing that in chronic pain states there is a kind of hypoactivity of endorphinergic mechanisms. Groups in which electrical stimulation of PAG (series 2) and S (series 3) was carried out showed an increase in ir b–E. The hypoactivity of the endorphine system observed in the animals with the chronic pain syndrome could be reversed by PAG stimulation (series 4). Control series 5 to 8 confirmed the reliability of the experimental method employed.

SERIES		1	2	3	4	5	6	7	8
GROUP	1	N	N	N	P	N	N	N	N
	2	P	PAGS	SS	P+PAGS	P-SH	PAGS-SH	SS-SH	GS
MEAN	1	10.6	7.9	11.	8.7	7.3	7.5	9.3	12.3
	2	6.2	21.7	18.3	17.3	8.8	9.5	11.1	14.6
S.E.	1	1.5	2.5	2.1	2.	2.4	2.1	4.2	2.5
	2	1.1	7.8	4.2	6.2	2.7	1.4	3.8	5.4

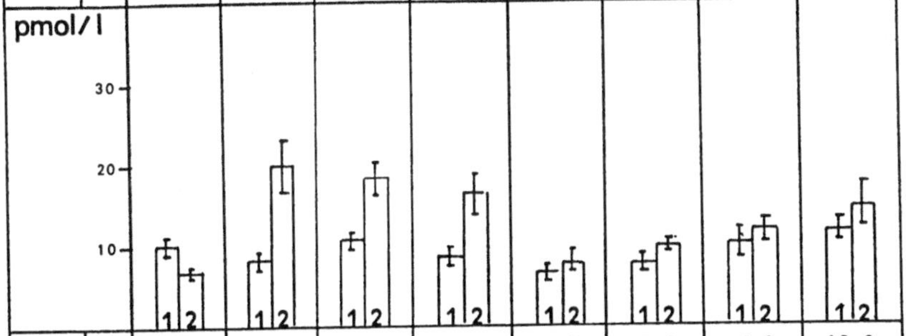

Fig. 1. Histogram of ir-beta-endorphin plasma levels

From these results and previous work by other authors, the relation between ACTH and beta-endorphin can be recognized. Stimulation-produced analgesia could be, at least in part, due to the activation of the stress response, thus providing a rationale for the aforementioned neuroaugmentative techniques.

References

1. Albe-Fessard, D., Nashold, B. S., jr., Lombard, M. C., Yamaguchi, Y., Boureau, F., Rat after dorsal rhizotomy. A possible animal model for chronic pain. In: Adv. in Pain Res. and Ther., vol. 3 (Bonica, J., Liebeskind, J., Albe-Fessard, D., eds.), pp. 761—766. New York: Raven Press. 1979.
2. Richardson, D. E., Analgesia produced by stimulation of various sites in the human beta-endorphin system. Appl. Neurophysiol. *45* (1982), 116—122.
3. Watson, S. J., Barchas, J. D., Li, C. H., Beta-lipotropin: localization of cells and axons in rat brain by immunocytochemistry. Proc. Natl. Acad. Sci. U.S.A. *74* (1977), 5155—5158.

Acta Neurochirurgica, Suppl. 33, 505—506 (1984)

Chronic VPM Thalamic Stimulation in Facial Anaesthesia Dolorosa Following Trigeminal Surgery

J. Broseta[1], **P. Roldán, G. Masbout,** and **J. L. Barcia-Salorio**

Keywords: Anaesthesia dolorosa; trigeminal surgery; pain; neurostimulation.

Various somatosensory areas have been stimulated to control deafferentation pain with general good results. Among them, there was general agreement about the efficacy of electric stimulation of ventroposteromedialis (VPM) thalami nucleus to this aim. On this base, in seven cases presenting with severe and resistent facial anaesthesia dolorosa following failed trigeminal surgery (two Frazier's technique and five selective thermolesion) were treated with chronic VPM stimulation. Using conventional stereotactic techniques, a four contact flexible electrode was implanted in this area. The target coordinates were: 9 mm behind the AC–PC midpoint, —1 to 1 mm up-down the AC–PC line and 8–9 mm lateral to midline. When electric paresthesias were evoked in the original dysesthesic area, the electrode was fixed and the percutaneous extensions withdrawn through the skin. A trial period of two weeks was established to determine the relief of facial dysesthesias. During this time, the patient was stimulated 3–5 periods daily on 30 minutes. 0.1 msec pulse duration, a rate from 80 to 120 Hz, according to patient's comfort and voltage at paresthesic threshold were used as electric parameter. After the trial period, as all our patients presented a positive dysesthesic relief, the system was chronically internalized.

Table 1 showed the general data of the patients before the VPM stimulation.

Table 2 illustrated the long-term results after a mean follow-up of 2 years. Despite the general initial benefit, that allowed the

[1] Department of Neurosurgery, Hospital Clínico Universitario, Valencia, Spain.

Table 1. *General Data of the Patients*

Case	Age/sex	Original pain	Operation	Years of dysesthesia	Location
1	62/F	R·V_1	Frazier	6 years	R·V_1
2	65/F	R·V_1–V_2	Thermolesion	3 years	R·V_1
3	71/F	R·V_1–V_2	Frazier	9 years	R·V_1
4	65/M	L·V_1–V_2–V_3	Thermolesion	2 years	L·V_1–V_2–V_3
5	56/F	R·V_1–V_2–V_3	Thermolesion	4 years	R·V_1–V_2
6	63/F	R·V_1	Thermolesion	5 years	R·V_1
7	69/F	L·V_1–V_2	Thermolesion	8 years	L·V_1–V_2

Table 2. *Results*

Case	Initial result	Stimulation tolerance	Follow-up	Long-term result	Dopamine administration
1	Excellent	19 months	3 years	Poor	Negative
2	Excellent	11 months	$2^1/_2$ months	Fair	?
3	Good	6 months	$2^1/_3$ years	Poor	Negative
4	Good	9 months	2 years	Poor	Negative
5	Fair	10 months	$1^2/_3$ years	Poor	Negative
6	Excellent	9 months	1 year	Poor	Negative
7	Good	3 months	1 year	Poor	Negative

patients to return to a normal life, after a mean period of 10 months a stimulation tolerance appeared, where the patients presented similar complaints as in the preoperative situation. The stimulation tolerance was resistent to dopamine oral administration. With the time, the situation worsened when the patient complained of dysesthesias in contralateral upper limb (2 cases) and upper and lower limb (1 case), without presenting any electrode displacement.

As conclusion, in our hands, VPM stimulation has not been as satisfactory as initially promised when results were long-term considered.

Acta Neurochirurgica, Suppl. 33, 507—510 (1984)

Recent Progress in the Treatment of Trigeminal Neuralgia: Glycerol into the Trigeminal Cistern and Percutaneous Gasserian Compression by Means of Fogarty's Catheter

B. Fraioli[1], **L. Ferrante, A. Santoro,** and **G. Di Giugno**

Summary

Out of 712 patients suffering from trigeminal neuralgia operated on between 1955 and December 1982, the preliminary results of two series of 32 and 30 patients respectively, the former treated by the introduction of glycerol into the trigeminal cistern and the latter by percutaneous compression of the Gasserian ganglion and the retrogasserian roots are presented. Both of these methods were effective and facial sensation was preserved in the majority of cases. Percutaneous Gasserian compression is preferred by the authors, mainly because its simplicity.

Keywords: Trigeminal neuralgia; glycerol; Gasserian ganglion compression.

Introduction

The technique of controlled differential thermocoagulation undoubtedly represents an advances in the treatment of trigeminal neuralgia, as is shown by the vast series reported in the last few years by various authors, including ourselves[2,3]. The only real criticism of this technique is that it does not completely preserve facial sensitivity and that a large number of patients complain of paraesthesia after treatment. However our conviction that trigeminal neuralgia should be treated by minor surgery, and this only after treatment with Carbamazepine has proven ineffective, has led us to carefully observe new forms of treatment of trigeminal neuralgia over the last two years and to build up our experience both in the technique of injection of glycerol into the trigeminal cistern and in that of percutaneous compression of the Gasserian ganglion by mean of a Fogarty's catheter.

[1] Neurosurgical Institute of the Rome University, Viale dell'Università no. 30, I-00185 Roma, Italy.

Methods

For the introduction of glycerol into the trigeminal cistern we have followed the technique described by Håkanson[4].

Compression of the Gasserian ganglion and the retrogasserian roots was carried out without need of general anaesthesia by means of endotracheal intubation as previously reported by other authors[1]. After endovenous injection of 2cc of a drug containing fentanyl and droperidol we proceeded with the percutaneous introduction of a needle into the foramen ovale so that tip of the needle did not exceed the foramen by more than half a centimeter. The needle must allow the passage of a 4 F Fogarty's catheter which is then inflated by introducing "Iopamiro 300" whilst the patients is put to sleep for a few minutes by endovenous injection of pentothal. In our experience, compression should last for 4–5 minutes as longer times have been associated with facial anaesthesia, even though transitory. The use of smaller catheters, particularly 2 F and 3 F, was not very effective.

Results

The results in 32 patients treated with glycerol were, on the whole, satisfactory. In particularly, success was obtained in 23 out of 29 cases of essential trigeminal neuralgia and it should be noted that in 4 of the 6 failures observed the instillation of glycerol was into Gasserian ganglion but not into the trigeminal cistern. The treatment was unsuccessful in 2 cases of neuralgia in multiple sclerosis and 1 case of post-herpetic neuralgia. With concern the facial sensation, it was completely preserved in about $^3/_4$ of the cases but in one patients marked hemifacial hypoaesthesia occurred after the introduction of glycerol into the trigeminal cistern and 3 months later he showed anaesthesia and initial keratitis.

Table 1 shows that encouraging results were obtained in the series of 30 patients treated with percutaneous compression of the Gasserian ganglion and the retrogasserian roots. Treatment was particularly successful in patients suffering from essential trigeminal neuralgia in the majority of whom facial sensation was completely preserved, without any significant complications. Success was obtained in only one of two patients with trigeminal neuralgia in multiple sclerosis.

Discussion

The relatively short observation period of our two series probably doesn't give an exact idea of the number of relapses but it should be noted that both methods were found to cause little stress

Table 1. *Results in 30 Patients Treated by Percutaneous Gasserian Compression*

	N. patients	Success	Failure	Relapses	Normal sensation	Hypoaes-thesia	Paraesthesia which required transitory antianxiety medication	Follow-up
"Essential" trigeminal neuralgia	22	17*	5**	—	15	7	1	
"Essential" trigeminal neuralgia already treated by other techniques	6	5*	1***	—	5	1	—	Averaging: From 4 to 8 months
Trigeminal neuralgia in multiple sclerosis	2	1	1	1	1	1	—	
Total	30	23	7	1	21	9	1	

* Treated with 4 F Fogarty's catheter, except 4 patients.
** Treated with 2 F or 3 F Fogarty's catheter.
*** Treated with 3 F Fogarty's catheter.

to the patients and to be repeatable; moreover, the Gasserian compression technique was particularly easy to perform.

As far as the facial sensation is concerned, this was completely preserved in the majority of cases and none of the patients developed painful anaesthesia following both procedures. As it was easier to perform and because of the anaesthesia and keratitis occurred in the already mentioned patient treated with glycerol into the trigeminal cistern, we prefer at present, the method of percutaneous compression of the Gasserian ganglion and the retrogasserian rootlets. However, it is obvious that more large experience are necessary for a definitive choice.

Lastly, we believe that thermocoagulation cannot be considered enterely outdated, especially as the two recent techniques presented were effective only in about 80% of the cases of essential neuralgia and were little effective in trigeminal neuralgia of the multiple sclerosis.

References

1. Bricolo, A., Dalle Ore, G., La microcompressione percutanea gasseriana per la nevralgia del trigemino: risultati preliminari. Com. al XXXI. Congresso Nazionale di Neurochirurgia. Bollettino d'Informazione *2*, 29—30. Società Italiana di Neurochirurgia (Ed.). 1982.
2. Fraioli, B., Controlled differential thermocoagulation in the treatment of trigeminal neuralgia. J. Neurosurg. Sci. *22* (1978), 71—76.
3. Guidetti, B., Fraioli, B., Refice, G. M., Modern trends in surgical treatment of trigeminal neuralgia. J. Max. Fac. Surg. *7* (1979), 315—319.
4. Håkanson, S., Trigeminal neuralgia treated by the injection of glycerol into the trigeminal cistern. Neurosurg. *9* (1981), 638—646.

Acta Neurochirurgica, Suppl. 33, 511—514 (1984)

Controlled Radiofrequency Thermocoagulation of Trigeminal Ganglion in the Treatment of Trigeminal Neuralgia, Hemifacial Spasm, and Facial Neuralgia

Y. Kanpolat[1,*], **N. Avman**[1], **H. Z. Gökalp**[1], **E. Arasil**[1], **E. Ozkal**, and **M. Selçuki**[1]

Summary

The authors present the results of the radiofrequency thermocoagulation of trigeminal ganglion in the treatment of trigeminal neuralgia, hemifacial spasm and various kinds of facial neuralgias. 370 procedures have been performed in 326 cases between 1974–1982.

Keywords: Radiofrequency thermocoagulation; trigeminal neuralgia; hemifacial spasm; facial neuralgia.

Introduction

Radiofrequency thermocoagulation (RFTC) of the trigeminal ganglion is widely used in the treatment of trigeminal neuralgia (TN). On the contrary very few reports have been presented on the value of RFTC in the treatment of chronic facial neuralgias[4]. Cushing had described coexistence of hemifacial spasm and TN (tic douloureux). Encouraging results of trigeminal ganglion RFTC in the treatment of tic douloureux have driven us to perform the same procedure in the treatment of pure hemifacial spasm in order to break the afferent arcus of trigemino-facial reflex[1].

Methods, Material and Results

Between 1974–1982 controlled RFTC of trigeminal ganglion has been performed in 326 patients with 370 procedures.

---

[1] Department of Neurosurgery, University of Ankara, School of Medicine, Ankara, Turkey.

* Mailing address: Tıp Fakültesi Hastahanesi, Nöroşirürji Kliniği, Dikimevi, Ankara, Turkey.

The procedure was performed in three different group of patients:

I. Trigeminal neuralgia: The procedure was performed in 306 TN cases. In this group, 256 patients had idiopathic TN (tic douloureux). 290 procedures were performed in 256 cases. 240 patients (93.7%) were pain free after the first RFTC. In 5 cases (2.1%) RFTC was ineffective and they were treated by intracranial surgery. In 256 cases of TN, 17 patients have recurrences or unsatisfactory results of previous intracranial surgery (17 retrogasserian root sections and 4 posterior fossa explorations). In 16 of these 17 patients the paroxysmal pain relieved by RFTC. In one case with anesthesia dolorosa neither posterior fossa exploration and sensorial root section nor RFTC were effective.

In the symtomatic group, 50 patients with functional deficits (motor, sensory, reflex) of 5th nerve, further examinations were done (brain scan, CT, etc.). In 31 patients no significant pathology was found. In only 19 cases, various pathologies had been found like: carcinoma of face in 8 cases, multiple sclerosis in 3 cases (2 cases have bilateral neuralgia), multiple operated chronic sinusitis in two cases and leucemia, cerebellopontine tumor, Bell's plasy, fracture of zygoma and Gradenigo syndrome in one case. In this symptomatic group, 45 cases were pain free after first RFTC. In 5 of 6 recurrences, pain was relieved following multiple RFTC, but in one case RFTC was ineffective.

II. Hemifacial spasm: 8 hemifacial spasms were treated by RFTC (one of them had bilateral spasms). In two cases, the spasm was present with moderate TN. One case had no spasm in the follow-up period of 4 years. In other cases, the spasm was controlled by RFTC for one year in one patient, 6 months in two patients and three months in last two patients. The two patients could not be followed.

III. Chronic facial neuralgias: In 12 cases, we have used RFTC to control the unilateral chronic facial pain. These patients did not respond to all other types of treatment. 4 patients had cluster headache (Horton). We have used 5 RFTC in Horton group. In three patients pain attacks were relieved after the procedure. In one of them, the pain attack was returned to medically controlled condition after two procedures.

A female patient's chronic migraineous neuralgia was relieved after RFTC.

Other forms of atypically unilateral chronic facial neuralgias were controlled in 7 patients by 9 RFTC procedures.

In 370 procedures main complications were as follows:

6th nerve palsy has been observed in two patients, 3rd nerve palsy also observed in other two patients (0.6%), which were transient and recovered in 7 days. In 9 cases we have observed trigeminal motor weakness (2.8%), recovered in 2–3 months. Lost or diminished corneal reflex has been observed in 24 cases (7.3%) and in only one of them keratitis was seen (0.3%). Anesthesia dolorosa was found in 6 cases (1.8%). One of 7 arterial punctures during the procedure had developed carotido-cavernous fistula which has been treated by ICA trapping.

In one case we have observed nasopharingeal CSF leakage, 4 hours after the procedure which has been verified by isotope cisternography and was spontaneously healed 2 days after RFTC.

Discussion

As far as the rates of mortality and complications are concerned, RFTC seems to be an effective, safe and simple method in the treatment of TN. In the standard lesion parameters RFTC causes scar tissue in the ganglion which effects nerve fibers at all sizes[2,6,7]. The method is widely used in the treatment of TN. In our experience the same procedure is effective in selected cases of unilateral chronic facial neuralgias, which are resistant to all other types of treatment. RFTC of trigeminal ganglion should be done as the last choice. In 8 cases we have done RFTC in the treatment of hemifacial spasm. This was the first application of RFTC of trigeminal ganglion in the literature[1]. Long term follow-up of our patients revealed that this application is effective but survival period is too short. As a concluding remark, we advise controlled RFTC lesion to facial nerve a few millimeters in front of stylomastoid foramen or microvascular decompression of nerve in posterior fossa. In TN patients, we usually prefer moderate hypoalgesic lesion levels to anesthesia dolorosa. This is why we have higher recurrence rates but markedly lower anesthesia dolorosa incidence as compared to classical literature[3,5].

References

1. Kanpolat, Y., Saveren, M., Erdoğan, A., R. F. Thermocoagulation of the Gasserian ganglion in the treatment of the hemifacial spasm. The Turkish Otorhinolaryngology Bul. *2* (1977), 169—178.

2. Kanpolat, Y., Onol, B., Experimental percutaneous approach to the trigeminal ganglion in dogs with histopathological evaluation of radiofrequency lesion. Acta Neurochir. (Wien), Suppl. *30* (1980), 363—366.
3. Loveren, V. H., Tew, M. J., Keller, T., Nurre, A. M., A 10-year experience in the treatment of trigeminal neuralgia. J. Neurosurg. *57* (1982), 757—764.
4. Maxwell, E. R., Surgical control of chronic migraineous neuralgia by trigeminal ganglio-rhilysis. J. Neurosurg. *57* (1982), 459—466.
5. Siegfried, J., Percutaneous controlled thermocoagulation of Gasserian ganglion in trigeminal neuralgia. Experiences with 1,000 cases. In: The Cranial nerves (Samii, M., Janetta, J. P., eds.), pp. 322—330. Berlin-Heidelberg-New York: Springer. 1981.
6. Smith, H. P., McWhorter, J. M., Chella, V. R., Radiofrequency neurolysis in a clinical model. Neuropathological correlation. J. Neurosurg. *55* (1981), 246—253.
7. Uematsu, S., Percutaneous electrothermocoagulation of spinal nerve trunk, ganglion and rootlets. Current technique in operative neurosurgery (Schmiedek, H. H., Sweet, W. H., eds.), pp. 469—490. New York: Grune and Stratton. 1977.

Acta Neurochirurgica, Suppl. 33, 515—520 (1984)

Percutaneous Thermolesion of the Glossopharyngeal Nerve: Results and Anatomo-physiological Considerations

G. Salar[1], **V. Baratto**[1], **C. Ori**[2], **I. Iob**[1], and **S. Mingrino**[1]

With 2 Figures

Summary

The authors report their experience in the treatment of symptomatic and essential neuralgia of the 9th cranial nerve by percutaneous radiofrequency thermocoagulation at the foramen jugulare. Neuroanatomical and neurophysiological aspects of this technique are also discussed.

Keywords: Neuralgia; glossopharyngeal; radiofrequency; rhizotomy.

Introduction

Percutaneous thermolesion of the 9th cranial nerve has been employed during the last two years for the treatment of essential and symptomatic glossopharyngeal pain. In the present report, after a brief explanation of immediate and late results of this technique, we take into consideration particularly neuroanatomic and neurophysiological problems appeared during the various phases of the procedure and the early postoperative period.

Material

Eight patients with glossopharyngeal neuralgia, 3 essential and 5 symptomatic (from tumours of the tonsillar and lingualis regions) were included in our series.

All the patients were male, mean age 56 years.

[1] Institute of Neurosurgery and [2] Institute of Anesthesia and Resuscitation, University of Padua, Via Giustiniani, 5, I-35100 Padova, Italy.

Method

The surgical procedure consisted of a percutaneous thermolesion by radiofrequency impulses at the level of the foramen jugulare. The foramen was reached by the lateral-cervical approach described by Bonica[1] rather than through the anterior-lateral way proposed by Lazorthes[6].

The correct needle position was controlled either by cranial base X-rays demonstrating the foramen jugulare and by low voltage electrical stimulation (0.2–0.4 V), which induces paresthesias at the level of the retropharynx and the internal acoustic meatus. The whole procedure was carried out under local anesthesia and continuous blood pressure and ECG monitoring. The thermic lesion, which followed in every cases the electrical stimulation in the absence of vagal responses, was performed at temperatures of 60–65 °C applied not more than 1–2 minutes.

Results

All our patients experienced an immediate and satisfactory result on pain symptomatology. In fact pain disappeared completely in the 3 cases with essential neuralgia, while it was significantly reduced in the 5 cases with symptomatic pain, although a residual slight painful sensation remained in the tonsillar area.

All the patients of the two groups were then controlled by a late follow-up from 4 to 16 months; in the 3 patients with essential symptomatology no recurrence of pain was noted. Of the 5 cases with symptomatic pain 2 died respectively 4 and 5 months after surgery with a good reduction of the pain, which was always controlled by minor analgesic drugs. Only in one case the neuralgia recurred twice requiring further surgical treatment. 16 months after the first procedure, the third recurrence of pain occurred.

No disturbances of speech or of deglutition from vagal damage, nor lesion of the 11th at the foramen jugulare or the 7th cranial nerves during penetration of the needle-electrode were noted. In one case the jugular vein was penetrated.

Before the thermic lesion, all our patients underwent electrical stimulation of the nervous structures interested during the penetration of the needle-electrode. In our experience the correct position of the electrode is confirmed by the appearance of paresthesias (swarming sensation) at the tonsillar and retropharyngeal regions, evoked by low voltage electrical stimulation (0.2–0.3 V).

Five patients reported also paresthesias at the external acoustic meatus, but never at the ala auris. Increasing the voltage, in 4 cases motor responses from the laryngeal muscles were evoked, reported as a quivering in the throat, without speech alterations. During low voltage electrical stimulation, slight bradycardia was noted in 3 patients, corrected by small changes of the position of the electrode in 2 cases, or, in one patient, by complete replacement of the electrode.

During thermocoagulation, vagal response occurred in other 2 patients, characterized by hypotension and bradycardia for 40–50 seconds, regressed after interruption of the lesion (Fig. 1).

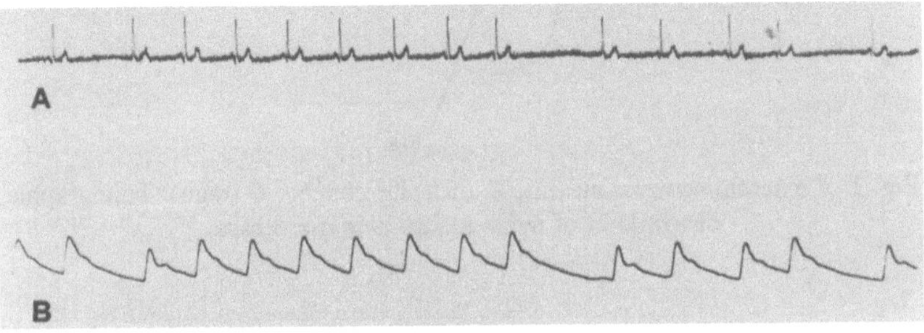

Fig. 1. Vagal response observed during r.f. thermolesion at 65 °C: there is a transient slowing of heart rate (*A*) and a slight hypotension (*B*)

In another case, on the contrary, bradycardia and hypotension were followed by convulsion and heart arrest, which needed reanimation with complete regression of symptoms.

Involvement of the 11th cranial nerve was never noted during electrical stimulation or after the lesional phase of the procedure.

After the surgical procedure, alteration of painful sensitivity was evaluated by the pin-pick test on the skin territories innervated by the glossopharyngeal and vagus nerves. A correct evaluation of the tonsillar and pharyngeal regions sensitivity was not carried out for the technical problems connected. In all patients one or more areas of hypo-analgesia at the external acoustic meatus or at the concha auris were found. These sensory disturbances, more evident at the end of the thermocoagulation, showed a partial tendency to decrease 24–48 hours after the surgical procedure.

Immediately after thermocoagulation we noted an alteration in the painful sensation at the posterior edge of the external acoustic meatus in 5 cases, of the anterior border in 3. In 6 patients

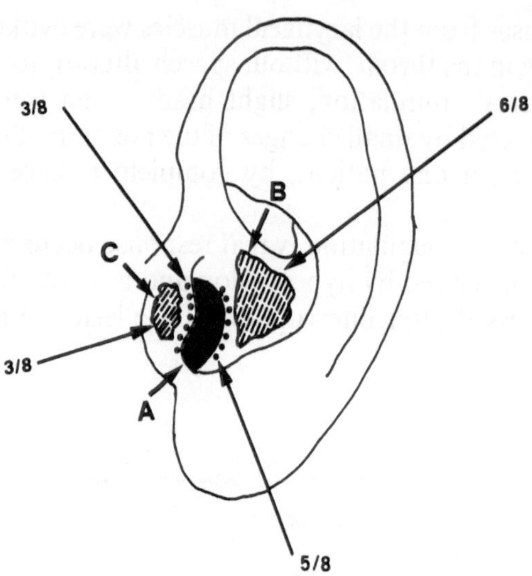

Fig. 2. *A* external acoustic meatus, *B* auricular concha, *C* tragus. Topographic distribution of hypo-analgesia in our 8 cases

involvement of the skin of the auricular concha, but never of the helix, antihelix, scapha, or lobulus auriculae; in 3 cases the tragus was also involved (Fig. 2).

Conclusions

Immediate and late surgical results demonstrate that percutaneous thermolesion is effective in the treatment of glossopharyngeal pain, particularly for essential forms; also symptomatic cancer pain is improved, patients requiring only minor analgesics and are free of pain on deglutition and speech. In addition, this technique, for its simplicity, low surgical risks and rare postoperative complications, may be carried out before other traditional and more invasive surgical procedures [2, 5]. In particular, later-cervical way seems to us more simple than the anterior-lateral, expecially in the presence of skull base tumours which can hamper the progression of the needle. In accordance with Isamat *et al.* [4], we considered the presence of paresthesias induced in the tonsillar region and the acoustic meatus during low voltage electrical stimulation an essential sign for correct position of the electrode at the foramen jugulare.

The appearence of transient hypotension and bradycardia, without postoperative disturbances of speech and deglutition, indicates a transient and quickly reversible involvement of the vagus, caused probably by heat diffusion from the tip of the needle to the adjacent nervous structures[4].

The topographic distribution of hypo-analgesia at the level of the external acoustic meatus and the auricular concha after the lesion has, in our opinion, peculiar interest.

According to some anatomical description[3,8,9] the glossopharyngeal nerve provides sensitive branches also only for the tympanic cavity through the nerve of Jacobson.

The vagus nerve originates the auricular nerve, innervating the posterior part of the external meatus, the concha and the medial part of the ear. Other authors[7,10] extend the area innervated by the glossopharyngeal nerve to a small part of the auricular concha.

Our constant observation of an alteration of pain sensitivity at the concha and at the external acoustic meatus could be—according to the opinion of some neuroanatomists cited above—expression of a functional damage to the vagus nerve. However, it is difficult to explain the persistence of the sensory damage as the only expression of vagal involvement while no motor nor visceral symptoms are present. In addition, none of our patient showed, even for short periods, neither alterations in speech and deglutition, nor sensory disturbances beyond the concha or at the medial part of the ear.

In conclusion, if a persistent vagal damage can be excluded, the sensitive area of the 9th cranial nerve at the concha and the external acoustic meatus must be wider than the neuroanatomical data previously assumed from the literature.

References

1. Bonica, J. J., Il dolore. Diagnosi, prognosi, terapia, pp. 217—220 (it. ed.). Milano: Vallardi. 1959.
2. Dandy, W. E., Glossopharyngeal neuralgia (tic douloureux). Its diagnosis and treatment. Arch. Surg. *15* (1927), 193—214.
3. David, M., Pourpre, H., Neurochirurgie, pp. 795—796. Paris: Ed. Flammarion. 1961.
4. Isamat, F., Ferràn, E., Acebes, J. J., Selective percutaneous thermocoagulation rhizotomy in essential glossopharyngeal neuralgia. J. Neurosurg. *55* (1981), 575—580.
5. Laha, R. K., Jannetta, P. J., Glossopharyngeal neuralgia. J. Neurosurg. *47* (1977), 316—320.

6. Lazorthes, Y., Verdie, J. C., Radiofrequency coagulation of the petrous ganglion in glossopharyngeal neuralgia. Neurosurgery *4* (1979), 512—516.
7. Lechevalier, B., Houtteville, J. P., Schupp, C., Atteinte isolée des nerfs crâniens. Encycl. Méd. Chir., Paris, Neurologie, I-1976, 17085 B-10.
8. Mumenthaler, M., Neurological diagnosis of caudal cranial nerves lesions. In: The Cranial Nerves (Samii, M., Jannetta, P. J., eds.), pp. 593—596. Berlin-Heidelberg-New York: Springer. 1981.
9. Testut, L., Jacob, O., Trattato di Anatomia Topografica, Vol. 1, pp. 311—321. Torino: UTET. 1967.
10. White, J. C., Sweet, W. H., Pain and the Neurosurgeon, pp. 285—289. Springfield, Ill.: Ch. C Thomas. 1969.

Acta Neurochirurgica, Suppl. 33, 521—525 (1984)

Percutaneously Implantable Chronic Electrode for Radiofrequency Stimulation of the Gasserian Ganglion. A Perspective in the Management of Trigeminal Pain

M. Meglio[1]

With 2 Figures

Summary

The author describes a method for percutaneous implant of a chronic electrode into the Gasserian ganglion. Such electrode, after a percutaneous test period, can be coupled to a subcutaneous receiver for chronic stimulation. The implanting procedure does not require any incision in the face.

No technical problems have been encountered in the first five patients treated with this method for trigeminal pain.

Keywords: Percutaneous electrode stimulation; Gasserian ganglion; trigeminal pain.

Introduction

Meyerson and Håkansson[2] first reported in 1980 a method of stimulation of the Gasserian ganglion via bipolar plate electrode sutured to the dura over the ganglion exposed through a subtemporal approach. We describe here a percutaneous technique of implantation of a chronic stimulating electrode into the Gasserian ganglion. Our electrode lead after a percutaneous test period can be coupled to a radio frequency unit for permanent stimulation. We also present our preliminary experience in the first five patients.

---

[1] Istituto di Neurochirurgia, Università Cattolica del Sacro Cuore, Largo A. Gemelli, 8, I-00168 Roma, Italy.

Material and Method

The electrode designed for trigeminal ganglion stimulation consists of a platinum iridium, stylet operated lead. At the tip of the lead is the contact area. To prevent dislodgement two sets of tines are locate at 5 and 10 mm from the tip of the electrode. After removing the stylet, the lead has an helically curved section designed to prevent traction on the tip with the movement of the mandible. The lead can be cut at the desired length so it can be easily attached to the temporary extension for the test period and than to the receiver extension in a second operation. The electrode is inserted under fluoroscopic control through a 15 gauge thin wall needle (inside diameter 1.50 mm placed into the foramen ovale) according to the technique described by Härtel[1] with the tip of the electrode at or close to the level of the clivus (Fig. 1 A–B). Electrical stimulation should evoke paresthesias over the painful area with very low current intensities (less than 0.5 V, 100 Hz, 1 msec duration); a small incision (1.5 cm) is than made in the submandibular region about 1 cm from the margo mandibulae and two to four cm from the midline (Fig. 1 C). A subcutaneous tunnel passing over the edge of the mandibular bone is created from the submandibular incision to the point of insertion of the needle (Fig. 1 D). To avoid a skin incision in the face two blunt instruments are passed together in the subcutaneous tunnel until they touch the needle. One catches the electrode when the needle is removed and is needed to hold it in place while the other pulls the distal extension of the electrode in the tunnel over the edge of the mandible and down toward the skin incision (Fig. 1 E). The electrode is now cut at the proper length and connected to the temporary extension tunnelled under the skin away from the point of incision. After the efficacy of the procedure has been tested, the submandibular skin incision is reopened and the temporary extension is removed. Another incision is made at the site chosen for receiver placement. The receiver extension is tunnelled to the lead end and connected to it. The receiver is placed in a subcutaneous pocket, the wounds are sutured. The receiver has an indifferent electrode built in and connected to its positive pole (Fig. 1 F).

We have treated with this technique five patients (Fig. 2 A). Three of them were affected by typical trigeminal pain repeatidly recurring after thermocoagulation (2 cases) and retrogasserian rhyzotomy (1 case). Our fourth patient had postherpetic facial pain with some involvement of the cervical regions and had reported only temporary benefit from VPM-thalamic stimulation. The last patient developped facial pain as a consequence of a middle fossa tumor compression over the ganglion. Pain did not subside after tumor removal, nor after percutaneous thermocoagulation of the ganglion. In all our patients there was some degree of sensory disturbance in the trigeminal area.

Stimulation was applied by the patients themselves as needed at 60–100 Hz, 0.1 msec, at the threshold value for paresthesiae with an external transmitter mod. 3522 Medtronic.

Results

A remarkable pain relief was achieved in all the patients without any detectable sensory loss (Fig. 2 B). In two of them the induction

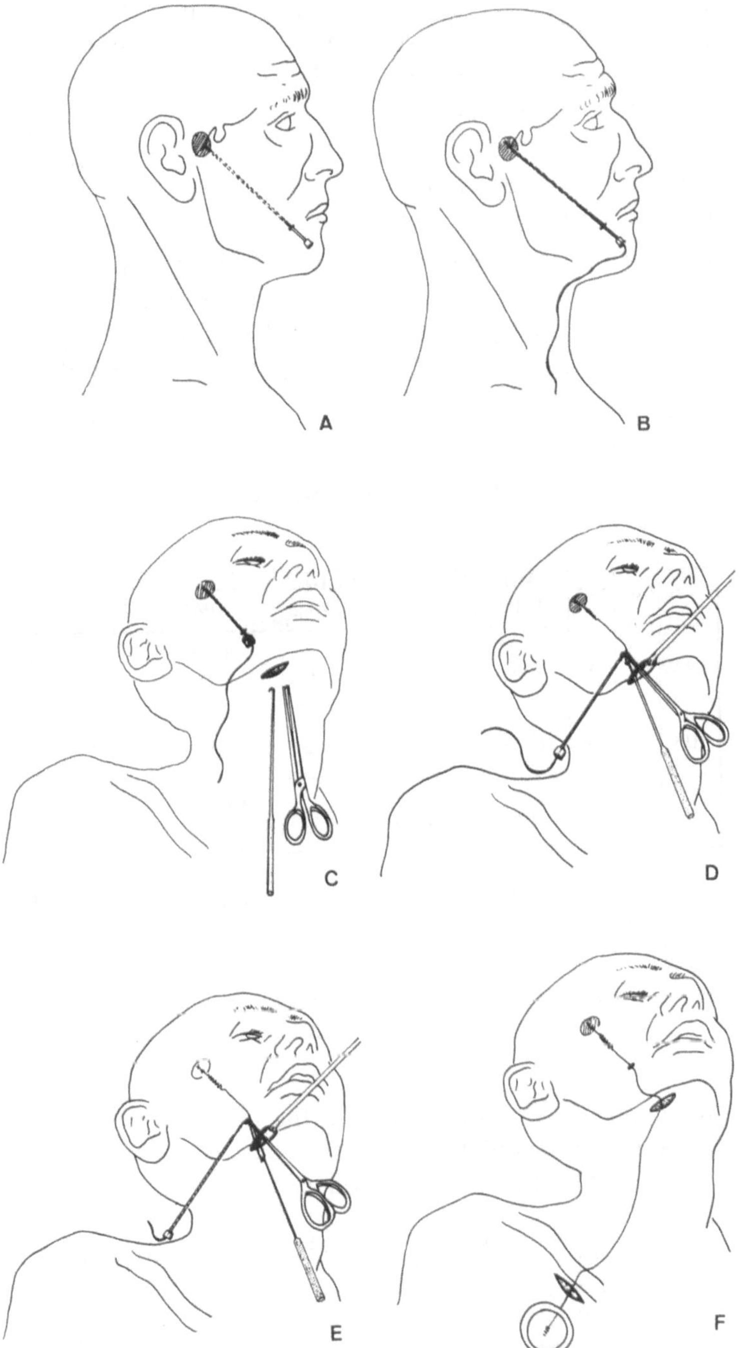

Fig. 1. Procedure of implant of the Gasserian ganglion electrode (see text)

Pz.	AGE	SEX	ETIOLOGY OF PAIN	DISTRIB. OF PAIN	DURAT. OF PAIN	PREVIOUS TREAT.	SENSORY DISTURB.
A. S.	71	M	UNKNOWN	II III L	7	THERMOC.	SLIGHT HYPAESTH.
U. E.	69	M	UNKNOWN	III L	2	THERMOC.	SLIGHT HYPAESTH.
B. M.	74	F	UNKNOWN	I II III R	12	NEUROTOM. PERIP. BLOCKS RETROGASS. RHIZOTOMY	MARKED HYPAESTH. HYPALG.
C. M.	78	M	POSTHERP.	I-II-III C_1-C_2 R	2	ACUPUNCT. PERIP. BLOCK THAL. STIM.	HYPERAES. HYPERALG.
DB. G.	56	F	COMPR. BY MIDL. FOSSA TUMOR removed	II III L	2	THERMOC.	HYPAESTH. HYPALG.

Fig. 2 A. Patients studied

Pz.	AGE	SEX	PAIN RELIEF %	INDUCTION TIME	STIMUL. TIME min.	POST STIM. TIME	FOLLOW UP months
A.S.	71	M	100	IMMEDIATE	1	HOURS DAYS	18
U.E.	69	M	50-75	MINUTES	20	HOURS	9
B.M.	74	F	100	IMMEDIATE	5	HOURS DAYS	7
C.M.	78	M	50	MINUTES	5	MINUTES HOURS	0,5
DB.G.	56	F	100	MINUTES	20	HOURS	2

Fig. 2 B. Results

time for analgesia was very short, in the other three it required several minutes of stimulation. The effect outlasted the stimulation in all the cases. Our first patient is still using the stimulator after 18 months.

In one patient (C. M.) the electrode had to be removed after the percutaneous test period because of a suspected meningeal reaction; this patient is now scheduled for reimplant.

In none of our patient we have noted any electrode dislodgement nor any technical failure of the equipment.

References

Härtel, F., Die Behandlung der Trigeminusneuralgie mit intrakraniellen Alkoholeinspritzungen. Deutsch. Z. Chir. *126* (1914), 429—552.

Meyerson, B. A., Håkansson, S., Alleviation of Atypical Trigeminal Pain by Stimulation of the Gasserian Ganglion with an Implant Electrode. Acta Neurochir. (Wien) Suppl. *30* (1980), 303—309.

Acta Neurochirurgica, Suppl. 33, 527—528 (1984)

The Use of Highly Detailed Three Dimensional Neuroanatomical Images in the Placing of Cerebral Stimulating Electrodes for Pain *

C. Giorgi [1], G. Garibotto [2], U. Cerchiari [3], G. Broggi [1], and A. Franzini [1]

Stereotactic implantion of stimulating electrodes in the thalamic sensory relais nuclei has proved to be effective in the treatment of chronic pain [1-3].

This "invisible" target procedure falls into the category of stereotactic operations in which the target location involves a quantitative correlation between the measurements obtained from the patient's images and an anatomical atlas. The introduction of CT performed in stereotactic conditions and the development of digital signal processing of neuroanatomical images make this correlation easier and more reliable [6].

In a previous paper [5] we described the threedimensional digital processing of neuroanatomical images obtained from the Schaltenbrand and Wahren Atlas [7]. The original images after digitalization, interpolation and low pass filtering were presented on a color graphic terminal. Three dimensional display of diencephalic volumes was possible, and sections were presented according to any arbitrary orientation to identify the anatomy along any surgical probe trajectory. Color coding allowed the identification of structures in planes different from the familiar orientation presented in conventional imaging techniques. In order to optimize the processing of these images, a computational technique has been introduced [4], based on the description of three

* This work was supported by C.N.R. grants 81.0173411 and 81.0171911.

[1] Istituto Neurologico "C. Besta", Div. Neurochirurgica, Via Celoria N. 11, I-20133 Milano, Italy.

[2] 3-M Italia, Div. Ricerche, Ferrania (SV), Italy.

[3] Istituto Naz. dei Tumori, Div. di Fisica Sanitaria, Milano, Italy.

dimensional structures by means of a skeleton model. The skeleton is described as the locus of points inside a three dimensional object, located at a minimum distance from at least two elements of the object surface. If these points are expanded into spheres with a radius equal to this distance, the original object can be recovered without distortion.

Rotation, translation and scale factors can be applied to the computational models of the structures, after identification and orientation of the patient's anatomy.

Identification of a sufficiently large number of reference points on images derived from the patient are required in order to decrease the statistical error in transferring the position of the target area selected on the atlas to the patient's anatomy.

At present the final electrode position is selected largely according to neurophysiological responses. Significant improvement of the quality of anatomical information derived from the patient has been achieved in the research activity on intraoperative computerized tomography currently under way at the Department of Radiology of New York University with the participation of our group.

References

1. Broggi, A., Franzini, G., Giorgi, C., Servello, D., Crenna, P., Carenini, L., SEP utilization in chronic thalamic stimulation for deafferentation pain. A preliminary study. Acta Neurochir. (Wien) (in press).
2. Hosobuchi, Y., Adams, J. E., Rutkin, B., Chronic thalamic stimulation for the control of facial anaesthesia dolorosa. Arch. Neurol. *9* (1973), 158—161.
3. Mazars, G. J., Intermittent stimulation of nucleus ventralis posterolateralis for intractable pain. Surg. Neurol. *4* (1975), 93—95.
4. Garibotto, G., Tosini, R., Description and classification of 3-D objects. IEEE Computer Society Press *82* (1982), 833—835.
5. Giorgi, C., Garibotto, G., Garozzo, S., Micca, G., Piretta, G., Three dimensional processing of a stereotactic brain atlas. Appl. Neurophysiol. *45* (1982), 419—425.
6. Koslow, M., Abele, M. G., Griffith, R. C., Mair, G. A., Chase, N. E., Stereotactic surgical system controlled by computed tomography. Neurosurgery *8* (1981), 72—82.
7. Schaltenbrand, G., Wahren, W., Atlas for stereotaxy of the human brain. 2nd Ed. Stuttgart: Thieme. 1974.

Section IV

Miscellaneous

Acta Neurochirurgica, Suppl. 33, 531—534 (1984)

Quantification of Thalamic EEG by the Shape-factor Intensity (SFI) Method

E. R. Heikkinen[1], **P. H. Eskelinen,** and **S. H. M. Nyström**

With 1 Figure

Summary

A new EEG quantification method based on detection of signal intensity and shape-factor was applied to stereotactic ventrolateral thalamotomy in treating Parkinson's disease. Signal groups that probably were derived from opposing hyperactive discharges could be demonstrated as well as their disappearance after the therapeutic coagulation. Usefulness of the method for investigating of thalamic electrophysiology and for assessment of extent of the coagulation is discussed.

Keywords: EEG quantification; thalamus; Parkinson's disease.

Introduction

Unitary recordings from the human thalamus have revealed rhythmic discharges synchronous to Parkinsonian tremor. The discharges do not respond to peripheral nor volitional or mental effort[1]. Results of multiple unit activity and thalamic EEG recordings depend mainly on the degree of general arousal of the patient[2].

The purpose of the present study was to evaluate usefulness of the new EEG quantification method; 1. in investigating of thalamic electrophysiology in Parkinson's disease, and 2. in assessing the extent of the therapeutic lesion.

---

[1] Department of Neurosurgery, Oulu University Central Hospital, SF-90220 Oulu 22, Finland.

Clinical Material and Methods

Ventrolateral thalamotomy was carried out on eight patients suffering from medically refractory Parkinson's disease by using a Laitinen stereotactic apparatus and a RFG-5 S lesion generator system. Tremor and rigidity as well as drug-induced dyskinesias dominated the clinical symptoms. A Kaiser type 8-pole depth electrode was used for bipolar recording of thalamic EEG. Analog registration of EEG and recording on magnetic tape for collecting data to a PDP-11/23 minicomputer were done simultaneously. The data were processed on-line in some instances. The new EEG quantitation method, SFI analysis, developed by one (P.H.E.) in our group was utilized. This method is based on detection of all processes separated by extreme values of the signal and on grouping them according to intensity of the signal and according to signal shape-factor. The latter is affected by duration and speed of change of the signal. Sampling frequency was 100 per second. The EEG was recorded in 1–2 minute periods at rest and during various tasks.

Results

A significant and persistent clinical improvement in tremor and rigidity was achieved in all the cases with no major surgical complications.

A typical distribution of EEG signals, a SFI map, is shown in Fig. 1 A. Two types of signal populations can be distinguished: one with increasing intensity but decreasing shape factor ("neck" on the map) and another with simultaneously increasing intensity and shape-factor (upper "clavicle" on the map). This type of signal distribution could be constantly registered throughout the resting periods prior to the coagulation.

Active movements of the arms were reflected on the SFI map as a decrease in coherence of slow and intensive signals and as a more homogenous distribution of faster and weaker signals. Active movements of the legs caused similar but smaller changes. Calculation performance representing a left hemisphere function and imaging visual stimuli as a right hemisphere function did not cause any absolutely convincing alterations. Also the SFI maps recorded during peripheral sensory stimuli and during conversation were similar to those at rest.

The SFI maps registered after the coagulation were totally different from the preoperative ones (Fig. 1 B): The signals at rest or during various tasks consisted of low-intensity waves showing no explicit groups. Only during active movements of the arms or legs one could identify scattered outlines of the typical preoperative configurations.

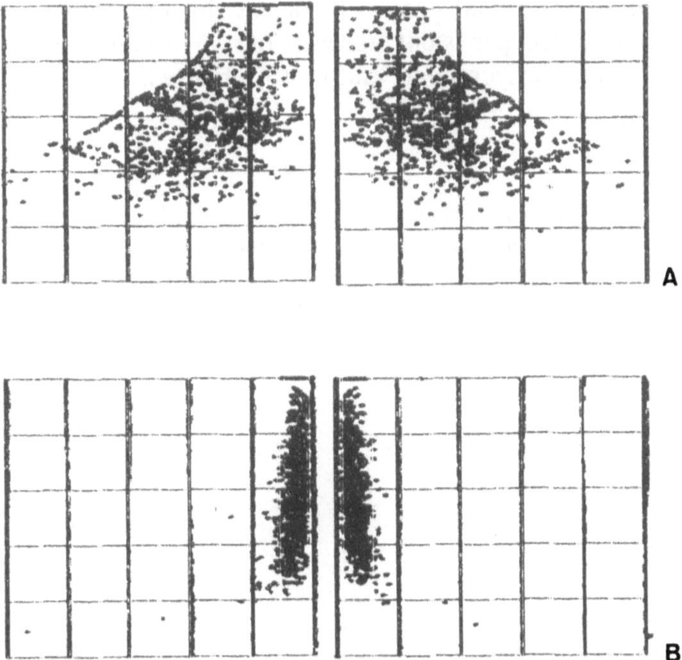

Fig. 1. Shape-factor intensity quantification of thalamic EEG prior to (A) and after (B) the coagulation. Signals registered at rest during one minute from the non-dominant right ventrolateral nucleus. Ordinate = Intensity (200 to 0 microvolts on the left and 0 to 200 microvolts on the right). Abscissa = Shape-factor (origo 0, top 1)

Discussion

Mapping the signals of thalamic EEG into various groups according to their intensity and shape-factor reveals signal patterns which behave opposite to each other. The patterns may represent the opposing nigro-striatal dopaminergic and cholinergic neurons, known to be in imbalance in Parkinson's disease. Also a relation to increased alpha motor activity and increased inhibition of gamma motor activity may have to be taken into account. As known, these components are suggested to be pathologically altered in parkinsonism. Therapeutic coagulation nearly totally abolished those signal patterns that probably are derived from hyperactively functioning neurons.

More detailed analysis of the SFI maps is in progress to confirm their usefulness for peroperative assessment of the extent of the coagulation. The final goal is to detect thalamic EEG changes which guarantee persistent absence of the tremor but exclude untoward neuropsychologic and motor changes.

References

1. Ohye, Ch., Saito, Y., Fukamachi, A., Narabayashi, H., An analysis of the spontaneous rhythmic and non-rhythmic burst discharges in the human thalamus. J. Neurol. Sci. *22* (1974), 245—259.
2. Velasco, M., Velasco, F., Olvera, A., Effect of task relevance and selective attention on components of cortical and subcortical evoked potentials in man. Electroenceph. clin. Neurophysiol. *48* (1980), 377—386.

Acta Neurochirurgica, Suppl. 33, 535—537 (1984)

Deep Brain Stimulations in Cases of Prolonged Post-traumatic Unconsciousness

F. Cohadon[1], **E. Richer, A. Rougier, Ph. Deliac,** and **H. Loiseau**

Keywords: Deep-brain stimulation; post-traumatic coma; permanent vegetative state.

In some patients in a state of prolonged post-traumatic unconsciousness (PTU), the absence of functional recovery over a long period of time could be due to a lack of upward non specific activation on the cortical fields. Indeed in the majority of such cases primary, or more often secondary, traumatic lesions of the upper brain stem do exist and are likely to interrupt the rostral projections of the midbrain activating system. A few number of cases have been reported[1–4] in which deep brain stimulations (DBS) of the non specific nuclei of the diencephalon and related structures have been attempted in order to provide artificial activation of the cortex with the hope of enhancing functional recovery. This report will consider 6 cases of PTU in which DBS of centrum medianum thalami has been tried.

Methods

Stimulation electrodes (Medtronic inc. Minneapolis U.S.A.) designed for DBS in pain problems (teflon coated platinum wires; 4 stimulation surfaces of 1 mm length separated by 2 mm spacings) have been implanted unilaterally through a coronal approach using a modified Talairach apparatus. The target was centrum medianum (CM) on the right side according to stereotactic coordinates of Talairach atlas. Stimulation was provided intermittently $^{1}/_{4}$ h/h, afterwards permanently from 8 a.m. to 8 p.m. Parameters were settled below the threshold of adversive and/or hypertonic reactions (squarewave impulses, more often 5 ms, 5 to 10 volts, 50 Hz).

---

[1] Service de Neuro-chirurgie A, C.H.U. Pellegrin Tripode, F-33076 Bordeaux, France.

Results of DBS have been checked weekly through a specially designed performance scale arbitrarilly coding vegetative functions, relational possibilities, dystonic pattern and goaldirected motor performances.

Cases

DBS has been proposed in a serie of 6 severe brain injuries fulfilling the following criteria:

1. Severe initial post-traumatic coma (Glasgow coma scale 5–3) with acute midbrain syndrome (decerebrate rigidity, abolition of oculo-cephalic responses).
2. PTU without any improvement over long period of time (4 to 15 months); akinetic mutism, axial tonic disturbances, eyes open, no evidence of communication whatsoever; EEG: diffuse slow wave pattern; evoked potential: long latency, simplified pattern; CT scan: large ventricular dilatation with normal ICP (1 case: normal CT scan).
3. Devoted families well aware of the predictable outcome, prepared to help the nursing staff in intensive rehabilitation management, well informed of the aim, scope and limitations of DBS.

Results

In 3 cases DBS pursued over 2 months brought no appreciable changes whether in clinical responses or in electrophysiological patterns. DBS was then removed. With 4 months to 2.5 years follow up, these patients are still in a permanent vegetative state. In 3 cases DBS brought a clear cut improvement of the overall situation: 1. vegetative functions are rapidly influenced (oral feeding becomes possible, bronchial hypersecretion is reduced, pulmonary infection disappears...); 2. a definite improvement of consciousness and relational possibilities is reached after 2 to 4 weeks and progresses steadilly; 3. motor functions are much less influenced: axial tonic disturbances are slightly modified; goal directed motricity remains very poor with limbs movements of limited amplitude.

Conclusion

DBS applied in selected case of prolonged post-traumatic unconsciousness. 1. In some patients yield no appreciable changes in electrophysiological pattern and clinical state. In these cases the diagnosis of permanent vegetative state with very poor chances of further recovery may be accepted and intensive management may be discontinued. 2. In some patients lead to unequivocal enhancement of both electrophysiological pattern and clinical responses. Stabilisation of vegetative disorders, recovery of some degree of interpersonal relationship and motor goal-directed behaviour is constant. Tonic disturbances are less attenuated.

If these results are confirmed DBS could be used earlier in the evolution of PTU with the aim of assessing the likelihood of some degree of ultimate recovery of cortical functions. Among a host of problems raised by this technique the more difficult in our opinion is as follows: is it ethically sound and practically worthwhile to move a given patient from a state of purely vegetative life to a status of half-way recovery in which rather poor performances and relational possibilities are likely to bring to both the patient and his family even more suffering and distress.

References

1. Hassler, R., Dalle Ore, G., Dieckmann, G., Bricolo, A., Dolce, G., Behavioural and EEG arousal induced by stimulation of unspecific projection systems in a patient with post-traumatic appallic syndrome. Electroenceph. clin. Neurophysiol. *27* (1969), 306—310.
2. Hassler, R., Dalle Ore, G., Bricolo, A., Dieckmann, G., Dolce, G., EEG and clinical arousal induced by bilateral long-term stimulation of pallidal systems in traumatic vigil coma. Electroenceph. clin. Neurophysiol. *27* (1969), 689—690.
3. MacLardy, T., Ervin, F., Mark, V., Attempted Inset-electrodes. Arousal from traumatic coma: neuropathological findings. Trans. Amer. Neurol. Assoc. *93* (1968), 25—30.
4. Sturm, V., Kühner, A., Schmitt, H. P., Assmus, H., Stock, G., Chronic electrical stimulation of the thalamic unspecific activating system in a patient with coma due to midbrain and upper brain stem infarction. Acta Neurochir. (Wien) *47* (1979), 235—244.

Acta Neurochirurgica, Suppl. 33, 539—541 (1984)

Selective Posterior Rootlet Section in the Treatment of Spastic Disorders of Infantile Cerebral Palsy: Immediate and Late Results

B. Fraioli[1], **C. Zamponi**[1], **L. Baldassarre**[2], and **G. Rosa**[1]

Keywords: Posterior rootlet section; spasticity.

Introduction

Over the last thirteen years we have accumulated a vast experience[5] in all the most important methods proposed by various authors for the treatment of spastic disorders of infantile cerebral palsy, such as stereotactic dentatolysis or pulvinolysis, C_1–C_4 posterior cervical rhizotomies or cronic paleocerebellar stimulation[4].

In our experience, the best results are stretched with the surgical procedure introduced by us[1] as far back as 1975, under the name of "partial posterior rootlet section". This operation has been presented under the name of "selective posterior rootlet section"[2,3].

The purpose of this paper is to report the immediate and long-term results obtained with this operation in a series of 44 spastic patients operated on from January 1973 to December 1976 who were all controlled, with 3 exceptions, in the early part of 1983.

Material and Method

The patients who underwent surgical treatment ranged from 4 to 16 years of age. Twenty-two suffered from spastic quadriplegia, 20 from diplegia and 2 from hemiplegia.

The surgical technique which we employed, illustrated in detail in previous publications[1,2], essentially consists of the section of only the dorso-medial part of

[1] Neurosurgical Institute of the Rome University and [2] Infantile Neuropsychiatric Department of Ospedale Bambino Gesù of Rome, Roma, Italy.

each sensory rootlet corresponding to the spastic muscles. With the aid of the operating microscope, half or two-thirds of each rootlet is cut, at 1 mm from its junction with the spinal cord, from the dorso-medial side to the ventro-lateral side. Surgery was performed from L_1 to S_1 in 31 patients, bilaterally in all cases except 2; from D_{12} to S_1 in 12 and from D_{11} to S_1 in one other, all bilaterally.

Results

For what concerns the immediate functional results, 30 patients improved considerably after operation, thanks to the disappearance or notable reduction of spasticity in the lower limbs, consisting, from a clinical point of view, in the disappearance of hyperadduction or crossing of the lower limbs, of hyperextension and intrarotation, of equinism and also of the arching of the trunk. On the other hand, there was only a modest improvement in 12 patients and no improvement in 2 others; this was partly due to the psychic conditions of the patients who hardly co-operated at all; partly to insufficient cutting of the rootlets, to be assumed from the persistence of spasticity, even if reduced, and partly to the fact that several of the patients presented tendineo muscular retractions which were by then permanent.

The long-term results have shown to be stable on an average observation period of 7 years. The 30 patients who had clearly improved immediately after operation have shown further improvement, due to the fact they have been better able to utilize the physiotherapy. In particular, it should be noted that 4 patients became independent when walking and 9 others became able to walk with supports. None of the patients have shown deficits of esterocettive sensitivity. Proprioceptive sensitivity has been accurately examined in 33 patients and fount to be normal, to be pointed out that the sense of position of the lower limbs and toes, tactile discrimination and pallesthesia were preserved, particularly in those patients who, neurologically, showed a lack of increase of the stretch reflexes and in particular a lack of tendon reflexes and, clinically, the complete regression of the disorders caused by spasticity.

Discussion

The partial section of the posterior rootlets is not a selective operation because it does not selectively cut the I a fibres which constitute the afferent arch of the stretch reflex. Nonetheless, it can be called selective as it has clinically shown itself capable of abolishing the increase of the stretch reflexes, that is spasticity, in absence of neurological disturbances, particularly estero-proprioceptive sensation. This fact, in our view, could merit a neurophysiological study of its own.

The indications for this operation are constituted by patients suffering from para-tetraspasticity who show, during the assisted erect position, equinism, hyperadduction or crossing of the lower limbs, hyperextension and intrarotation, provided that the level of paresis is sufficient to allow then to hold up at least their body weight. Although we have never come across a reduction in the capability to remain standing, immediately or some time after operation, we do not advise the operation for those patients who show a marked paresis of the extensor muscles, namely those who cannot even hold up their body weight, when in the assisted erect position. We also consider that the operation is rarely suitable for patients who have been, for many years, autonomous in the erect position and in deambulation, that is patients who present stabilized compensatory behaviour, such as flexion of the pelvis and the knees, where permanent contractions are often present.

References

1. Fraioli, B., Guidetti, B., La rizotomia posteriore parziale e una nuova tecnica, la radicolotomia posteriore parziale, nel trattamento della spasticità tonica. Riv. Pat. Nerv. Ment. *99* (1975), 118—135.
2. Fraioli, B., Guidetti, B., Posterior partial rootlet section in the treatment of spasticity. J. Neurosurg. *46* (1977), 618—626.
3. Fraioli, B., Guidetti, B., Selektive partielle Radiculotomia posterior in der Therapie der Spastizität. Zbl. Neurochir. *40* (1979), 319—326.
4. Fraioli, B., Baldassarre, L., Refice, G. M., Chronic paleocerebellar stimulation in dystonia and athetosis. J. Neurosurg. Sci. *24* (1980), 99—103.
5. Guidetti, B., Fraioli, B., Neurosurgical treatment of spasticity and dyskinesias. Acta Neurochir. (Wien) Suppl. *24* (1977), 27—39.

Acta Neurochirurgica, Suppl. 33, 543—546 (1984)

Clinical and Electrocardiographic Improvement of Ischemic Heart Disease After Spinal Cord Stimulation

S. Sandric[2], M. Meglio[1], F. Bellocci[2], A. S. Montenero[2], E. Scabbia[2], and V. D'Annunzio[1]

With 1 Figure

Keywords: Spinal cord stimulation; ischemic heart disease; electrocardiogram; functional sympathectomy.

Electrocardiographic (ECG) follow-up study was performed in 16 patients before and after spinal cord stimulation (SCS) for different chronic neurological disturbances. Four patients had on ECG signs of ischemic heart disease. Two of them had a history of myocardial infarction with residual chest pain on exercise in spite of adequate medical treatment (Table 1).

SCS was applied via percutaneously implanted epidural electrodes as described elsewhere[1]. Stimulation parameters were 60 to 120 Hz, 0,1–1 msec pulse duration, voltage at threshold for paraesthesiae. All the patients with ECG signs of myocardial ischemia showed a remarkable improvement with SCS (Fig. 1). In one of them (case 4) the effect became evident during the first stimulation. In all cases it was progressive with time. In three patients the ECG became normal respectively after one month (case 3) and after two months (case 2) of SCS. Patients two and three did not complain anymore chest pain since the beginning of SCS. No evidence of ECG changes during the period of SCS was observed in the twelve patients who had a normal ECG tracing before SCS. As shown by Schwartz and coll. experimental surgical sympathectomy reduces the incidence of arrhytmias associated

[1] Istitutes of Neurosurgery and of [2] Cardiology, Catholic University, Roma, Italy.

Table 1. *Clinical, Electrocardiographic and SCS Data Before and After Stimulation*. PVD = Peripheral vascular disease. MS = Multiple sclerosis

Case	Sex	Age	Electrode vertebral level	Indication for SCS	ECG before SCS	after SCS	Angina pectoris before SCS	after SCS	Medical treatment before SCS	after SCS
1	M	44	D 7 D 9	neurogenic bladder in MS	diffuse negative T-waves	T-waves normalized	absent	absent	no	no
2	M	69	D 12	leg pain in PVD	ST-segment depression V 4-5-6	ST-segment normalized	present	absent	β-block. agents nitrates	no
3	M	65	D 8	leg pain in PVD	ST-segment depression Deep negative T-waves V 3-4-5-6	ST-segment normalized T-waves slightly improved	present	absent	β-block. agents nitrates	no
4	F	44	D 10	neurogenic bladder in MS	negatives T-waves V 1-2-3	T-waves normalized	absent	absent	no	no

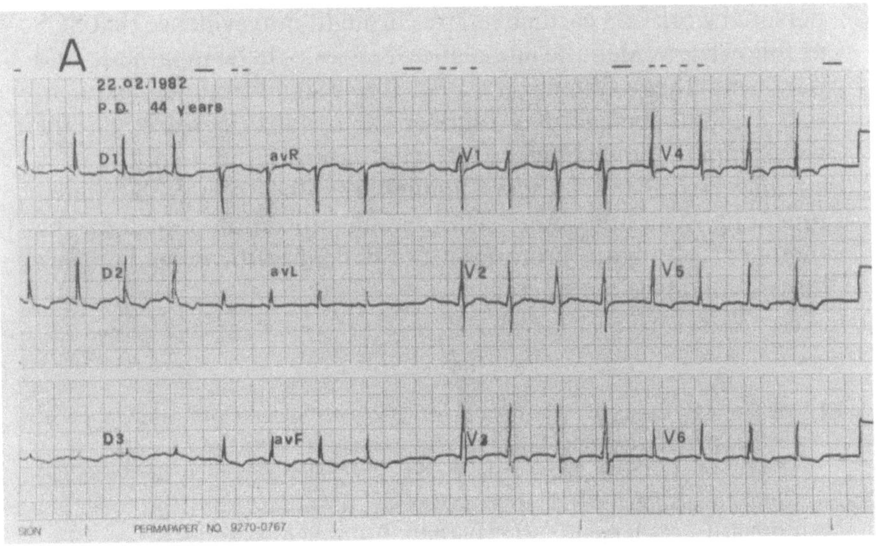

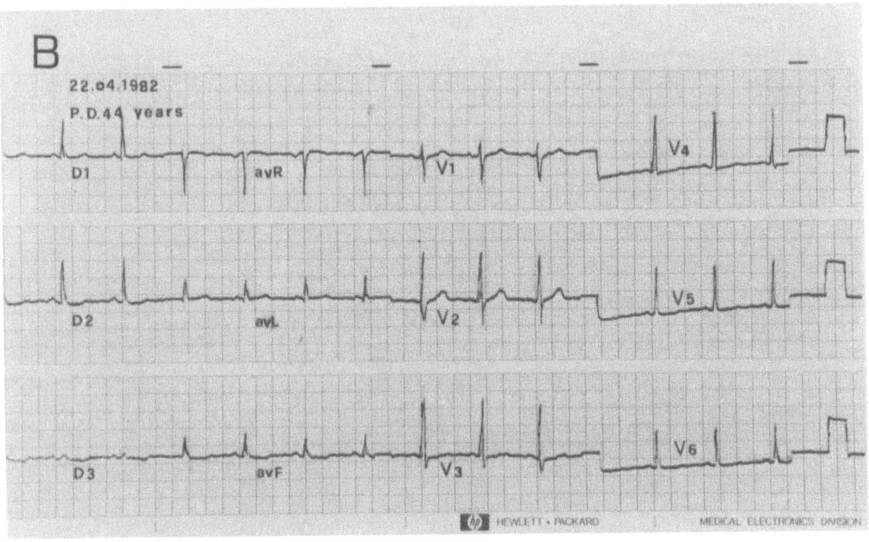

Fig. 1. P.D. 44 years old man with neurogenic bladder due to multiple sclerosis. ECG tracing—(A) before SCS—diffuse myocardial ischemia, negative T-waves—(B) two months after SCS T-waves normalized

with transient coronary occlusion and increases the capability of the coronary bed to dilate at rest and during exercise[3]. Previous personal work[2] on cardiac reflexes brought into evidence that SCS is followed by definite imbalance between the sympathetic and parasympathetic systems; it is related to a significant depression of the sympathetic activity and/or a certain increase of the parasympathetic activity. For what above, the hypothesis is advanced that the present findings are due to a SCS related functional sympathectomy. The possible utilization of SCS for the treatment of angina pectoris in the patients with ischemic heart disease might be considered.

References

1. Meglio, M., Cioni, B., Personal experience with Spinal Cord Stimulation in chronic pain management. Appl. Neurophysiol. *45* (1982), 195—200.
2. Meglio, M., Cioni, B., Sandric, S., Evaluation of cardiac activity during Spinal Cord Stimulation. In: Indications for Spinal Cord Stimulation (Hosobuchi, Y., Corbin, T., eds.), pp. 67—71. München: Excerpta Medica. 1981.
3. Schwartz, P. J., Lowell Stone, H., Left stellectomy in the prevention of ventricular fibrillation caused by acute myocardial ischemia in conscious dogs with anterior myocardial infarction. Circulation *62* (1980), 1256—1265.

Acta Neurochirurgica, Suppl. 33, 547—551 (1984)

Third Ventricular Width and Thalamo-capsular Laterality

E. Hitchcock[1] and **J. Cadavid**

Summary

One hundred and eleven sequential "normal" CAT scans have been reviewed and ventricular dimensions and thalamo-capsular laterality measured.

1. There is no direct correlation between third ventricular width and age (after 15 years).

2. Male third ventricular mean width (4.8 mm) is slightly greater than female (4.1 mm).

3. There is a wide variation of thalamo-capsular laterality.

Pre-operative CAT scan measurements are helpful in stereotactic thalamic surgery.

Keywords: CAT scan; anatomical structures; coordinates stereotaxic surgery.

Introduction

Intracranial stereotactic targets are mostly determined by reference to ventricular landmarks, in particular the length and width of the third ventricle. The increasing use of computed tomography in stereotactic surgery and the interfacing of stereotactic instrumentation and computed axial tomograms encourages an examination of the value and accuracy of ventricular measurements in CAT scanning.

Clinical contrast studies with air encephalography or air or contrast ventriculography have been widely used as a basis for measurement, Peltonen[10] and others. Ventricular size has also been estimated by echoencephalography (Grumme[5], Huber *et al.*[9], Feurlein and Dilling[4] and others).

The basis for many measurements has been anatomical preparations which have the disadvantage of shrinkage.

[1] Department of Neurosurgery, University of Birmingham, U.K.

Mundinger noted statistically significant difference between third ventricular width at X-ray and at post-mortem (although distensional collapse can occur in contrast studies). Computed axial tomography has been used to measure changes in the size of the lateral ventricles (Barron *et al.*[3], Gyldensted and Kosteljanetz[6]). Hahn and Rim[7] computed frontal ventricular dimensions on normal computed tomography and Sklar *et al.*[11] estimated lateral ventricular size from CAT measurements noting a linear relationship between ventricular size and brain elasticity. Arimitsu *et al.*[2] discussed white/grey matter differentiation in computed tomography.

The internal capsule is one of the more clearly defined features of CAT scanning and the relationship of the internal capsule to the third ventricle is an important aspect of stereotactic measurement. Hardy *et al.*[8], using stereotactic stimulation techniques established a definite relationship between the width of the third ventricle and the position of the medial border of the internal capsule. Their results indicated that the thalamo-capsular border varied directly with the width of the third ventricle. The disadvantage of shrinkage met in anatomical preparations or distentional collapse in contrast studies are such that the study of the thalamo-capsular border by CAT scanning appeared likely to produce useful information.

Method

359 sequential CAT scans produced by EMI 1010-1007 were examined in patients with neurological symptoms but without organic intracranial lesions reported or subsequently revealed. 111 of these satisfied the criteria of good quality, minimal angulation, normal subarachnoid space, and a clearly visible internal capsule.

These unmagnified scans were examined and the pallidal limit of the internal capsule outlined with a sharp pencil. Although electronic methods of measurements are available because of the inherent difficulty in defining a sharp border it was found not to materially improve the accuracy achieved by this simple method.

A reduced (2 : 1) centimetre grid was placed over the scan and viewed through a magnifiying lens. Using the known diameter of the visible CAT scan cone it was possible to relate measurements to the grid divisions, the magnification being 1 : 4.45. Measurement was made with reproducible accuracy to 0.25 mm.

The following reference points were noted.

1. The mid-point of the foramen of Monro in its anterior portion.
2. The mid-point of the posterior end of the third ventricle, if clearly visible, or the mid-point of lamina quadrigemina or the most anterior point of the pineal gland.

3. The distance from the mid-point of the third ventricle to the internal capsule was measured in its anterior, middle and posterior portions. The greatest width of the third ventricle was noted also the presence or absence of a massa intermedia.

In 20% of scans the third ventricle appeared in only one section taken at mid-point including a massa intermedia and lying within the thalamic height of 20–25 mm. However, no sections selected above the foramen of Monro, below the anterior commisure or posteriorly above or below the pineal. Thus the selected sections were all within the middle third of the thalamic height, approximately 15 mm above the AC/PC line or in the FM/PC line.

Results

Third ventricular width. The greatest width for the patient sample varied from 2.27 mm to 9.08 mm with a mean of 4.5 mm and a large standard deviation of 1.9. 65 of the 111 patients had a massa intermedia. No positive or negative correlation could be found between ventricular width and the presence or absence of the massa intermedia. The mean width of the third ventricle in males was 4.8 mm and in females 4.1 mm with a range for each from 2.27 to 9.08 but with a large standard deviation of 1.9 for each group. No definite correlation could be found between third ventricular width and age.

Third ventricular width and thalamo-capsular border. No positive correlation could be found between the ventricular width and the laterality of the capsule in either its anterior middle or posterior portion.

The mean distance from the mid-line to the thalamo-capsular border was 10.7 (SD 2.4) in the anterior capsule and 22.7 (SD 2.8) at mid-capsule. In the posterior portion of the capsule the mean distance was 35 (SD 4.3). The 99% confidence intervals were anterior capsule 10.2–11.0, middle capsule 22.2 23.2, posterior capsule 34.3–35.8.

Of the 111 patients 36 had symmetrical distances both anteriorly and posteriorly for each hemisphere. 42 were only symmetrical anteriorly and 33 were unsymmetrical both anteriorly and posteriorly.

Discussion

These measurements confirm the observations of a number of other authors using different methods. Hardy *et al.*[8] and Andrew and Watkins[1], amongst others. Our results show that in patients with "normal" CAT scans and no gross evidence of cortical atrophy or increased subarachnoid space or hydrocephalus the ventricular width varies within the limits described with no definite relationship to age. Our results also show that there is no correlation between ventricular width and thalamo-capsular border with either symmetrical or asymmetrical brains suggesting that the practice of adding to the Z co-ordinates an amount which takes into account ventricular width is grossly unreliable. Assuming laterality of the thalamo-capsular border is a reasonable indicator of thalamic bulk and assuming that the normal relationships of thalamic nuclei are retained within the limits of human variation it is evident that our common practice of using empirical lateralities for selected targets could be greatly improved by careful measurements of thalamic dimensions obtained at pre-operative CAT scanning. These together with electro-physiological recording should enhance the accuracy of the thalamotomies performed for any purpose.

Comparison of CAT scan measurements with other measurements based on a variety of different techniques showed considerable agreement so that even with the definition afforded by the older CAT scanners thalamic/capsular measurements appeared to be useful especially considering the very large standard deviations. Increasing definition with the newer CAT scans will undoubtdly make these measurements more accurate and more valuable in stereotactic procedures. The pre-operative measurement of thalamocapsular distance may be useful in subsequent stereotactic procedures and may also be used in systems where the CAT scan and stereotactic instrument is interfaced and measurements related directly to the stereotactic system can be made. At the present time the CAT definition does not appear sufficiently good to dispense with contrast ventriculography but the improved definition between white and grey matter afforded by NMR scanning holds greater promise.

Acknowledgements

We are grateful to the staff of the CAT scan Unit at the Midland Centre For Neurosurgery And Neurology for their help in collecting material and to Mrs. V. Turner for typing the manuscript.

References

1. Andrew, J., Watkins, E. S., Human Thalamus And Adjacent Structures. Baltimore: Williams and Wilkins Co. 1969.

2. Arimitsu, T., DiChiro, G., Brooks, R. A., Smith, P. B., White-Grey Matter Differentiation in Computed Tomography. J. Comp. Assist. Tomogr. (Computed Tomography) *1* (4), 1977.
3. Barron, S. A., Jacobs, L., Kinkel, W. R., Changes in size of normal lateral ventricles during aging determined by computerized tomography. Neurology *26* (1976), 1011—1013.
4. Feurlein, W., Dilling, H., Das Echo-Encephalogramm des 3. Ventrikels in verschiedenen Lebensaltern. Arch. Psychiat. und Z. ges. Neurologie *209* (1967), 137—147.
5. Grumme, T., Die Breite der 3. Hirnkammer vom Frühgeborenen bis ins 10. Dezennium. Fortschr. Neurol. Psychiat. *45* (1977), 223—268.
6. Gyldensted, C., Kosteljanetz, M., Measurements of the normal ventricular system with computer tomography of the brain. A preliminary study on 44 adults. Neuro-radiology *10* (1976), 147—149.
7. Hahn, F. J. Y., Rim, K., Frontal ventricular dimensions on normal computed tomography. Amer. J. Roentgenol. *126* (1976), 593—596.
8. Hardy, T. L., Bertrand, G., Thompson, C. J., Position of the Medial Internal Capsular Border in Relation to Third-Ventricular Width. Appl. Neurophysiol. *42* (1979), 234—247.
9. Huber, G., Betz, H., Kleinoder, I., Echoencephalographische Untersuchungen der 3. Hirnkammer bei einer männlichen Normal-Bevölkerung. Nervenarzt *39* (1968), 82—84.
10. Peltonen, L., Pneumoencephalographic studies on the third ventricle of 644 neuropsychiatric patients. Acta Psych. Scand. *38* (1962), 15—34.
11. Sklar, F. H., Diehl, J. T., Beyer, C. W., Kemp Clark, W., Brain elasticity changes with ventriculomegaly. J. Neurosurg. *53* (1980), 173—179.

Acta Neurochirurgica, Suppl. 33, 553—557 (1984)

Stereotactic Cryosurgery in a CT Scanner

J. Boëthius[1], **T. Greitz**[2], **R. Kuylenstierna**[3], **M. Lagerkranser**[4], **P. G. Lundquist**[3], **T. Ribbe**[5], and **H. Wiksell**[6]

With 5 Figures

Keywords: Stereotactic cryosurgery; CT scan.

Introduction

Small deep seated tumors constitute a surgical problem. They are often difficult to find with conventional techniques and the amount of brain tissue which must be destroyed to reach the tumor may be fairly large. Ideally they should be treated stereotactically, but it is difficult to create a stereotactic lesion, which is sufficiently large to cover the tumor. The present communication describes a method to use stereotactic cryosurgery. The procedure was done in the CT-scanner in order to make it possible to monitor the size of the lesion intraoperatively.

Technical description: The patient was mounted in a base plate as previously described[1]. A craniotomy was performed in the operating room and the patient was brought down to the scanner. The base plate was mounted on a special support on the scanner table. A CT localizing frame was adapted and the stereotactic coordinates were determined[1]. The localizing frame was removed and a modified Leksell instrument was mounted on the base plate. The instrument was set according to the coordinates and adjusted so that the probe would pass through the craniotomy. A biopsy was performed. The Leksell instrument was now removed from the base plate without disturbing its setting. The patient was removed from the scanner and a new base plate was put in the special support (Fig. 1). In order to make it possible to remove the Leksell frame and arch, which would

Departments of [1] Neurosurgery, [2] Neuroradiology, [3] Otorhinolaryngology, [4] Anaestesiology, [5] Medical Engineering, Karolinska Institutet, S-10 401 Stockholm, Sweden, and [6] The Royal Technical Highschool, S-10 401 Stockholm, Sweden.

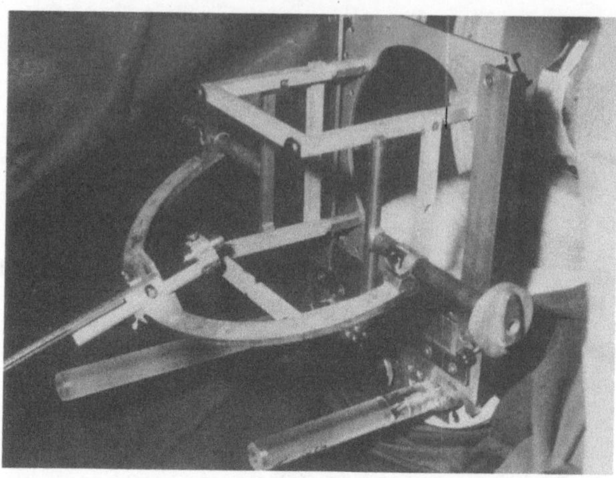

Fig. 1. The patient has been removed from the scanner and a new base plate has been put in the special support. Note the two perspex rods fixed to the base plate support

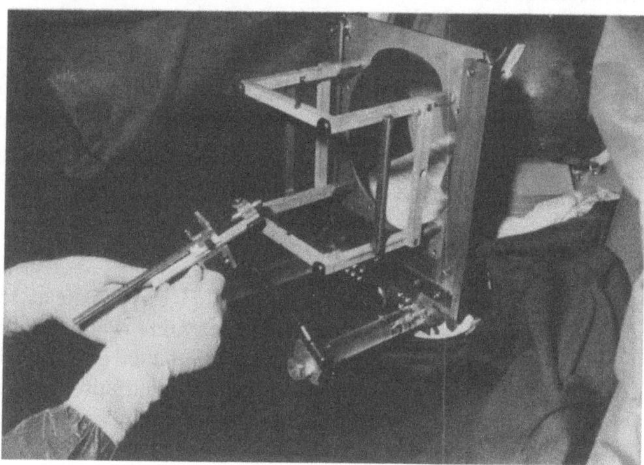

Fig. 2. Swan-halses form a rigid attachment between the base plate holder and the probe holder

cause artefacts on the CT while still retaining the probe orientation the following method was used. The unchanged Leksell instrument was mounted in the empty base plate. Two perspex rods were fixed to the base plate support (Fig. 1). A pair of "swan-halses" were fixed to the perspex rods and fastened to the probe holder of the Leksell instrument with the screws. When the swan-halses were tigthened they formed a rigid attachment between the base plate holder and the probe holder (Fig.

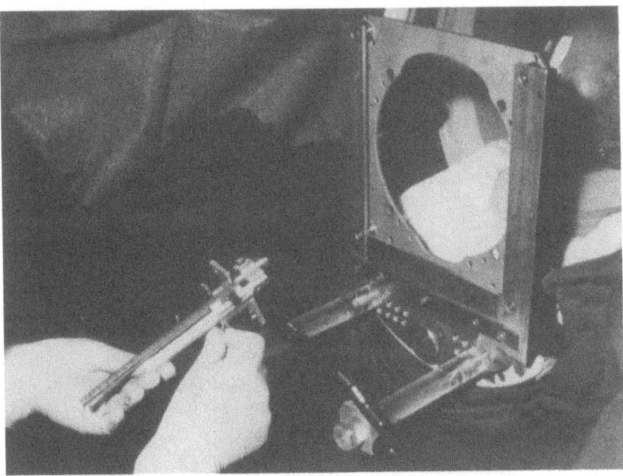

Fig. 3. The stereotactic instrument has been removed from the base plate leaving the perspex rods and the swan-halses as the sole support of the probe holder

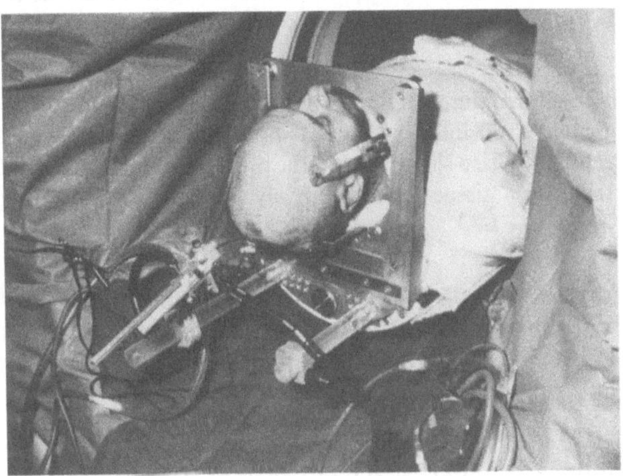

Fig. 4. The patient is repositioned in the base plate holder

2). The arch was removed carefully from the probe holder and so was the Leksell instrument leaving only the Leksell probe holder rigidly fixed to the base plate support und thus retaining the orientation it had when it was fixed in the Leksell instrument (Fig. 3). The base plate was then removed and the patient who still carried his base plate was again reattached to the base plate holder (Fig. 4). The cryoprobe could now be introduced through the craniotomy and brought down to

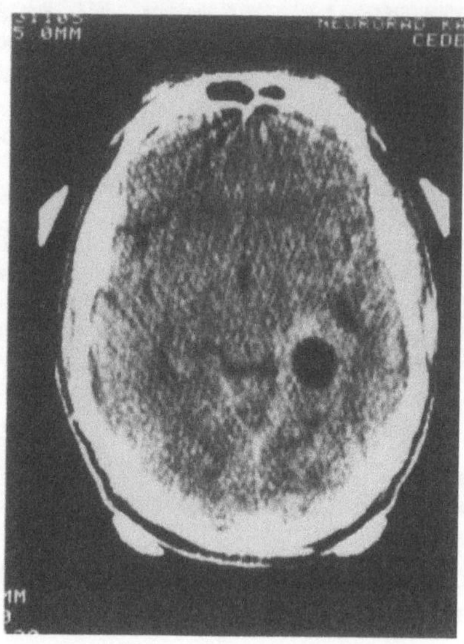

Fig. 5. Intra operative CT scanning showing localization of the ice of the cryolesion which shows up as a circular region of low density

the previously selected stereotactic position. The freezing could be performed and providing the probe was introduced from above and the scanner table adjusted to give a CT section localized slightly below the tip of the probe was possible to see the extent of the frozen tissue intraoperatively without any disturbing artefacts (Fig. 5).

General consideration: When the cryolesion thaws, there is a phase of capillary bleeding. This bleeding subsides spontaneously after a certain time. It is therefor advisable to keep the cryoprobe in place for 15–20 minutes after the lesion has been done in order to minimize this problem. This phase of a capillary bleeding makes it counter indicated to perform a cryolesion which at any part can be expected to reach the ventricular system. If it is necessary to pass through the ventricular system in order to reach a deep seated target it is advisable to have an outer canula through which the cryoprobe is inserted. This precaution should diminish the risk that the bleeding could follow the insertion track and in this way escape out into the ventricular system. It ought to be possible to evacuate at least part of the necrotisized tissue by a suction tube introduced through such an outer canula. We have not tried this in actual practice.

Ice will form for about one to one and a half centimeter out from the wall of the cooling body of the cryoprobe. Thus the diameter of the cryoprobe determines the size of the cryolesion.

The procedure is lengthy and difficult for the patient. However it is still advisable to perform it under local anesthesia since one then has the possibility to check if there are any neurological side effects. If the cooling is then immediately interrupted these deficits will subside.

Acknowledgement

This work was supported by grants from Karolinska Institutets fonder and stiftelsen Minerva.

Reference

1. Boëthius, J., Bergström, M., Greitz, T., Stereotactic computerized tomography with a GE 8800 scanner. J. Neurosurg. *52* (1980), 794—800.

Acta Neurochirurgica, Suppl. 33, 559—565 (1984)

A New Stereotactic Instrument Which Can Be Used in Conjunction With Open Surgery

J. Boëthius[1] and **T. Ribbe**[2]

With 6 Figures

Keywords: Stereotactic instrument.

Introduction

Since the introduction of stereotactic neurosurgery a number of well known stereotactic instruments have been constructed, some of which have been brought to an amazing degree of estetical and mechanical perfection. These instruments were all constructed in the era preceeding the introduction of the new imaging techniques. The type of information produced by these techniques has made it meaningfull and desirable to have an instrument which can easily be used in conjunction with open surgery. Most older instruments also show some dead angles and some restrictions on the number of possible probe trajectories. These disadvantages have been felt to be sufficiently grave to validate the construction of a new instrument. This instrument was constructed to fulfill the following demands: 1. Compatibility with open microsurgery. 2. Minimum of restraints on possible probe trajectories. 3. Minimum of dead angles. 4. Possibility of continuous feed-back from the stereotactic X-ray picture *e.g.* localization of an arbitrary point in the brain on the X-ray picture.

The general construction principle of the instrument is similar to the one used by Riechert with a special phantom for target setting from which the probe holder is moved to a patient ring.

---

[1] Department of Neurosurgery, Södersjukhuset, Karolinska Institutet, S-10401 Stockholm, Sweden.

[2] Department of Medical Engineering, Karolinska Institutet, S-10401 Stockholm, Sweden.

Technical description: The instrument is built to be used together with the base plate system previously described[4]. This base plate system has been further developed and by now constitutes the backbone of an integrated diagnostic stereotactic system which allows localisation with conventional radiography and CT- and PET-scanning[1-3].

Fig. 1 shows the instrument mounted on the base plate which is fixed to a skull with aluminium bars. The instrument consists of a ring which is mounted on the base plate with four feet. On the top of the ring a number of screw holes are drilled, one at every 15th degree, which are used to mount the probe carrier. The probe carrier is also seen in Fig. 1. It consists of an adjustable support which can be locked in position and which, at its outer end carries the probeholder. The probeholder can be moved up and down to adjust the penetration depth of the probe.

The phantom is shown in Fig. 2. Its upper part consists of a ring identical to the one mounted on the base plate. Below the ring there is a device for setting the target position. This device consists of the target pointer, which can be adjusted with three millimetre scales along the three main axes. The target pointer can be set in any position inside the ring.

Practical applications: The coordinates are set with the aid of special frames[1,2] which are mounted on the base-plate during the diagnostic procedure[1,2]. That being done the frame is replaced with the instrument which fits into the same holes in the base-plate as the frames.

Biopsies along a predetermined trajectory: The trajectory is laid out on the stereotactic X-ray picture by determining the target point and one other arbitrary point along the trajectory. That having been done, the target point is set on the phantom (Fig. 3). A marker is mounted on the ring pointing at the target indicator (Fig. 3). The target indicator is now moved to the other point along the trajectory (Fig. 4). Finally, the probe is mounted on its adjustable support and adapted in such a way that its tip touches the pointer which indicates the target point while its shaft touches the target indicator which indicates the point along the trajectory (Fig. 4). The probe is now ready to be used and the probe carrier is removed from the phantom ring and placed in the analogous position on the patient ring. A craniotomy is done at the site indicated by the probe, whereafter the probe is passed down along its predetermined trajectory (Fig. 5).

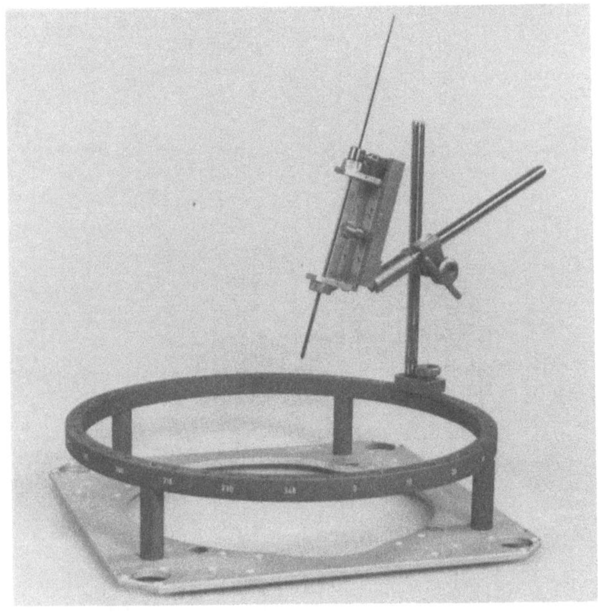

Fig. 1. Instrument with probe carrier mounted on base-plate

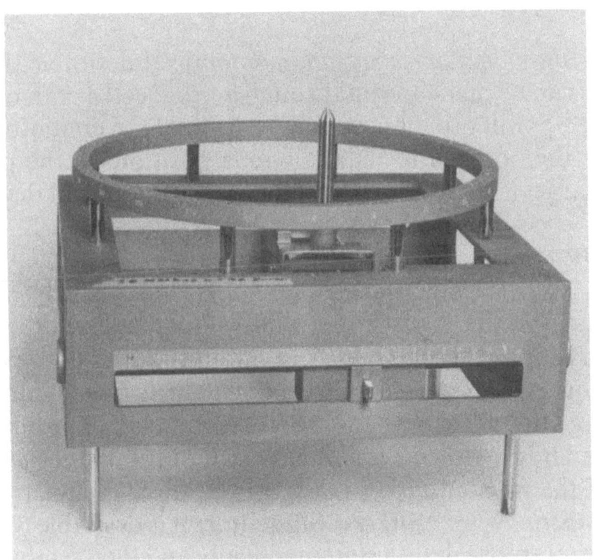

Fig. 2. Phantom with ring and mechanical device for setting stereotactic coordinates

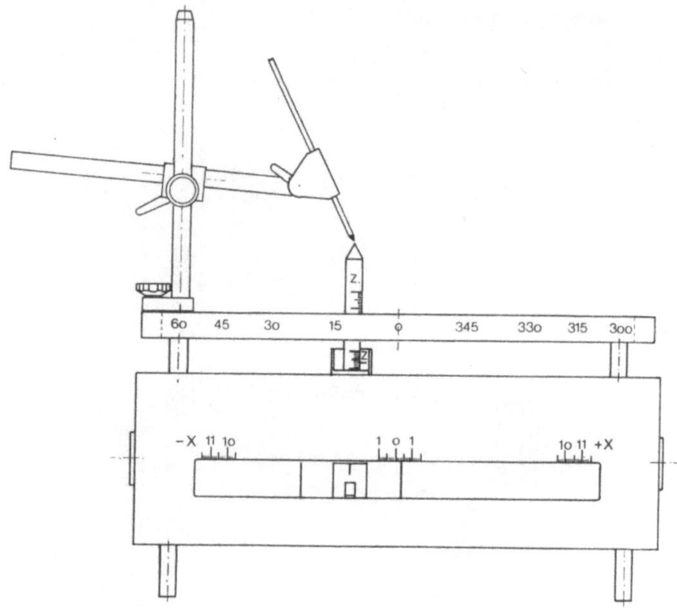

Fig. 3. The target is set on the phantom and the target position is saved by marking it with a pointer

Biopsy through a preselected craniotomy: If desirable the probe trajectory can be made to run through a preselected craniotomy by mounting a pointer to indicate the position of the craniotomy. The pointer is then moved to its analogous position on the phantom ring, the target indicator is set to indicate the target and the probe is mounted as described above.

Identification of a "real life" structure on CT: Sometimes it is desirable to acertain during an operation which structure corresponds to the radiograph. The stereotactic coordinates of such a structure are determined by mounting the pointer on the patient ring so that its tip touches the structure. The pointer is then moved to the phantom and the stereotactic coordinates are determined by moving the target indicator of the phantom to touch the tip of the pointer and reading off the three millimetre scales.

Stereotactic "open" surgery: Sometimes it is desirable to localize a small intracerebral lesion stereotactically and then remove it with open surgery. The stereotactic localization is done as described above. By moving the probe down towards the skull, the center of a

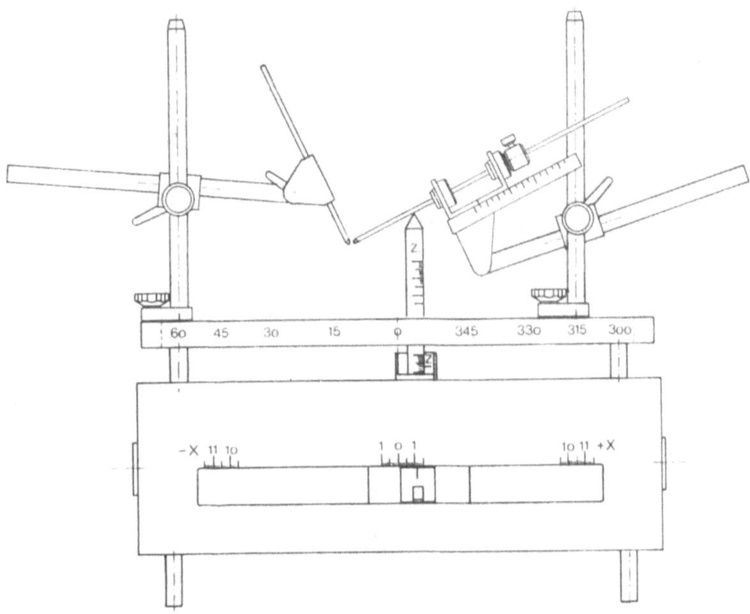

Fig. 4. A second point on the trajectory is indicated with the target indicator and the probe holder is mounted so that the probe hits the target while the probe shaft touches the second point on the probe trajectory

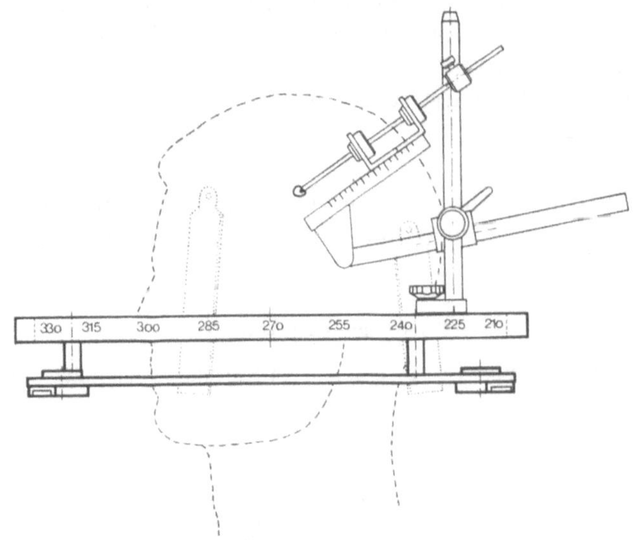

Fig. 5. The probe holder is moved from the phantom to the analogous position on the patient ring for the intervention

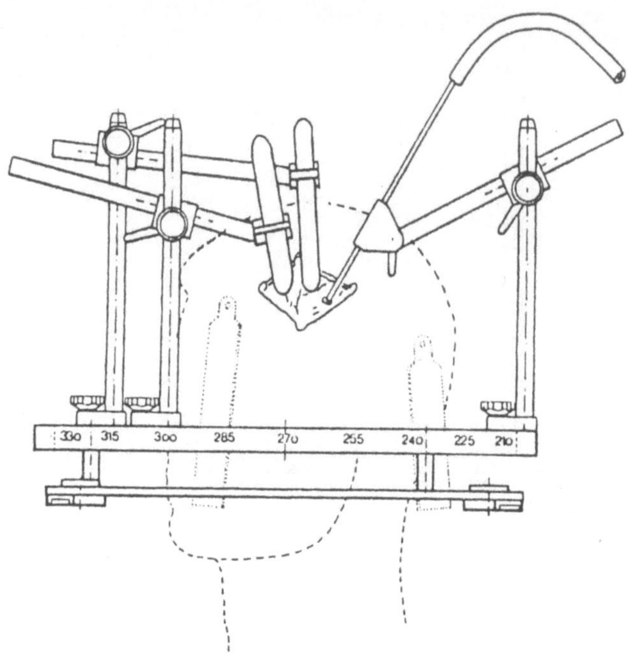

Fig. 6. Retractors and suction tube mounted on the instrument for open surgery

conventional craniotomy is indicated. The probe is pushed through brain tissue to the lesion. The probe is followed with microsurgical techniques down to the lesion, which is then removed. The patient ring can be used to carry retractors and other surgical instruments (Fig. 6).

The instrument has been in use for some months. It has been easy to handle and the members of the department have found it simple and reliable.

Acknowledgement

This work was supported by grants from Karolinska Institutets fonder and Minervastiftelsen.

References

1. Bergström, M., Boëthius, J., Eriksson, L., Greitz, T., Ribbe, T., Widén, L., Head fixation device for reproducible position alignment in transmission CT and positron emission tomography. J. Comput. Assist. Tomogr. *5* (1981), 136—141.

2. Bergström, M., Greitz, T., Ribbe, T., A method for stereotactic localization adapted for conventional and digital radiography. To be published.
3. Boëthius, J., Bergström, M., Greitz, T., Stereotactic computerized tomography with a GE 8800 scanner. J. Neurosurg. *52* (1980), 794—800.
4. Lewander, R., Bergström, M., Boëthius, J., Collins, V. P., Edner, G., Geitz, T., Willems, J., Stereotactic computer tomography for biopsy of gliomas. Acta Radiol. Diagn. *19* (1978), 867—888.

Acta Neurochirurgica, Suppl. 33, 567 (1984)

A Portable Computerized Tomographic Method for Tumor Biopsy

T. L. Hardy[1], **A. Lassiter,** and **J. Koch**

Keywords: Computer graphics; CT stereotaxic surgery; tumor biopsy; functional neurosurgery.

A system has been developed to store, manipulate, and selectively display computerized tomographic (CT) images in the operating theatre on a portable computer graphics display system. It is designed to aid the surgeon by presenting an on-line graphics display of stereotaxic probes superimposed on CT images. Graphic simulation of the operative procedure by this technique also avoids the extreme expense of a CT-dedicated stereotaxic system or the cumbersome use of a non-dedicated CT scanner for performing stereotaxic biopsies and other procedures. The system also has multiple color graphics capabilities which can be used to enhance tumor demarcation zones. Additional software subroutines allow volumetric determination of brain lesions and graphics overlaying of diencephalic brain maps for functional neurosurgical procedures.

---

[1] Department of Neurosurgery, Lovelace Medical Center and Research Foundation, Albuquerque, New Mexico, U.S.A.

Acta Neurochirurgica, Suppl. 33, 569—572 (1984)

Clinical Application of an Original Stereotactic Apparatus

F. Colombo[1] and **A. Zanardo**[2]

With 2 Figures

Introduction

Within the last years, many computer assisted stereotactic procedures have been developed. The next step toward a completely automatized operation would be the introduction of a new stereotactic system mechanized by servomotors[2]. The authors have built a computer driven stereotactic machine which allows the positionning of the probe carrier automatically according to the target coordinates[1].

Materials and Method

A completely new stereotactic apparatus had to be designed for two main reasons: 1. it is very difficult to plan servomotors and actuators controlling rotational displacement of small angles. Consequently stereotactic apparatuses working with polar coordinates system must be discarded. 2. Servomotors and coordinates readouts cannot be mounted on commercially available head frames. The existing room is restricted. Intraoperative X-ray must be possible. All mechanical gadgets must be mounted in distance from the operating field for reasons of asepsis.

The authors have solved the problem by building a new operating machine[1]. The probe carrier is fitted on top of two rotating arms and can be moved all around an ideal sphere centered to the target. The base supporting the rotating arms assembly can be shifted along three orthogonal slides (one for each coordinate). The positionning is controlled by digital readouts and operated by servomotors.

---

[1] Department of Neurosurgery, City Hospital, Viale Rodolfi, I-36100 Vicenza, Italy.

[2] Institute of Applied Mechanics, Padua University, Via Venezia, 1, I-35100 Padova, Italy.

Results

The first stereotactic robot was built only for evaluating the accuracy of the automatic positionning and was employed only on head phantoms.

The main shortcomings were the size of the apparatus and the necessity to have three high power (3.5 hp) electric motors in the base working with 220 Volts, 52 Hz A.C. that entails problems with insulation. On the other hand, the accuracy, with which the target was hit, was very high (0.1 mm). The second generation stereotactic apparatus has the three movements mounted on low friction roller bearings and can be moved by small 12 Volts D.C. motors. We are studying also the possibility to fit an hydraulic movement system which would avoid any electric power problem.

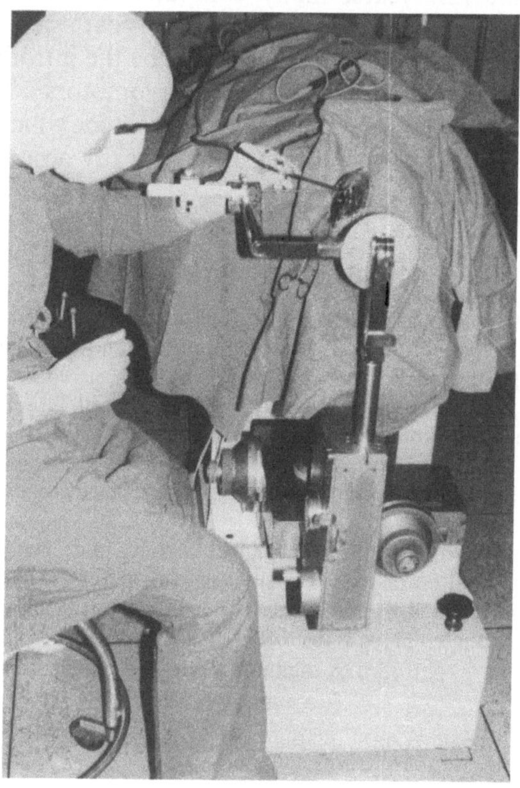

Fig. 1

The senior author has used this apparatus for more than 50 stereotactic operations of both "organic" and "functional" stereotactic neurosurgery with complete satisfaction.

Discussion

The main advantages inherent to the motorized procedure are:

1. It is possible to avoid any intraoperative calculation.

2. The accuracy of the probe is high, confirming the data obtained with the first experimental apparatus.

3. The two-arms probe carrier is very agile and versatile: frontal, temporal, occipital, suboccipital approaches are very easily performed. Working with stereoangiographies, the ncessary

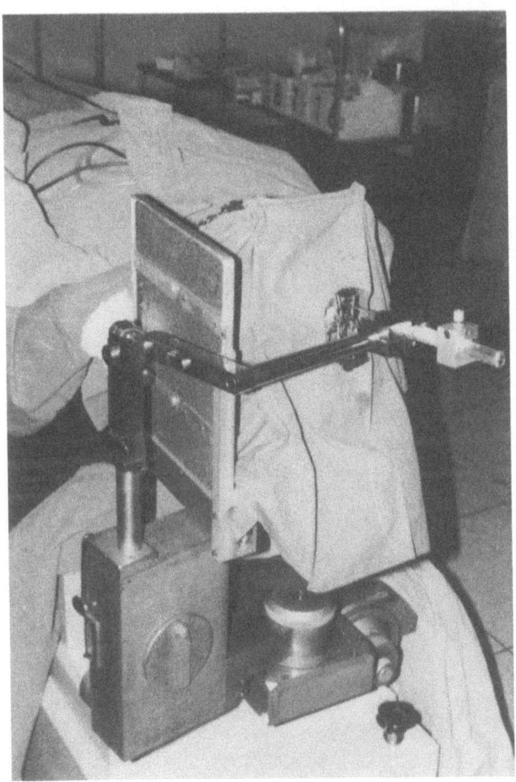

Fig. 2

horizontal approaches are simply done. So-called "open" stereotactic procedures are not disturbed by cumbersome probe carriers (Fig. 1).

4. In many cases the X-ray plates can be mounted inside the two arms assembly: this arrangement provides completely unobstructed stereo X-rays (Fig. 2).

References

1. Colombo, F., Angrilli, F., Zanardo, A., *et al.*, A universal method to employ CT spatial information in stereotactic surgery. Appl. Neurophysiol. *45* (1982), 352—364.
2. Kelly, P. J., Future possibilities in stereotactic neurosurgery. Surg. Neurol. *19* (1983), 4—9.

Acta Neurochirurgica, Suppl. 33, 573—575 (1984)

Advanced Intraoperative Imaging for Stereotaxis. The Surgical CT Scanner

L. D. Lunsford[1]

Keywords: Stereotactic instrument; CT scan.

Introduction

Earlier recognition and superior definition of intracranial pathology by computerized tomography (CT) have demanded the introduction of CT imaging into the operating room itself[1]. A CT scanner dedicated to improved surgical diagnosis and therapy has been combined with a compatible stereotaxic device to promote exploration, and removal or treatment of a wide spectrum of brain lesions.

Methods and Materials

The Leksell stereotaxic frame (AB Eleckta, Stockholm, Sweden) was used. A General Electric 8800 CT/T scanner (General Electrical Medical Systems, Milwaukee, Wisconsin, U.S.A.) was installed in an especially designed operating room. By reversing the usual placement of the CT scanner, full access to the head of the patient can be achieved after advancing the scanner pallet ("OR table") through the gantry aperture. Direct and television monitoring of the patient is possible during intraoperative imaging.

Results

Table 1 demonstrates the usages of the surgical CT scanner. In deep-seated lesions previously considered unapproachable by surgery, a firm histologic diagnosis was achieved in 96% of 100 consecutive cases. No mortality occurred and only 3 patients suffered transient neurologic impairments. Intraoperative

[1] Department of Neurological Surgery, University of Pittsburgh, Room 9402, Presbyterian Hospital, 230 Lothrop St., Pittsburgh, PA 15213, U.S.A.

Table 1. *Uses of the Surgical CT Scanner in Morphologic Brain Operations*

Usage	Type of procedure	No. cases	Comment
Diagnostic	Biopsy cyst puncture	100	Consecutive series, 96% diagnostic; mortality-0 transient morbidity-3
	Stable Xenon cerebral blood flow	3	Dynamic scanning; intraoperative precise blood flow determination
Therapeutic	Tumor removal	6	Stereotaxic craniotomy-3; percutaneous aspiration of colloid cysts-3
	Catheter placement/ drainage	5	Brain abscesses-3; deep non-neoplastic cysts-2
	Intracystic ^{32}P Beta irradiation	3 3	Craniopharyngioma; 20–30 krads to cyst wall
	^{125}I interstitial irradiation	3	Recurrent glioma or metastases; CT volume determination and isodose planning

measurement of cerebral blood flow using stable inhaled Xenon was performed to assess the effects of suspected vascular brain insults[2]. Small lesions located by stereotaxic CT were removed by either percutaneous techniques or by craniotomy. Intracystic irradiation of craniopharyngioma by ^{32}P has been performed in 3 cases. A program of interstitial irradiation by ^{125}I volume implantation of recurrent malignant gliomas was initiated using CT isodose planning.

Discussion

Intraoperative CT demonstrates that an advanced imaging tool improves intracranial surgery. A dedicated surgical CT scanner permits precise multiplanar determination of stereotaxic targets, calculation and variation of probe trajectories in advance, immediate verification of therapeutic efficacy and accuracy, and early recognition of potential complications. New applications of guided brain surgery are dependent on the development of CT as a therapeutic instrument.

References

1. Lunsford, L. D., Rosenbaum, A. E., Perry, J., Stereotactic surgery using the "therapeutic" CT scanner. Surg. Neurol. *18* (1982), 116—122.
2. Gur, D., Yonas, H., Wolfson, S. K., *et al.*, Xenon and iodine enhanced cerebral CT: A closer look. Stroke *12* (1981), 573—578.

Acta Neurochirurgica, Suppl. 33, 577—583 (1984)

Functional Stereotactic Surgery Utilizing CT Data and Computer Generated Stereotactic Atlas

P. J. Kelly[1], **B. Kall**[2], and **S. Goerss**[2]

With 5 Figures

Introduction

Stereotactic atlases attempt to relate the position of subcortical structures to intracranial landmarks detected by radiographic methods[7,8]. Considerable anatomic variability exists between individual brains. Subcortical structures have no consistent quantitative relationship to radiologically determined landmarks[1,3]. This variability increases in direct proportion to the distance the substructure lies from particular landmarks[8]. Although anterior-posterior and superior-inferior measurements from stereotactic atlases can be adjusted for variations in the intracommissural distance and thalamic height, there is no anatomical landmark detected by ordinary radiographic techniques which allows correction for medial lateral variability in the position of the internal capsule or the axial configuration of the thalamus and third ventricle. Fortunately, these structures are usually visualized on quality CT scans.

Even though large grey matter masses are apparent on CT scans, small nuclear subgroups, usually selected as stereotactic targets, are not. However, a computer generated stereotactic atlas can be stretched or contracted to fit within CT defined boundaries. This can be overlayed on reformatted CT slices, and used to subdivide and label specific grey matter masses into subnuclei and

[1] State University of New York at Buffalo, 2121 Main Street, Buffalo, NY 14214, U.S.A.

[2] Sisters of Charity Hospital, Buffalo, NY 14214, U.S.A.

fiber tracts. If the CT scan is obtained under stereotactic conditions, the stereotactic coordinates of a point selected from the CT sclice can then be calculated[2]. The following report will describe such a system.

Methods and Materials

Multiple points on the boundaries of individual substructures detailed on standard Schaltenbrand-Wahren stereotactic atlas[7] sections were digitized in reference to midcommissural and midline planes utilizing an X, Y digitizing board. The points are reconstituted as outlines within a two dimensional computer matrix. Thus, various portions of each atlas section can be transformed, stretched, contracted or rotated by computer to fit within designated structural boundaries.

Stereotactic CT scanning data is obtained on a GE 8800 CT scanning unit utilizing a method described elsewhere[2, 5, 6]. Briefly, the patient's head is fixed in a CT-compatible stereotactic head holder to which a CT localization system is attached (Fig. 1). The CT localizing system creates a series of nine (9) reference marks on each CT slice. These define a plane in space for each CT slice in reference to the stereotactic surgical frame. Five (5) millimeter overlapping CT sclices are obtained through the third ventricle. Following the CT scan, the archived CT data tape is input to an operating room computer system*. CT sclices are displayed on the Ramtek raster display terminal. A midline reconstruction is performed and the anterior and posterior commissures are identified. Utilizing the Arrange II® software, an oblique semihorizontal reconstruction at a 7° angle from the midpoint of the intercommissural line is generated (Fig. 2). The surgeon first digitizes the nine reference marks on the oblique reconstruction. The CT-defined boundaries of an area of surgical interest, or sector, are then traced by the surgeon utilizing cursor and trackball. For instance, in the case of thalamic structures, the surgeon traces the medial wall of the third ventricle, the superior colliculus and medial wall of the internal capsule (Fig. 3). The computer calculates the centers of gravity of the sector on the stereotactic atlas and of the area traced on the reformatted CT slice. The substructures within that sector are assigned polar coordinates. A polar stretch transformation is performed along multiple vectors drawn from the center of gravity to the designated boundary. The substructures wthin the computer generated atlas sector are stretched or contracted in order to fit within that area traced on the reformatted CT slice (Fig. 4). Several options are available at this point. The surgeon can retrieve a substructure name by positioning the cursor over any area within the designated CT region. Secondly, a substructure may be located by cursor by typing its name or abbreviation into the terminal (Fig. 5). Finally, stereotactic coordinates on the stereotactic instrument may be obtained by positioning the cursor over a substructure of interest and striking the deposit key.

---

* Independent Physician Diagnostic Console (IPDC) for GE 8800 CT scanning unit (data General Eclipse S 140 mainframe, Ramtek raster display terminal).

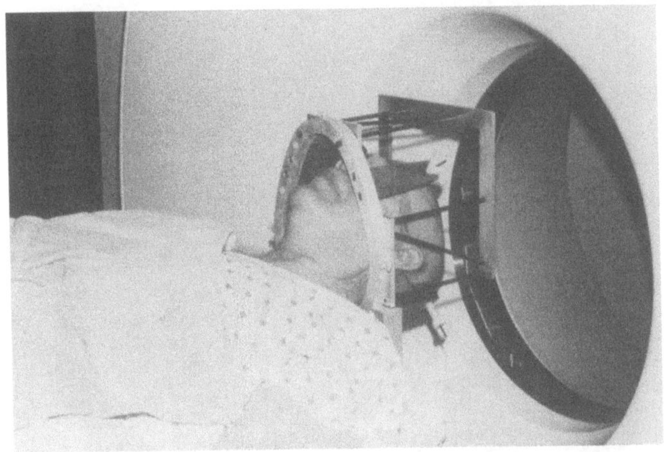

Fig. 1. CT compatible stereotactic head frame with localizing system

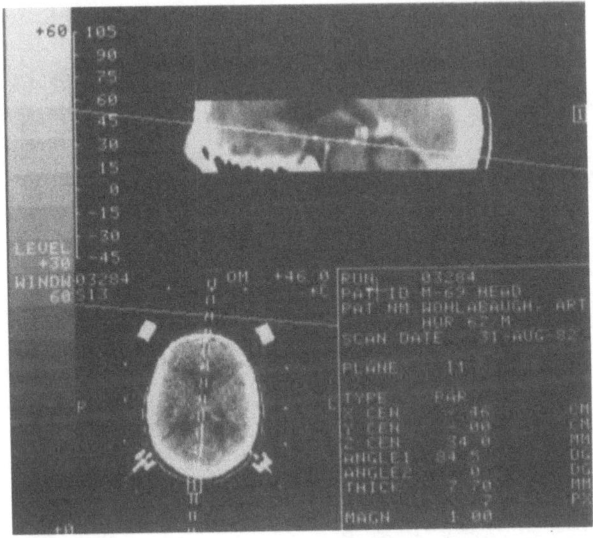

Fig. 2. Midline CT reconstruction with cursor line designating plane 7° oblique to intracommissural line

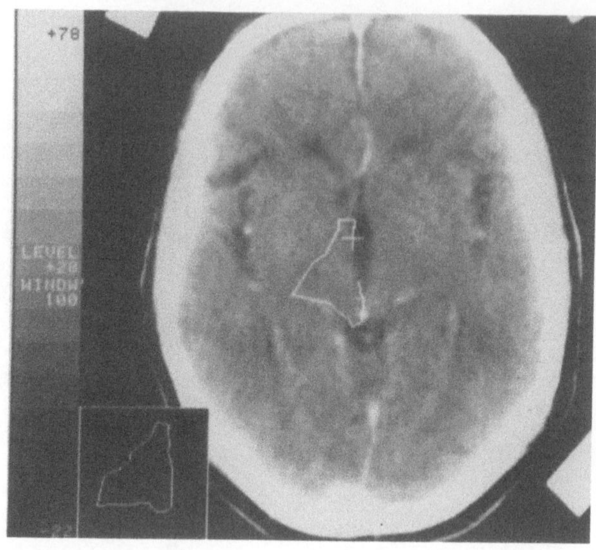

Fig. 3. Surgeon traces the outline of the thalamus on reformatted CT slice

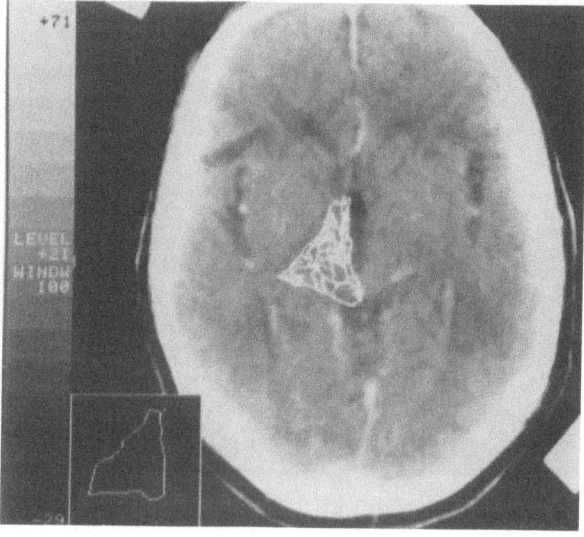

Fig. 4. The thalamic substructures from the computer generated atlas are scaled to fit within the CT defined thalamic boundaries

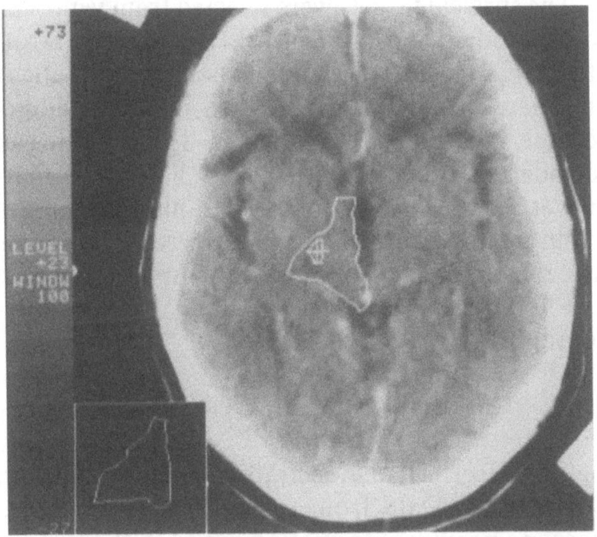

Fig. 5. The surgeon selects á substructure of interest. Its atlas defined boundary is traced by computer within the CT defined area of the thalamus

Results

As outlined in another publication[6], the CT-stereotactic atlas was used to augment the data base in five patients undergoing functional stereotactic procedures. Two (2) patients underwent thalamotomies for movement disorders and one underwent a mesencephalotomy for pain. Two additional patients had deep brain stimulating (DBS) electrode systems placed in sensory

Table 1. *Comparison of Target Sites Determined by CT-stereotactic Atlas and Ultimate Target Point Derived from Ventriculography and Microelectrode Recording in Five Patients*

Case		Diagnosis	Procedure	Average error
1	62 M	Parkinson's	VL Thalamotomy	4.3 MM
2	58 M	Parkinson's	VL Thalamotomy	2.4 MM
3	64 M	Pain	DBS in VCE	2.1 MM
4	63 M	Pain	Mesencephalotomy	1.6 MM
5	34 M	Pain	DBS in VCE	1.3 MM

thalamus. The surgical targets were selected from ventriculography and microelectrode recording control. The average error in X, Y and Z between CT targets selected by the stereotactic atlas program and the ultimate surgical target selected by venticulography and microelectrode recording are shown in Table 1. In case No. 1, microelectrode recording failed to give reliable information. The lesion site was selected from ventriculographic landmarks and the parkinsonian tremor returned after a few weeks. It is possible that, in this case, the target site determined by the CT-stereotactic atlas may have been more effective than that selected from ventriculography.

Discussion

The method described demonstrates one utility of a computer in stereotactic surgery. Data from two or more data bases can be superimposed to provide information useful to the surgeon during a stereotactic procedure. In the present report, CT data is reformatted in a plane which corresponds to the orientation of horizontal sections of a stereotactic atlas. The atlas section is scaled to fit within CT-defined boundaries. The atlas is used to label a CT slice by proportionally subdividing it into anatomical areas not discernable by ordinary CT imaging. A CT reference localization system is used to relate points selected from the labeled CT slice to settings on a stereotactic frame[6]. This CT localization system has been tested extensively and found to have an accuracy of ± 600 microns in X and Y and within the CT slice thickness in Z[2].

To some, it may be appealing to utilize such a system for determination of target points in neuroaugmentative or neuroablative procedures. However, it is our opinion that stereotactic CT scanning utilizing a computer generated atlas is only an additional piece of information which should be used to augment rather than replace the data base provided by positive contrast ventriculography and neurophysiologic localization methods[3,4].

References

1. Brierley, J., Beck, E., The significance in human stereotactic brain surgery of individual variation in the diencephalon and globus pallidus. J. Neurol. Neurosurg. Psychiat. *22* (1959), 286—298.
2. Goerss, S., Kelly, P. J., Kall, B., Alker, G. J., A computed tomographic stereotactic adaptation system. Neurosurgery *10* (1982), 375—379.

3. Kelly, P., Derome, P., Guiot, G., Thalamic spatial variability and the surgical results of lesions placed with neurophysiologic control. Surg. Neurol. *9* (1978), 307—315.
4. Kelly, P. J., Microelectrode recording for the somatotopic placement of stereotactic thalamic lesions in the treatment of parkinsonian and cerebellar intention tremor. Appl. Neurophysiol. *43* (1980), 262—266.
5. Kelly, P. J., Alker, G. J., Goerss, S., Computer-assisted stereotactic laser microsurgery for the treatment of intracranial neoplasms. Neurosurgery *10* (1982), 324—331.
6. Kelly, P. J., Kall, B. A., Goerss, S., Stereotactic CT scanning for the biopsy of intracranial lesions and functional neurosurgery. Appl. Neurophysiol. (in press).
7. Schaltenbrand, G., Wahren, W., Atlas for Stereotaxy of the Human Brain. Stuttgart: G. Thieme. 1977.
8. Van Buren, J., Maccubbin, D., An outline atlas of human basal ganglia with estimation of anatomical variants. J. Neurosurg. *19* (1962), 811—839.

3. Kelly, P. J., Derome, P., Guiot, G.: Thalamic spatial variability and the surgical results of lesions placed with neurophysiologic control. Surg. Neurol. 9 (1978), 307—315.
4. Kelly, P. J.: Microelectrode recording for the somatotopic placement of stereotactic thalamic lesions in the treatment of parkinsonian and cerebellar intention tremor. Appl. Neurophysiol. 43 (1980), 262—266.
5. Kelly, P. J., Alker, G. J., Goerss, S.: Computer-assisted stereotactic laser microsurgery for the treatment of intracranial neoplasms. Neurosurgery 10 (1982), 324—331.
6. Kelly, P. J., Kall, B. A., Goerss, S.: Stereotactic CT scanning for the biopsy of intracranial lesions and functional neurosurgery. Appl. Neurophysiol. (in press).
7. Schaltenbrand, G., Wahren, W.: Atlas for Stereotaxy of the Human Brain. Stuttgart: G. Thieme, 1977.
8. Van Buren, J., Maccubbin, D.: An outline atlas of human basal ganglia with estimation of anatomical variants. J. Neurosurg. 19 (1962), 811—839.

ACTA NEUROCHIRURGICA

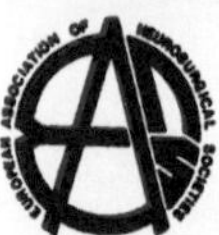

Official Organ of the European Association of Neurosurgical Societies

Clinical and scientific literature increases in an exponential form every year. In the neurological sciences scarcely a year passes without the addition of at least one new journal, and for the clinical neurosurgeon expanding his fields of contact in Europe, an established European journal which covers the field of neurosurgery and touches in its interest the basic sciences and neurology as well, is of inestimable value. For many years ACTA NEUROCHIRURGICA has endeavoured to fulfill this function. It has consistently offered an excellent level of reproduction and in recent years has provided an English language editing service enabling the uniform production of this European journal in a language common to most European readers. It is the official bulletin of the European Association of Neurosurgical Societies and publishes reports of meetings of these member societies. Scientific links between the European nations are now closer than they have ever been.

Teaching courses organized by the European Association have brought young neurosurgeons from a wide variety of Eastern and Western European countries together in common study groups and Acta offers them an opportunity to acquaint themselves with each others work as the years progress. No academic can afford to neglect a wide literature search, but here is a journal that brings the most up-to-date coverage of significant research and clinical work in Europe on Neurosurgery, which will be of interest to neurologists and basic neuroscientists and carries facets of interest to surgeons in related disciplines.

The surgery of the ear, orthopaedic surgery, particularly in relation to spinal problems, and the management of trauma and intracranial pressure are all covered in the course of a years publication of Acta and no European neurosurgeon can regard his bookshelves as complete without it.

Subscription Information:

1984: Vols. 70—73 (4 issues each)
Per vol. DM 198,—, S 1.420,—, plus carriage charges

New:
Special price for individual members of a society affiliated with the E.A.N.S.:
Per vol. DM 89,—, S 639,—, plus carriage charges*

* Such orders should be placed directly with Springer-Verlag, P.O. Box 367, Mölkerbastei 5, A-1011 Wien, Austria

Prices for *Back Volumes* are available on request.

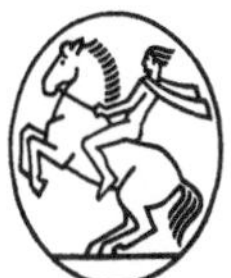

Springer-Verlag Wien New York